Controversies in Managing the Progressive Collapsing Foot Deformity (PCFD)

Editor

CESAR DE CESAR NETTO

FOOT AND ANKLE CLINICS

www.foot.theclinics.com

Consulting Editor
CESAR DE CESAR NETTO

September 2021 • Volume 26 • Number 3

ELSEVIER

1600 John F. Kennedy Boulevard • Suite 1800 • Philadelphia, Pennsylvania, 19103-2899

http://www.theclinics.com

FOOT AND ANKLE CLINICS Volume 26, Number 3
September 2021 ISSN 1083-7515, ISBN-978-0-323-79457-2

Editor: Lauren Boyle
Developmental Editor: Arlene B. Campos

Foot and Ankle Clinics (ISSN 1083-7515) is published quarterly by Elsevier, Inc., 360 Park Avenue South, New York, NY 10010-1710. Months of issue are March, June, September, and December. Periodicals postage paid at New York, NY, and additional mailing offices. Subscription price per year is $344.00 (US individuals), $741.00 (US institutions), $100.00 (US students), $371.00 (Canadian individuals), $778.00 (Canadian institutions), $100.00 (Canadian students), $479.00 (international individuals), $778.00 (international institutions), and $215.00 (international students). To receive student/resident rate, orders must be accompanied by name of affiliated institution, date of term, and the *signature* of program/residency coordinator on institution letterhead. Orders will be billed at individual rate until proof of status is received. Foreign air speed delivery is included in all *Clinics* subscription prices. All prices are subject to change without notice. **POSTMASTER:** Send address changes to *Foot and Ankle Clinics*, Elsevier Health Sciences Division, Subscription Customer Service, 3251 Riverport Lane, Maryland Heights, MO 63043. **Customer Service: 1-800-654-2452 (US and Canada). From outside of the United States and Canada, call 314-447-8871. Fax: 314-447-8029. E-mail: JournalsCustomerService-usa@elsevier.com (for print support); JournalsOnlineSupport-usa@elsevier.com (for online support).**

Reprints. For copies of 100 or more, of articles in this publication, please contact the Commercial Reprints Department, Elsevier Inc., 360 Park Avenue South, New York, NY 10010-1710. Tel.: 212-633-3874; Fax: 212-633-3820; E-mail: reprints@elsevier.com.

Editorial Advisory Board

Contributors

CONSULTING EDITOR

CESAR DE CESAR NETTO, MD, PhD
Orthopaedic Foot and Ankle Surgeon, Director of the UIOWA Orthopedic Functional Imaging Research Laboratory (OFIRL), Assistant Professor, Department of Orthopaedic and Rehabilitation, University of Iowa, Carver College of Medicine, Iowa City, Iowa, USA

EDITOR

CESAR DE CESAR NETTO, MD, PhD
Orthopaedic Foot and Ankle Surgeon, Director of the UIOWA Orthopedic Functional Imaging Research Laboratory (OFIRL), Assistant Professor, Department of Orthopaedic and Rehabilitation, University of Iowa, Carver College of Medicine, Iowa City, Iowa, USA

AUTHORS

ALEXEJ BARG, MD
Professor and Head of Foot and Ankle Surgery Section, Department of Orthopaedics, Trauma and Reconstructive Surgery, University of Hamburg, Senior Attending Surgeon, Department of Trauma and Orthopaedic Surgery, BG Hospital Hamburg, Hamburg, Germany; Adjunct Full Professor, Department of Orthopaedics, University of Utah, Salt Lake City, Utah, USA

ERIC M. BLUMAN, MD, PhD, FAAOS
Vice Chairman, Brigham Health Orthopedics, Associate Professor of Orthopedics, Harvard Medical School, Boston, Massachusetts, USA

LORRAINE A. BOAKYE, MD
Brigham Health Orthopedics, Boston, Massachusetts, USA

NICHOLAS D. CASSCELLS, MD
Assistant Professor of Orthopaedics, Georgetown University, Department of Orthopaedic Surgery, MedStar Georgetown University Hospital, Washington, DC, USA

FELIPE CHAPARRO, MD
Foot and Ankle Surgeon, Hospital San José, Foot and Ankle Surgeon, Clinica Universidad de los Andes, Santiago, Chile

MICHELLE M. COLEMAN, MD, PhD
Emory University School of Medicine, Atlanta, Georgia, USA

MATTHEW S. CONTI, MD
Orthopaedic Surgery Resident, Academic Training Department, Hospital for Special Surgery, New York, New York, USA

ALEXANDER W. CRAWFORD, MD
Department of Orthopedic Surgery, Oklahoma University Health Sciences Center, University of Oklahoma College of Medicine, Oklahoma City, Oklahoma, USA

CESAR DE CESAR NETTO, MD, PhD
Orthopaedic Foot and Ankle Surgeon, Director of the UIOWA Orthopedic Functional Imaging Research Laboratory (OFIRL), Assistant Professor, Department of Orthopaedic and Rehabilitation, University of Iowa, Carver College of Medicine, Iowa City, Iowa, USA

SCOTT J. ELLIS, MD
Associate Professor of Orthopaedic Surgery, Foot and Ankle Service, Hospital for Special Surgery, New York, New York, USA

ALEXANDRE LEME GODOY-SANTOS, MD, PhD
Professor, Department of Orthopedic Surgery, Faculdade de Medicina, Universidade de São Paulo, Foot and Ankle Surgeon, Hospital Israelita Albert Einstein, São Paulo, Sao Paulo, Brazil

CHRISTOPHER E. GROSS, MD
Medical University of South Carolina, Charleston, South Carolina, USA

DANIEL GUSS, MD, MBA
Department of Orthopaedic Surgery, Foot and Ankle Service, Harvard Medical School, Massachusetts General Hospital and Newton-Wellesley Hospital, MGH-NWH Foot & Ankle Center, Waltham, Massachusetts, USA

GREGORY P. GUYTON, MD
Department of Orthopaedic Surgery, MedStar Union Memorial Hospital, Baltimore, Maryland, USA

AMGAD M. HALEEM, MD, PhD
Department of Orthopedic Surgery, Oklahoma University Health Sciences Center, University of Oklahoma College of Medicine, Oklahoma City, Oklahoma, USA; Department of Orthopedic Surgery, Kasr Al-Ainy Hospitals, College of Medicine, Cairo University, Cairo, Egypt

KAAN SULEYMAN IRGIT, MD
Associate Professor, Orthopedics and Traumatology, Marmara School of Medicine, İstanbul, Turkey

J. BENJAMIN JACKSON III, MD, MBA, FACS
University of South Carolina, Prisma Orthopaedics, Columbia, South Carolina, USA

ANISH R. KADAKIA, MD
Professor of Orthopedic Surgery, Fellowship Director – Orthopedic Foot and Ankle, Northwestern Medicine Department of Orthopedics, Chicago, Illinois, USA

PHILIP KAISER, MD
Department of Orthopaedic Surgery, Foot and Ankle Service, Harvard Medical School, Massachusetts General Hospital and Newton-Wellesley Hospital, MGH-NWH Foot & Ankle Center, Waltham, Massachusetts, USA

ATANAS ZHIVKOV KATSAROV, MD, PhD
Associate Professor, Ortomedica Clinic, Sofia, Bulgaria

MICHAEL J. KELLY, MD
Department of Orthopaedic Surgery, MedStar Georgetown University Hospital, Washington, DC, USA

KURT KRAUTMANN, MD
Northwestern Medicine Department of Orthopedics, Chicago, Illinois, USA

FRANCOIS LINTZ, MD, MSc, FEBOT
Department of Foot and Ankle Surgery, Ramsay Healthcare Clinique de l'Union, Saint-Jean, Toulouse, France

PILAR MARTÍNEZ-DE-ALBORNOZ, MD
Orthopaedic Foot and Ankle Unit, Orthopaedic and Trauma Department, Hospital Universitario Quirónsalud Madrid, Faculty Medicine UEM, Madrid, Spain

MANUEL MONTEAGUDO, MD
Orthopaedic Foot and Ankle Unit, Orthopaedic and Trauma Department, Hospital Universitario Quirónsalud Madrid, Associate Professor, Orthopaedics, Faculty Medicine UEM, Madrid, Spain

CARSTEN SCHLICKEWEI, MD
Senior Attending Surgeon, Department of Orthopaedics, Trauma and Reconstructive Surgery, University of Hamburg, Hamburg, Germany

ELI L. SCHMIDT, BS
Department of Orthopaedics and Rehabilitation, University of Iowa, Carver College of Medicine, Iowa City, Iowa, USA

AKACHIMERE C. UZOSIKE, MD, MPH
Brigham Health Orthopedics, Boston, Massachusetts, USA

Contents

Preface: Big Shoes to Fill in Foot and Ankle Clinics of North America, but They are Definitely Pointed in the Right Direction xv

Cesar de Cesar Netto

What Are the Updates on Epidemiology of Progressive Collapsing Foot Deformity? 407

Alexandre Leme Godoy-Santos, Eli L. Schmidt, and Felipe Chaparro

Progressive collapsing foot deformity is one of the most controversial topics in foot and ankle surgery. Much research has been done regarding anatomy, biomechanics, and etiology behind this complex deformity and there is interest in studying metabolic or genetic conditions that could influence the development of this multifactorial disorder. Relevant anatomy includes osseous and soft tissue structures. Several risk factors like obesity, genetics, and flat foot during childhood have been proposed in literature. It occurs 3 times more often in women, the peak incidence happening at age 55, and is more common in white, obese, diabetic, rheumatic, and hypertensive patients.

Progressive Collapsing Foot Deformity: Should We Be Staging It Differently? 417

Lorraine A. Boakye, Akachimere C. Uzosike, and Eric M. Bluman

This article cursorily reviews the history of classification systems for pathologic flatfoot deformity in the adult and also critically reviews the recent introduction of a classification system intended to improve on the deficiencies of prior systems. The article concludes by offering suggestions for further work in evolving even more utilitarian systems for the staging and treatment of adult flatfoot disorder.

Is Advanced Imaging a Must in the Assessment of Progressive Collapsing Foot Deformity? 427

Francois Lintz and Cesar de Cesar Netto

Advanced imaging modalities have, in very recent years, enabled a considerable leap in understanding progressive collapsing foot deformity, evolving from a simple confirmation of clinical diagnostic using basic measurements to minute understanding of soft tissue and bone involvements. MRI and weight-bearing cone-beam computed tomography are enabling the development of new 3-dimensional measurement modalities. The identification of key articular and joint markers of advanced collapse will allow surgeons to better indicate treatments and assess chances of success with conservative therapies and less invasive surgical procedures, with the hope of improving patient outcomes.

Progressive Collapsing Foot Deformity. Is There Really a Johnson and Strom Stage I? **443**

Manuel Monteagudo and Pilar Martínez-de-Albornoz

Video content accompanies this article at http://www.foot.theclinics.com.

Johnson and Strom stage I posterior tibialis tendon dysfunction presents with pain and swelling but preserved function and no deformity. Diagnosis is clinical. Pathomechanics explains the overloading of the tendon that may be worsened by a tight gastrocnemius, but systemic inflammatory disease may also be responsible for a stage I condition. Medial heel wedged orthoses are effective in most patients. Surgery usually consists of an open/endoscopic tenosynovectomy. In cases of complete tendon rupture, flexor digitorum longus tendon transfer may be considered. Stage I patients with a higher risk of progression—inflammatory conditions, excessive laxity, obese—may benefit from a "prophylactic" medializing calcaneal osteotomy.

Tendon Transfer versus Allograft Reconstruction in Progressive Collapsing Foot Deformity **465**

Michael J. Kelly and Nicholas D. Casscells

The posterior tibial tendon (PTT) is the principal dynamic stabilizer of the medial longitudinal arch of the foot. The basic goal of surgically reconstructing PCFD is to restore the foot's medial longitudinal arch, often through a combination of bony and soft tissue procedures. While the FDL transfer has long been the gold standard for reconstruction, allograft reconstruction of the PTT has recently been increasing in popularity.

Calcaneal Osteotomies in the Treatment of Progressive Collapsing Foot Deformity. What are the Restrictions for the Holy Grail? **473**

Carsten Schlickewei and Alexej Barg

Video content accompanies this article at http://www.foot.theclinics.com.

The progressive collapsing foot deformity is a complex three-dimensional deformity, including valgus malalignment of the heel. The medial displacement calcaneal osteotomy is an established surgical procedure reliably resulting in an efficient correction of the inframalleolar alignment. However, complications are common, including undercorrection of underlying deformity, progression of hindfoot osteoarthritis and/or deformity, and/or symptomatic hardware.

The Importance of the Medial Column in Progressive Collapsing Foot Deformity: Osteotomies and Stabilization **507**

Christopher E. Gross and J. Benjamin Jackson III

Adult acquired flatfoot deformity is a complex pathologic condition that requires considerate and thoughtful surgical solutions. Medial column procedures are often supplemented by a medializing calcaneal osteotomy and/or a lateral column lengthening because of the complex nature of progressive collapsing foot deformity and its resultant peritalar instability.

Other osteotomies and fusions include a Cotton osteotomy and first tarsometatarsal fusion.

I am Afraid of Lateral Column Lengthening. Should I Be? **523**

Alexander W. Crawford and Amgad M. Haleem

Lateral column lengthening has long been used in conjunction with other soft tissue and bony procedures to correct the midforefoot abduction seen in class B progressive collapsing foot deformity. The effectiveness of this osteotomy to restore the physiologic shape of the foot has been used by foot and ankle surgeons around the world to provide functional improvement for patients suffering from this disease. The overall low complication rates, low nonunion rates, and improved radiographic and functional outcomes provided by lateral column lengthening make this a valuable option for the treatment of class B progressive collapsing foot deformity.

Flexible Progressive Collapsing Foot Deformity: Is There Any Role for Arthroereisis in the Adult Patient? **539**

Kaan Suleyman Irgit and Atanas Zhivkov Katsarov

Over the last two decades there is a growing interest in the adult literature for subtalar joint arthroereisis. Parallel to this interest, there have been improvements in the design and biomechanics of the implant, although the main indication of subtalar joint arthroereisis in adults is not clear. Most studies show significant improvement in postoperative clinical scores and visual analog scores. Sinus tarsi pain, being the most common complication, is the main determinant of clinical satisfaction. This review focuses on the role and complications of subtalar joint arthroereisis in the adult population.

Surgical Management of Musculotendinous Balance in the Progressive Collapsing Foot Deformity: The Role of Peroneal and Gastrocnemius Contracture **559**

Philip Kaiser and Daniel Guss

Surgical treatment of progressive collapsing foot deformity (PCFD) relies on understanding the dynamic and deforming musculotendinous structures that contribute to hindfoot valgus, forefoot abduction, forefoot varus, and collapse or hypermobility of the medial column. Equinus commonly is seen in PCFD and consideration should be given to isolated gastrocnemius or Achilles lengthening. Although transfer of the flexor digitorum longus tendon is performed in PCFD attributed to dysfunction and pathology of the posterior tibialis tendon (PTT), retention of PTT is an area for further research. The peroneus brevis, which contributes to hindfoot imbalance in chronic cases, is a possible component of tendon rebalancing.

Spring and Deltoid Ligament Insufficiency in the Setting of Progressive Collapsing Foot Deformity. An Update on Diagnosis and Management **577**

Kurt Krautmann and Anish R. Kadakia

The spring ligament and deltoid ligament are important stabilizers of the medial ankle. Together, they form a complex along the medial ankle and foot that is critical to stability of both the ankle and the medial longitudinal arch. Incompetence of the spring and deltoid ligament is a component of both the early and late stages of progressive collapsing foot deformity. As the importance of this medial ligament complex has been recognized, repair and reconstruction of these ligaments have progressively evolved, initially as separate reconstructions, and more recently as combined techniques.

Spare the Talonavicular Joint! The Role of Isolated Subtalar Joint Fusion in the Treatment of Progressive Collapsing Foot Deformity **591**

Matthew S. Conti and Scott J. Ellis

Surgical management of progressive collapsing foot deformity continues to evolve. Previous studies have demonstrated that fusion of the talonavicular joint results in limited hindfoot motion and, therefore, may accelerate adjacent-joint arthrosis. Recent literature has supported using alternative arthrodesis constructs that spare the talonavicular joint, such as naviculocuneiform or isolated subtalar fusions, which may maintain some hindfoot motion through the talonavicular joint yet adequately address a patient's deformity. Concomitant reconstructive procedures may be used in addition to subtalar fusion to address severe deformities. Isolated subtalar fusions may be considered in cases of sinus tarsi or subfibular impingement deformities.

Is Arthrodesis Sufficient in the Setting of Complex, Severe and Rigid Progressive Collapsing Foot Deformities? **609**

Michelle M. Coleman and Gregory P. Guyton

Arthrodesis of the hindfoot is typically used for the correction of severe and arthritic progressive collapsing foot deformity. Concomitant bony or soft tissue procedures may be helpful in patients with congenital abnormalities including the ball-and-socket ankle or congenital vertical talus. Dysplasia of the hindfoot bones may be more common than previously recognized, and corrective procedures or alterations in technique may need to be performed during hindfoot arthrodesis to account for bony deformity. Intraarticular osteotomies, extraarticular osteotomies, tendon lengthening, and tendon transfer procedures may be used in specific instances to aid in deformity correction and improve overall function.

FOOT AND ANKLE CLINICS

FORTHCOMING ISSUES

December 2021
Foot Ankle Deformity in the Child
Maurizio De Pellegrin, *Editor*

March 2022
Alternatives to Ankle Joint Replacement
Woo-Chun Lee, *Editor*

June 2022
Managing Complications of Foot and Ankle Surgery
Scott Ellis, *Editor*

RECENT ISSUES

June 2021
Deltoid-Spring Ligament Complex and Medial Ankle Instability
Gastón Slullitel and Roxa Ruiz, *Editors*

March 2021
Advances in the Treatment of Athletic Injury
Mark S. Myerson, *Editor*

December 2020
Controversies in Acute Trauma and Reconstruction
Jorge Filippi and German Joannas, *Editors*

RELATED SERIES

Foot and Ankle Clinics
Orthopedic Clinics
Clinics in Sports Medicine

Preface

Big Shoes to Fill in *Foot and Ankle Clinics of North America*, but They are Definitely Pointed in the Right Direction

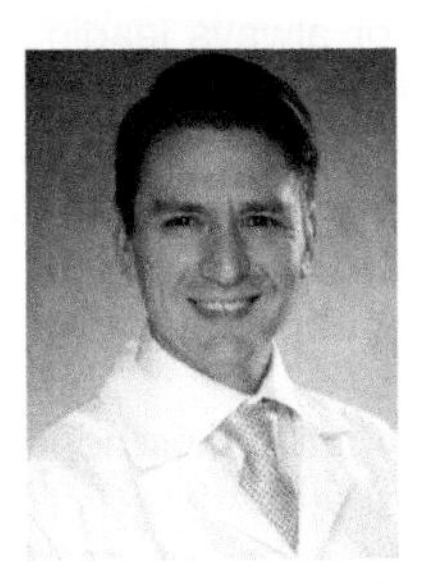

Cesar de Cesar Netto, MD, PhD
Editor

When I was asked by Dr Myerson to serve as the Guest Editor for this issue of *Foot and Ankle Clinics of North America* back in mid-2019, I was ecstatic! I consider it a huge honor and responsibility to write high-quality review articles for this prestigious journal. As one can imagine, serving as guest editor of an issue on Progressive Collapsing Foot Deformity was more than I could hope for. I enjoyed every step of the process, starting with considering the essential subjects to be covered, discussing possible leading titles, and selecting the right people to author the articles. It was indeed a rewarding, enjoyable, and interactive process. During my interactions with Dr Myerson and the Editorial Team, I quickly noticed the love and passion they have for the journal and the intense and zealous amount of time and effort they put into every single issue. The whole experience was inspiring and energizing for me.

Several months later, when Dr Myerson selected me to lead the journal after his venerable 25-year tenure as the Consulting Editor, I would not be able to describe the mix of emotions I experienced. Surprise and happiness were first. I've always been a strong proponent of dreaming big, the "sky is the limit" type of thing, but even still, I could never have imagined or expected this invitation was coming. Satisfaction and pride were also there. We all admire Dr Myerson for his countless accomplishments and successful clinical, surgical, academic, and mentorship careers. But *Foot and Ankle Clinics of North America* is indisputably among his most important legacies in the Orthopaedic Foot and Ankle Community. It would have been a unique honor to even be considered for the position. Anxiety and fear came right after. Replacing the unreplaceable. The arduous task and huge challenge

Foot Ankle Clin N Am 26 (2021) xv–xvi
https://doi.org/10.1016/j.fcl.2021.06.007
1083-7515/21/© 2021 Published by Elsevier Inc.

of filling Dr Myerson's shoes. Calmness and relief followed, since as expected from this unique leader of our field, he told me he would be by my side and showing me the way, as he has done throughout his entire life and career, supporting and guiding the countless fellows/surgeons/clinicians he trained over the years.

I can promise Dr Myerson, the editorial team, all the authors, readers, and followers of the journal that I will give my best to keep the journal at the forefront of Foot and Ankle Surgery.

Dr Myerson set the bar high, and I'll need all of you reading this editorial to support and partner with me and with the journal to continue the brilliant work he started.

I want to thank Dr Myerson on behalf of the entire Orthopaedic Foot and Ankle Community for his 25 years of service and devotion to the journal. Thank you so much for trusting me with this opportunity of a lifetime and for always leading the way, pointing in the right direction. I would also like to thank all my mentors from the University of Sao Paulo, Johns Hopkins University, the University of Alabama at Birmingham, Hospital for Special Surgery, and Medstar Union Memorial Hospital. Without the teaching and support of our mentors, we don't get anywhere. Last, but not least, I want to share this career achievement with my wife, Sabrina, my daughters, Manuela and Juliana, as well as my parents and sister.

I am looking forward to interacting with the National and International Orthopaedic Foot and Ankle Surgery Community. Without all of you, the *Foot and Ankle Clinics of North America* would not represent what it represents. So, let's keep on the great path Dr Myerson carefully laid and work toward the future, starting now!

I hope you all enjoy this issue on Progressive Collapsing Foot Deformity, with outstanding articles from respected authors on the subject.

My best regards,

Cesar de Cesar Netto, MD, PhD
Orthopaedics and Rehabilitation
University of Iowa
200 Hawkins Drive
Room 01066 JPP
Lower Level
Iowa City, IA 52242, USA

E-mail address:
cesar-netto@uiowa.edu

What Are the Updates on Epidemiology of Progressive Collapsing Foot Deformity?

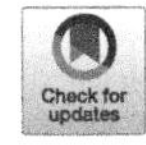

Alexandre Leme Godoy-Santos, MD, PhD[a,b,*], Eli L. Schmidt, BS[c], Felipe Chaparro, MD[d,e]

KEYWORDS

• Epidemiology • Etiology • Flatfoot • Progressive collapsing foot deformity • PCFD

KEY POINTS

- A key element in understanding osseus etiology is the subtalar and talonavicular joint complex. Recent imaging techniques have led us to a better understanding.
- Posterior tibial tendon, plantar fascia, interosseus ligament, and spring ligament complex represent the key soft tissue elements in maintaining foot architecture.
- The real prevalence of flatfoot deformity is unknown. A recent systematic review showed that no universally accepted criteria for diagnosing pediatric flat foot was found within the existing literature.

INTRODUCTION

Progressive collapsing foot deformity (PCFD) is one of the most controversial topics in foot and ankle surgery. Reviews normally focus on different surgical approaches depending on alterations presented, which are highly variable and make decision making a difficult task. In recent years, considerable research has been done regarding the anatomy and biomechanics behind this complex deformity and some interest has been put on studying metabolic or genetic conditions that could influence the development of this multifactorial disorder. Still, there remains no uniform approach either in the evaluation process or in the treatment strategies. This is in light

[a] Department of Orthopedic Surgery, Faculdade de Medicina, Universidade de São Paulo, Rua Dr Ovídio Pires de Campos 333, Cerqueira Cesar, Sao Paulo, Sao Paulo 05403-010, Brazil; [b] Hospital Israelita Albert Einstein, São Paulo, Sao Paulo, Brazil; [c] Department of Orthopaedics and Rehabilitation, University of Iowa, 200 Hawkins drive, Iowa City, IA 52242, USA; [d] Hospital San José, Santiago, Chile; [e] Clinica Universidad de los Andes, Avenida Plaza 2501, Las Condes, Santiago 7620157, Chile

* Corresponding author. Rua Dr Ovídio Pires de Campos 333, Cerqueira Cesar, Sao Paulo, Sao Paulo 05403-010, Brazil.

E-mail address: alexandrelemegodoy@gmail.com

Foot Ankle Clin N Am 26 (2021) 407–415
https://doi.org/10.1016/j.fcl.2021.05.006

of new arising technologies that could increase our knowledge and change classical concepts in dealing with this multifocal and multiplanar deformity.

ANATOMY AND BIOMECHANICS

The pathophysiology leading to flatfoot deformity is multifactorial and poorly understood. Terminology referring to deformity has been one of the first confounding issues. Normally PCFD is used synonymously with posterior tibial tendon dysfunction, but it is important to notice that, although degeneration of the tendon can be present, the tendon is only one of the overloaded and degenerated soft tissue structures on the medial aspect of the foot and ankle.[1,2]

The new terminology, "progressive collapsing foot deformity" (PCFD)[3,4] potentially better describes the pathologic progressive cases, in which the deformity and symptoms progress over time, affecting osseous and soft tissue structures.

Osseus and Articular Elements

A key element in understanding PCFD pathophysiology is related to the anatomy and deformity around the triple joint complex, including the concept of peritalar subluxation (PTS).[5] Recent imaging techniques have led us to a better understanding of underlying deformities that can predict and increase the chances of PCFD.[6]

In the past few years, we have witnessed a vertiginous advance in the assessment and understanding of this topic, mostly related to weight-bearing computed tomography (WBCT) imaging. Apostle and colleagues[7] described that patients with symptomatic PCFD had an increased valgus orientation in the subtalar posterior facet, studied by simulated WBCT, a finding that could represent an anatomic predisposition to PTS of the hindfoot and could be an important element in PCFD development in some patients.

Arthur Manoli[8] described remodeling of the calcaneocuboid (CC) joint in patients with PCFD, showing that all studied patients had some degree of change in the CC joint, concordant with the amount of deformity observed.

Walley and colleagues[9] measured the lateral column length of subjects with PCFD compared with healthy patients with conventional non-WBCT scan and found that, on average, the lateral column was shorter in patients with PCFD. The concept of lateral column shortening is very controversial and not supported by the literature in adult patients with no pediatric deformity.

Soft Tissues

Gastrocsoleus complex

In the presence of gastrocsoleus complex contracture, during the gait the foot moves to the heel prematurely and increases the overload of body weight on the plantar fascia, midfoot, and metatarsal heads. Midfoot pronation associated with forefoot supination and abduction can occur to compensate for limited ankle dorsiflexion and may increase forces in the talonavicular, medial naviculocuneiform, and medial cuneiform-first metatarsal joints and medial soft tissues.[10–12]

Although Arangio and colleagues[12] identified that the arm of the hindfoot valgus moment was increased in symptomatic PCFD with contracture of the gastrocsoleus complex when compared with controls, Tryfonidis and colleagues[13] found that patients with PCFD with perolateral dorsolateral subluxation, decreased medial arch height, and forefoot abduction may be caused by insufficiency of the medial soft tissues with normal posterior tibial tendon and without the presence of contracture of the gastrocsoleus complex.

There is a reasonable rationale for the relationship between gastrocsoleus contracture and PCFD pathomechanics; however, it remains controversial because most studies related to this topic show a low level of evidence.[8–13]

Posterior tibial tendon

The posterior tibial tendon (PTT), plantar fascia, and spring ligament complex play a key role in maintaining foot architecture. PTT dysfunction is part of a myriad of pathologic events happening in PCFD, but there is general agreement that this dysfunction cannot be the sole factor that leads to PCFD.[1,2] In this respect, the real importance of PTT dysfunction in PCFD is not fully understood. During walking, contraction of the PTT generates locking of the transverse tarsal joint and allows the forward propulsion force of the gastrocsoleus complex to be translated to the metatarsal heads. When the PTT fails, the unlocked transverse tarsal joint allows this force to be exerted over the midfoot, allowing medial longitudinal arch collapse. Degenerative disease of the PTT is multifactorial and could be age-related.[8,9] Trnka[14] described different etiologic factors that could be involved in PTT dysfunction pathogenesis, from inflammatory synovitis to degenerative trauma. Lately, importance has been given to the study of genetic or metabolic variations that could be involved. Most studies examining the effect of metabolic changes on tendon homeostasis have been undertaken for rotator cuff tendinopathy. Reasonably, these metabolic alterations have a systemic effect, altering not only shoulder tendons but others, like PTT, as well. Metabolic syndrome[15] is a cluster of clinical findings, including hypertension, insulin resistance, dyslipidemia, and obesity, which determine an increased risk for cardiovascular diseases. Metabolic syndrome is also associated with other, less widely known changes, such as musculoskeletal pathology. Diabetes has long been linked to PCFD[16] by epidemiologic studies, but in the past few years through basic science research, we have begun to better understand this process. In a recent literature review, Nichols and colleagues[16] described factors that affect tendon homeostasis both clinically and at a cellular level, expanding on the role of diabetes in the pathologic process. In these patients, it is common to find functional impairments like loss of movement and structural abnormalities, including loss of collagen organization, tendon thickening, and calcification, all of which may increase the chance of tendon rupture and impair tendon healing. These alterations are collectively described as diabetic tendinopathy.

Other metabolic syndrome manifestations are also associated with tendon pathology. The association between obesity and PTT pathology is well known.[17,18] For instance, obesity may influence both PTT dysfunction pathogenesis and results after surgical management.[19] Interestingly, no correlation was found between body weight and pronated feet. Kun-Chung Chen and colleagues[20,21] analyzed 1748 children looking for relevant factors influencing flatfoot in preschool-aged children by visual inspection for flat foot, Beighton score, body mass index (BMI), and demographic parameters. Pita-Fernández and colleagues[18] conducted a cross-sectional study including 1002 random volunteers to determine flatfoot prevalence. They found a 19% prevalence of flat foot deformity, and a positive correlation with age, female gender, and BMI.

Dyslipidemia is another alteration seen during metabolic syndrome that has also been linked to PTT dysfunction pathogenesis, and changes in cholesterol level and its treatment have been suggested to impair tendon function.[22,23] Taylor and colleagues[22] reviewed the relationship between hypercholesterolemia and tendon pathology. They described recent research showing that the release of proinflammatory cytokines and upregulation of matrix-degrading proteins in hypercholesterolemic conditions leads to an increase in tendon stiffness and elastic modulus that influences tendon biomechanical and healing properties and could be implicated in a higher rupture risk. Not only could cholesterol level alteration be affecting tendon metabolism, but also its treatment has been implicated in tendon pathology. The use of statins in managing cholesterol levels has been associated with an increased risk of tendon rupture[23] by affecting tendon remodeling through its action over collagen metabolism.

Tendinopathy can be the presenting complaint in hypothyroidism, and symptomatic relief can be obtained by appropriate management of the primary thyroid deficiency.[24]

Some patients may develop PTT dysfunction and PCFD without any identifiable risk factor, suggesting that individual characteristics, including genetic inheritance, play an important role in tendinopathy.[25] In the past few years, there has been an increased interest in studying a possible relationship between genetic predisposition with PCFD development. The matrix metalloproteinases (MMPs) are responsible for the degradation and removal of collagen and could play an important role in the tendinopathy process. Molecular changes in extracellular matrix (ECM) and MMP polymorphism may influence the risk of developing PTT degeneration and PCFD.[26] The literature has shown 95% of collagen type I and small amounts of collagen types III, IV, and V in PTT extracellular matrix in normal PTT.[27] These collagen percentages allow elastic and mechanical resistance to PTT through parallel bundles on the tendon structure. Increased percentages of collagen types III and V (both molecules responsible for the elasticity of the tendon tissue) and decreased percentages of the alpha 1 and 2 chains of collagen type I (responsible for building thick fibers that give resistance to the tendon tissue) have been observed in the ECM of posterior tibial tendinopathy in patients with PCFD, and could be a possible explanation for decreased resistance and elasticity of the tendon tissue, leading to PTT degeneration and development of PCFD.[28] Genetic polymorphisms of MMP-1, MMP-8, and MMP-13 have been related to an increased risk for PTT tendinopathy and thereby PCFD development.[29]

All these metabolic and genetic alterations described previously are possible risk factors involved in PTT degeneration and PCFD development by imposing a progressive clinical burden to some patients with an anatomic predisposition to PCFD and "tip the scale" toward deformity development, but the importance of these risk factors in each individual patient is difficult to clinically determine.

Spring ligament complex

The role of other medial soft tissue structures in the development of PCFD is somehow controversial and has been given more importance recently in the literature.[2,6]

However, during those same years, most foot and ankle surgeons were prone to do "some kind" of medial soft tissue repair, with nearly half of them repairing the spring ligament.[30] Since those times, many investigations and advances have been done, and medial soft tissue repair is currently part of the repair algorithm for most surgeons.[31] This change is principally due to improvements in both anatomic and biomechanical knowledge on the subject, allowing for a better understanding of the crucial role that both the spring ligament complex, deltoid ligament, and interosseus talocalcaneal ligament play in the pathophysiology and stability of the deformity.[2]

The spring ligament complex is a group of ligaments connecting sustentaculum tali and navicular bone, with a main function of providing static stability to the talar head. It has 2 distinct ligamentous bands: the superomedial calcaneonavicular (SMCN) ligament and the inferomedial calcaneonavicular (ICN) ligament.[32] It is generally accepted that PTT degeneration in isolation is not capable of producing PCFD by itself, but can act as the trigger of a pathologic cascade that puts increased mechanical stress over the static medial stabilizers, which eventually fails, leading to progressive deformity and potential talonavicular deformity when there is a combined spring ligament complex degeneration.[1]

Studying specific contributions of each structure in the pathologic process is difficult, as they function as a group, and it is impossible to completely isolate one structure without affecting the function of the other. Anatomic studies have shown that the spring ligament complex is confluent with the superficial deltoid ligament, functioning as a unit for medial tibiotalar and talonavicular stability.[33]

Computer modeling strategies have been used recently to analyze the biomechanical behavior of medial soft tissue structures under deformity stress. Cifuentes-De la Portilla and colleagues[34] conducted a biomechanical study by foot computer modeling showing the specific amount of stress over each structure and found that both the PTT and the spring ligament have a principal role in avoiding hindfoot valgus, whereas the plantar fascia is the main tissue that prevents arch elongation. This approach offers an option in clinical research for quantifying tissue strain by expanding tools available for analyzing PCFD development, but further clinical studies are needed to validate their use.

ETIOLOGY AND EPIDEMIOLOGY

The real prevalence of PCFD is unknown, mainly because of poorly conducted clinical research studies and the lack of a strict definition of pathologic flatfoot deformity.

The Role of Pediatric Flatfoot on Etiology and Its Epidemiology

A recent systematic review by Banwell and colleagues[35] showed that no universally accepted criteria for diagnosing pediatric flat foot was found within the existing literature. As stated by Vincent Mosca,[36] a flatfoot has been defined subjectively as a weight-bearing foot with an abnormally low or absent longitudinal arch, which only takes into account the height of the arch within a population and not determinant features as pain or disability that this deformity may produce. This is a key element, as "normal variations" for arch heights may occur between people depending on age or ethnicity. Pediatric flat feet can be divided into flexible and rigid flatfoot deformity. Flexible flatfoot is physiologic and comprises nearly 95% of cases. On the other side, a rigid flatfoot has a restricted subtalar joint motion, normally due to underlying pathologies, such as tarsal coalition or a neuromuscular process, and is often associated with pain.[37] Which patients with a flexible flatfoot will become pathologic is unknown. The vast majority of clinical studies regarding this topic have been conducted in the child population, describing the normal foot development occurring at this age. The evolution of the medial longitudinal arch can occur over several years during childhood, with a broad spectrum of normal variations. Morley[38] found 97% of children younger than 18 months to have "flatfeet," which was persistent by the age of 10 in only 4% of the population. This result has been supported by clinical observation and epidemiologic studies throughout the years, supporting the general agreement that pediatric flatfoot generally resolves spontaneously during the first decade of life. As stated by Staheli and colleagues,[39] 54% of 3-year-old children had flat feet, a prevalence that decreases to 26% at the age of 6, showing a similar trend as previous studies and suggesting ages 3 to 6 years may be a critical period for the development of the medial longitudinal arch.[37] Yin and colleagues[40] conducted a cross-sectional epidemiologic study, including 1059 children aged 6 to 13 years, measuring the footprints according to the FootScan analysis and found that flatfoot percentage decreased from 39.5% at 6 years to 11.8% at 12 years, and the decrease reached a plateau at 12 to 13 years.

It is clear that the vast majority of flatfeet during childhood will become a “normal” foot during adulthood, and yet, persistent flatfoot during adulthood most commonly will behave as a normal foot, probably emphasizing the concept that a flatfoot appearance can be part of normality in a gaussian curve. Which flexible flatfeet during childhood will become symptomatic and could benefit from early treatment is yet to be elucidated.

POPULATION INCIDENCE STUDIES

Kohls-Gatzoulis and colleagues[41] investigated the prevalence of symptomatic posterior tibialis tendon dysfunction among 582 women older than 40. They found a prevalence of 6.6% of symptomatic flatfoot deformity. However, only 3.3% of the patients met the strict criteria to be included in the posterior tibialis tendon dysfunction and the rest of flatfeet cases were attributable to different etiologies (eg, Charcot arthropathy). Although it is possible to document different aspects of patients seeking medical attention due to foot problems, it is difficult to accurately measure the exact number of patients with asymptomatic flatfoot, who therefore go unnoticed. An improved understanding of the natural history of asymptomatic flatfoot into adulthood in needed to act on possible risk factors or initiate prophylactic treatment that could avoid progression into symptomatic flatfeet and prevent the development of more complicated deformities.

PCFD is 3 times more common in female individuals, with the peak incidence happening at the age of 55, and is more common in white, obese, diabetic, rheumatic, and hypertensive patients. It affects 3.3% of English women.[1,41]

FINAL CONSIDERATIONS

PCFD is one of the most controversial topics in foot and ankle surgery. In recent years, much research has been done regarding anatomy, biomechanics, and etiology behind this complex deformity, whereas some interest has been put on studying epidemiology and metabolic and genetic conditions that could influence the development of this multifactorial disorder.

Relevant anatomy elements include osseous and soft tissue structures. Regarding the bony anatomy, the most important elements are articular position/angulation and bone shape. On the other hand, soft tissue key elements are spring ligament complex, subtalar ligament complex, gastrocsoleus complex, and PTT.

CLINICS CARE POINTS

- Anatomy is a key element in PCFD pathophysiology.
- Pay attention to soft tissues and joint alignment.
- Take into account the characteristics of population susceptibility.
- Remember the metabolic and genetic conditions related to PCFD.

DISCLOSURE

The authors have nothing to disclose.

REFERENCES

1. Deland JT, de Asla RJ, Sung IH, et al. Posterior tibial tendon insufficiency: which ligaments are involved? Foot Ankle Int 2005;26(6):427–35.

2. de Cesar Netto C, Saito GH, Roney A, et al. Combined weightbearing CT and MRI assessment of flexible progressive collapsing foot deformity. Foot Ankle Surg 2020. https://doi.org/10.1016/j.fas.2020.12.003.
3. de Cesar Netto C, Deland JT, Ellis SJ. Guest editorial: expert consensus on adult-acquired flatfoot deformity. Foot Ankle Int 2020;41(10):1269–71.
4. Myerson MS, Thordarson DB, Johnson JE, et al. Classification and nomenclature: progressive collapsing foot deformity. Foot Ankle Int 2020;41(10):1271–6.
5. Ananthakrisnan D, Ching R, Tencer A, et al. Subluxation of the talocalcaneal joint in adults who have symptomatic flatfoot. J Bone Joint Surg Am 1999;81(8):1147–54.
6. de Cesar Netto C, Shakoor D, Roberts L, et al. Hindfoot alignment of adult acquired flatfoot deformity: A comparison of clinical assessment and weightbearing cone beam CT examinations. Foot Ankle Surg 2019;25(6):790–7.
7. Apostle KL, Coleman NW, Sangeorzan BJ. Subtalar joint axis in patients with symptomatic peritalar subluxation compared to normal controls. Foot Ankle Int 2014;35(11):1153–8.
8. Manoli A. Remodeling of the calcaneocuboid joint in the flatfoot. Foot Ankle Orthop 2017;2(3). 2473011417S000278.
9. Walley KC, Roush EP, Stauch CM, et al. Three-dimensional morphometric modeling measurements of the calcaneus in adults with stage IIB posterior tibial tendon dysfunction: a pilot study. Foot Ankle Spec 2019;12(4):316–21.
10. Rong K, Ge W-T, Li X-C, et al. Mid-term results of intramuscular lengthening of gastrocnemius and/or soleus to correct equinus deformity in flatfoot. Foot Ankle Int 2015;36(10):1223–8.
11. DiGiovanni CW, Langer P. The role of isolated gastrocnemius and combined Achilles contractures in the flatfoot. Foot Ankle Clin 2007;12(2):363–79, viii.
12. Arangio G, Rogman A, Reed JF 3rd. Hindfoot alignment valgus moment arm increases in adult flatfoot with Achilles tendon contracture. Foot Ankle Int 2009;30(11):1078–82.
13. Tryfonidis M, Jackson W, Mansour R, et al. Acquired adult flat foot due to isolated plantar calcaneonavicular (spring) ligament insufficiency with a normal tibialis posterior tendon. Foot Ankle Surg 2008;14(2):89–95.
14. Trnka HJ. Dysfunction of the tendon of tibialis posterior. J Bone Joint Surg Br 2004;86(7):939–46.
15. Samson SL, Garber AJ. Metabolic syndrome. Endocrinol Metab Clin North Am 2014;43(1):1–23.
16. Nichols AEC, Oh I, Loiselle AE. Effects of Type II diabetes mellitus on tendon homeostasis and healing. J Orthop Res 2020;38(1):13–22.
17. Holmes GB Jr, Mann RA. Possible epidemiological factors associated with rupture of the posterior tibial tendon. Foot Ankle 1992;13(2):70–9.
18. Pita-Fernández S, González-Martín C, Seoane-Pillado T, et al. Validity of footprint analysis to determine flatfoot using clinical diagnosis as the gold standard in a random sample aged 40 years and older. J Epidemiol 2015;25(2):148–54.
19. Soukup DS, MacMahon A, Burket JC, et al. Effect of obesity on clinical and radiographic outcomes following reconstruction of stage II adult acquired flatfoot deformity. Foot Ankle Int 2016;37(3):245–54.
20. Khan FR, Chevidikunnan MF, Mazi AF, et al. Factors affecting foot posture in young adults: a cross sectional study. J Musculoskelet Neuronal Interact 2020;20(2):216–22.

21. Chen KC, Yeh CJ, Tung LC, et al. Relevant factors influencing flatfoot in preschool-aged children. Eur J Pediatr 2011;170(7):931–6.
22. Taylor B, Cheema A, Soslowsky L. Tendon pathology in hypercholesterolemia and familial hypercholesterolemia. Curr Rheumatol Rep 2017; 19(12):76.
23. Gowdar SD, Thompson PD. Multiple tendon ruptures associated with statin therapy. J Clin Lipidol 2020;14(2):189–91.
24. Magnusson SP, Heinemeier KM, Kjaer M. Collagen homeostasis and metabolism. In: Ackermann PW, Hart DA, editors. Metabolic influences on risk for tendon disorders. Cham (Switzerland): Springer International Publishing; 2016. p. 11–25.
25. Godoy-Santos A, Ortiz RT, Mattar Junior R, et al. MMP-8 polymorphism is genetic marker to tendinopathy primary posterior tibial tendon. Scand J Med Sci Sports 2014;24(1):220–3.
26. Godoy-Santos A, Cunha MV, Ortiz RT, et al. MMP-1 promoter polymorphism is associated with primary tendinopathy of the posterior tibial tendon. J Orthop Res 2013;31(7):1103–7.
27. Satomi E, Teodoro WR, Parra ER, et al. Changes in histoanatomical distribution of types I, III and V collagen promote adaptative remodeling in posterior tibial tendon rupture. Clinics 2008;63(1):9–14.
28. de Araujo Munhoz FB, Baroneza JE, Godoy-Santos A, et al. Posterior tibial tendinopathy associated with matrix metalloproteinase 13 promoter genotype and haplotype. J Gene Med 2016;18(11–12):325–30.
29. Diniz-Fernandes T, Godoy-Santos AL, Santos MC, et al. Matrix metalloproteinase-1 (MMP-1) and (MMP-8) gene polymorphisms promote increase and remodeling of the collagen III and V in posterior tibial tendinopathy. Histol Histopathol 2018; 33(9):929–36.
30. Hiller L, Pinney SJ. Surgical treatment of acquired flatfoot deformity: what is the state of practice among academic foot and ankle surgeons in 2002? Foot Ankle Int 2003;24(9):701–5.
31. Deland JT. Spring ligament complex and flatfoot deformity: curse or blessing? Foot Ankle Int 2012;33(3):239–43.
32. Bastias GF, Dalmau-Pastor M, Astudillo C, et al. Spring ligament instability. Foot Ankle Clin 2018;23(4):659–78.
33. Campbell KJ, Michalski MP, Wilson KJ, et al. The ligament anatomy of the deltoid complex of the ankle: a qualitative and quantitative anatomical study. J Bone Joint Surg Am 2014;96(8):e62.
34. Cifuentes-De la Portilla C, Larrainzar-Garijo R, Bayod J. Analysis of the main passive soft tissues associated with adult acquired flatfoot deformity development: a computational modeling approach. J Biomech 2019;84: 183–90.
35. Banwell HA, Paris ME, Mackintosh S, et al. Paediatric flexible flat foot: how are we measuring it and are we getting it right? A systematic review. J Foot Ankle Res 2018;11:21.
36. Mosca VS. Flexible flatfoot in children and adolescents. J Child Orthop 2010;4(2): 107–21.
37. Carr JB 2nd, Yang S, Lather LA. Pediatric pes planus: a state-of-the-art review. Pediatrics 2016;137(3):e20151230.
38. Morley AJ. Knock-knee in children. Br Med J 1957;2(5051):976–9.

39. Staheli LT, Chew DE, Corbett M. The longitudinal arch. A survey of eight hundred and eighty-two feet in normal children and adults. J Bone Joint Surg Am 1987; 69(3):426–8.
40. Yin J, Zhao H, Zhuang G, et al. Flexible flatfoot of 6-13-year-old children: a cross-sectional study. J Orthop Sci 2018;23(3):552–6.
41. Kohls-Gatzoulis J, Woods B, Angel JC, et al. The prevalence of symptomatic posterior tibialis tendon dysfunction in women over the age of 40 in England. Foot Ankle Surg 2009;15(2):75–81.

Progressive Collapsing Foot Deformity: Should We Be Staging It Differently?

Lorraine A. Boakye, MD, Akachimere C. Uzosike, MD, MPH,
Eric M. Bluman, MD, PhD

KEYWORDS

- Classification system • Hindfoot • Flatfoot • Progressive collapsing foot deformity • AAFD • PTTD • PTTI • Peritalar Subluxation

KEY POINTS

- The PCFD work group nomenclature advances our ability to describe this deformity.
- Despite the advancement the PCFD nomenclature provides further refinements are needed.
- Future improvements should focus on a more intuitive and easily categorized framework.

INTRODUCTION

This article cursorily reviews the history of classification systems for pathologic "flatfoot deformity" in the adult and also critically reviews the recent introduction of a classification system intended to improve on the deficiencies of prior systems. The article concludes by offering suggestions for further work in evolving even more utilitarian systems for the staging and treatment of adult flatfoot disorder.

To be effective, orthopedic classification systems should not only provide a lucid delineation of different categories of pathologic condition but also demonstrate why the differences are clinically important. The clinical importance of the differences can be conveyed either intrinsically or overtly. The best staging systems also provide treatment options for each of the stages. Good examples of orthopedic systems that have high utility are the Schatzker classification of tibial plateau fractures,[1] the Enneking classification of musculoskeletal tumors,[2] the Salter-Harris classification of physeal fractures,[3] and the Refined Classification of adult flatfoot deformity.[4]

Review of "Flatfoot" Classification Systems

This article is not a comprehensive review of the classification and staging systems of "adult flatfoot"; however, it serves instead as a cursory overview useful in framing the current discussion.

Orthopedic Surgery, Brigham Health, 75 Francis Street, Boston, MA 02115, USA
E-mail address: ebluman@bwh.harvard.edu

Foot Ankle Clin N Am 26 (2021) 417–425
https://doi.org/10.1016/j.fcl.2021.06.002 foot.theclinics.com

Our understanding and secondarily our ways of describing and classifying this pathologic condition continues to evolve. At present, there have been at least 6 published classifications for adult flatfoot (**Table 1**). It is difficult to determine which of these systems is used most frequently. One can estimate the frequency of use, and perhaps secondarily the utility of these systems, based on the number of times each has been referenced in the scientific literature. This estimation would, however, necessitate adjusting for the length of time each has been in existence. The popularity of each system would therefore equate to the total citations of the article describing the system divided by the number of years since its publication. To our knowledge this has not been done before. However, using a publication-based metric may bias toward those classification systems with greater scientific utility and away from those with greater clinical utility. The Arbeitsgemeinschaft für Osteosynthesefragen classification of fractures is one system prone to this bias.[5]

The Progressive Collapsing Foot Deformity Workgroup

The latest classification system for "adult flatfoot" was published last year; this warrants a brief review. The progressive collapsing foot deformity (PCFD) classification was devised by a consensus group meeting on the subject held in New York City in 2019.[6] Experts from around the globe, many of whom have devoted substantial portions of their academic and clinical careers to the understanding and treatment of PCFD, were invited to be panel members. This new descriptor is accurate and will be used throughout the rest of this article.

Each panelist was asked to make a presentation about one facet of PCFD treatment (eg, medializing calcaneal osteotomy, hindfoot fusions, Cotton osteotomy, lateral column lengthening, ligamentous reconstruction, etc.). From these presentations and subsequent discussions additional consensus statements specific to each aspect were formulated and voted upon. These statements provided more specific treatment recommendations, although no algorithmic treatments were formulated.[6,11–18]

This group formulated 5 consensus statements that supported formulation of a novel classification scheme.[6] The first consensus statement was to adopt PCFD as nomenclature in lieu of previous terminology. There were several reasons for adopting this new nomenclature. Many of the terms used in previous nomenclature had inaccuracies as well as practical drawbacks. The most recent widely accepted nomenclature used adult-acquired flatfoot deformity (AAFD).[19] Although the AAFD descriptor did provide an improvement over prior nomenclature that improperly centralized the role of the posterior tibial tendon, it was not entirely accurate. Despite the fact that the vast majority of this pathologic condition is acquired in adulthood this is not always the case. Sometimes the deformity is present in childhood and only becomes

Table 1
Summary of the PCFD classification systems and associated features

Classification, Publication Year	#Stages	#Categories	Clinical Findings	Radiographic Findings	Treatment
Johnson & Strom,[7] 1989	3	3	Y	Y	N
Myerson et al,[8] 1997	4	4	Y	Y	Y
Bluman et al,[4] 2007	4	11	Y	Y	N
Raikin et al,[9] 2012	3	6	N	Y	N
Deland,[10] 2008	4	7	Y	Y	Y
Myerson et al,[6] 2020	2	242	Y	Y	N

pathologic in adulthood. The term flatfoot led to problems with reimbursement by third-party payers because they consider care of the flatfoot "routine" because many individuals have asymptomatic flatfeet. The descriptor "deformity" was retained because of its accuracy. The terminology was changed to "progressive" because this indicates the worsening of the pathologic components over time. "Collapsing" was substituted for "flat" for multiple reasons. One is that determinations of "flat" are subjective in that they are difficult to measure and standardize. Collapsing was also chosen because it better represents that the entire foot is becoming dysmorphic rather than just undergoing loss of the longitudinal arch. Last, many insurance underwriters will not reimburse diagnoses that incorporate flatfoot. These changes were agreed upon by the workgroup in unanimity. Similarly, the second position statement that current classification systems are incomplete or outdated was approved unanimously.

Position statement 3 proposed the inclusion of MRI findings in the new classification system. There was weak negative consensus on this with 67% of the panelists feeling that MRI should not be part of the new system.

The question of whether weight-bearing computed tomography (WBCT) should be incorporated into the new classification system was also considered in consensus statement 4. Only weak consensus was arrived at with 56% agreeing that it should be included; this is related to the current situation that most clinical locations do not have WBCT capabilities.

Strong consensus was arrived at for position statement 5. This statement proposed the adoption of a new classification system for staging of PCFD and to define treatment. Of 9 delegates 8 voted affirmatively, with 1 abstention.

The Progressive Collapsing Foot Deformity Classification System

The PCFD classification system is both anatomically and functionally based. The system categorizes deformities as either being flexible (stage 1) or rigid (stage 2). Only anatomy with deformity is annotated; that without deformity is signified by omission. The 5 deformity patterns focused on in the PCFD system are the hindfoot valgus, midfoot/forefoot abduction, forefoot varus/medial column instability, peritalar subluxation/dislocation, and ankle instability. **Table 2** summarizes the system. Using this system, a patient with flexible hindfoot varus, midfoot abduction through the transverse tarsal joint resulting in talar head uncoverage of 40%, passively correctable forefoot varus but without any ankle deformity, or subflbular impingement would be staged 1ABC using the PCFD system. This patient would be classified as IIB using the Refined Classification system.[20] A second example is the patient with rigid hindfoot valgus with an associated rigid forefoot varus without any significant uncoverage of the talar head whose deformity is complicated by a flexible ankle valgus deformity that results in subfibular impingement with the latter 2 components being relieved with passive correction. This patient would be staged as a 2ACD1E using the PCFD system; the Refined Classification system refers to this as a IVA deformity.

We congratulate the PCFD consensus working group. To our knowledge this is the first time that individuals of different academic blocs with significant interest and experience in the treatment of "adult flatfoot" have gathered to form a consensus on best practices for the diagnosis and treatment of this disorder; this is a major accomplishment in and of itself. This approach has leveraged in-depth clinical scientific evidence in combination with surgical experience the absence of which hampered previous efforts to create a comprehensive classification system. The PCFD Workgroup Collaboration has gone far to synthesize the fragmented, albeit focused, knowledge base into a more well-formed whole.

Table 2
PCFD classification 2020

	Stages of the Deformity	
Stage I		Flexible
Stage II		Rigid
	Types of Deformity (Classes- Isolated or Combined)	
	Deformity Type/Location	**Consistent Clinical/Radiographic Findings**
Class A	Hindfoot valgus deformity	Hindfoot valgus alignment Increased hindfoot moment arm, hindfoot alignment angle, foot and ankle offset
Class B	Midfoot/forefoot abduction deformity	Decreased talar head coverage Increased talonavicular coverage angle. Presence of sinus tarsi impingement
Class C	Forefoot varus deformity/medial column instability	Increased talus-first metatarsal angle Plantar gapping first TMT joint/NC joints Clinical forefoot varus
Class D	Peritalar subluxation/dislocation	Significant subtalar joint subluxation/subfibular impingement
Class E	Ankle instability	Valgus tilting of the ankle joint

Abbreviations; NC, naviculocuneiform; TMT, tarsometatarsal.
Consensus group classification of progressive collapsing foot deformity.

The PCFD Workgroup has highlighted and expanded upon concepts that were introduced in earlier classification systems; specifically, how the roles that abduction through the transverse tarsal joint and/or midfoot, forefoot supination and deformity, and complication by ankle involvement contribute to make this one of the most conceptually difficult and technically challenging conditions of the foot and ankle to treat.

This group astutely addressed a concern that has been discussed openly for some years, namely, that progression within "adult flatfoot" deformity does not necessarily follow a linear progression and may involve components of many of the previously described staging systems. Despite this recognition they incorporate the term "stage" in the classification terminology. Future classifications would do well to completely dispense with the term.

The Path Forward

Despite the Yeoman's work that the PCFD Workgroup has done, as well as that from others in the preceding 3 decades, there are still gaps remaining that need to be addressed. Careful evaluation of their publications brings this to light.

Consensus

Proper categorization of consensus group work within journals can be difficult—it is not original research but does not conveniently fit topical review criteria either. Although no new clinical data are presented, new concepts including a novel classification scheme and nomenclature are introduced.

A large number of orthopedic foot and ankle surgeons have written on the subject and provided valuable contributions. However, including all potential experts in this workgroup would have been unwieldy. As a result, somewhat arbitrary criteria were established to limit the number of participants and make the work group manageable. Inclusion criteria for invitees included authorship of at least 10 peer-reviewed publications on progressive collapsing flatfoot deformity.[20] After inclusion criteria were met there were 9 individuals empaneled to this work group. Experts generally agree that an ideal consensus group should include 9 to 12 members.[21]

We suggest that the organizers of future efforts use more inclusive criteria for workgroup members. There is no question that the consensus workgroup panelists are all experts in the diagnosis and treatment of PCFD. Perhaps, in addition to the total numbers of flatfoot-related articles published by an expert, the impact of each expert's contributions will be factored in. Assigning weight to an individual's publications by way of the number of times each has been cited is one simple way to achieve this. Although we recognize that there is no perfect way to assemble a consensus panel, additional discerning measures may add value to the workgroup process.

Broadening the scope of the work group would allow incorporation of even more individuals with substantive experience in the diagnosis and treatment of this disease process. One method that could have been used to broaden the input of experts would be to conduct one or more serial panels.[21] In this way the increased numbers and broadened scope would not make the workgroup unwieldy.

It is clear that the panel used a consensus method, but it is unclear exactly what or whether a described method was used. No materials and methods section is present in their article, but a careful reading of the article suggests that a modification of a nominal group technique was used.[20] Future iterations of such consensus groups could be made more rigorous through closer adherence to and description of accepted consensus methods.

The rate of future findings will likely be rapid. As such interim updates of experts in the field should be undertaken at regular intervals, perhaps every 5 to 10 years, to make sure that classification and treatment recommendations that arise from these developments are incorporated to iterative systems in a timely manner.

Imaging

This latest classification scheme comes at the advent of a new and what promises to be an exciting era in our understanding of the natural history and anatomic contributions to the pathology of PCFD. Although some work has examined the 3-dimensional relationships of the hindfoot in the past,[22,23] the development and widespread availability of WBCT will no doubt provide many new insights into the early stages of this deformity, as well as some hitherto unknown aspects of this deformity. The findings that will be made possible through this new technology will need to be incorporated into further refinement of the classification scheme.

There may be some parallels between the evolution of the PCFD classification system of the future and the evolution of classification systems for calcaneal fractures. With calcaneal fractures the initial classification systems were quite simple involving either joint depression or tongue-type fracture.[24] Obviously this was not sophisticated enough, but until CT became widespread we were not able to adequately delve into the nuances of calcaneal fractures. The CT-based Sanders classification system has become preeminent for these injuries because of its completeness in characterizing these injuries and efficacy in guiding surgical treatment of these injuries.[25]

Although a small majority of the PCFD Workgroup delegates supported incorporating WBCT findings into the classification system, questions regarding the availability of this technology led to some individuals to shy away from full endorsement. No workgroup member thought that the 3-dimensional information that this technology contributes is trivial.[12] As WBCT technology will very quickly become the standard method for imaging this deformity it should be incorporated into future iterations of PCFD classifications as soon as possible.

In the past, one of us (E.M.B.) has espoused that MRI of the patient with PCFD is not routinely necessary. We still believe this to be the case. However, with the new emphasis on both the deltoid and spring ligaments in earlier stages of the disease MRI may routinely provide value especially if future classification systems rely on the condition and location of ligamentous damage. In these cases, it may be beneficial to have MRI data, not only for diagnosis but also for assessing treatment options.[26]

Comprehensibility and Usability

Although the newly proposed PCFD classification and nomenclature makes sense, it does lack some of the intrinsic organizational simplicity that some of the other classifications have. Our understanding of the condition is becoming more complex, and it follows that future classification systems will necessarily mirror this. Previous systems built off Johnson & Strom's 3-stage classification. The iterative approach previously used allowed clinicians to build nuance into this initial simple framework.

The PCFD classification is simultaneously robust and lacking. Although conceptually simple and comprehensive in practice, the descriptors do not lend themselves to easy comprehension. In certain situations, the requirement to include every detail of the deformity in its notation renders it cumbersome (see examples cited earlier). An argument can be made that it fails to adequately describe nuanced aspects of the condition (the only descriptive options for each anatomic location are flexible or rigid).

This tradeoff of comprehensive accuracy at the expense of usability is reminiscent of the AO Classification of Fractures. The AO system is accurate and has a high interobserver reliability. However, it is unwieldy and digitizes named anatomic structures (eg, a noncomminuted transverse midshaft tibia-fibula fracture is designated 43-A3). For this reason, it is infrequently used in clinical discussions and has largely been relegated to research communications. It will be interesting to see if the PCFD classification suffers the same fate.

Future PCFD classifications would do well to use easily relatable abbreviations (eg, H, rather than A, for hindfoot) with a minimum number of characters/digits to spare users the effort of translating seemingly arbitrary symbols to obtain clinically useful imagery.

Classification nomenclature should be easy to follow and user friendly. Perhaps the most effective way to make these systems user friendly is for them to be structured with some intuitive scaffold, whether it be anatomically or severity based. As the PCFD Workgroup has used an anatomic organization we recommend that future iterations follow this convention but proceed in a linear fashion. Currently the classification system starts with hindfoot valgus deformity as Class A and then progresses distally until Class C (forefoot varus) whereupon the system jumps retrograde to peritalar subluxation as Class D and then again to ankle instability as Class E. The classification would be easier to remember and follow if it progressed in a single direction from ankle to forefoot.

Furthermore, the PCFD Workgroup has chosen to use arbitrary digits for representation of the different anatomic locations that they focus on. We believe that it would be more intuitive to substitute digits that logically represent the anatomic locations (eg, A, ankle; H, hindfoot; P, peritalar subluxation; Ab, abduction mid/forefoot; F, forefoot varus), and this could also be modified to an acronym if desired.

In addition, the workgroup's description of the deformities as either flexible or rigid is limiting. Flexible deformities can have either stable or unstable variants. The presence of significant arthritis within supple or unstable joints should also be noted. Inclusion of this within the classification system would make it more complete. One suggestion would be that the nature of the deformities be described along a spectrum progressing from supple and stable without deformity (normal, I), to supple and stable with deformity (II), to unstable (III), and ending with substantially arthritic and/or stiff (IV).

Crystallization of Treatment Recommendations

Another criticism is that the PCFD Workgroup did not crystallize a treatment algorithm for the framework of deformities that they have described. This, however, would not be entirely fair because many of the treatments that are currently being used have not been validated relative to each other in studies with high levels of evidence. In addition, the breadth of recognized deformity has increased significantly. In the Refined Classification there are 12 different deformities delineated.[20] With the PCFD classification there are theoretically 242 unique combinations of deformities. Without consolidation this panoply of possibilities could make formulation of comprehensive treatment recommendations a monumental task.

The most utilitarian classifications stand the test of time, even as new treatment options arise. The Sanders classification of calcaneal fractures is an example of this.[27] Early after its introduction many orthopedic foot and ankle surgeons recommended that a Sanders IV calcaneal fracture be treated with open reduction and internal fixation (ORIF) and primary subtalar fusion.[28] Two factors drove this recommendation. The first was the increased likelihood that such high-energy fractures would result in post-traumatic arthritis necessitating a subsequent fusion procedure. The second was the difficulty of going back through a lateral extensile approach to revise the initial joint sparing effort to a subtalar arthrodesis. Use of a standard sinus tarsi approach following a lateral extensile exposure would complete a triangle of scar at least theoretically placing the tissue within this triangle at risk of necrosis. With the subsequent popularization of the sinus tarsi approach for ORIF of calcaneal fractures and availability of fixation hardware designed for it more surgeons now attempt joint-sparing surgery for Sanders IV injuries than previously. This is due to several reasons, not the least of which was that it is much easier to perform a subsequent subtalar arthrodesis if necessary, through the previously used sinus tarsi incision. In this way the classification remains intact but the way many treat one severity class has evolved.

Considering PCFD, the corollary to this may be the addition of WBCT scan for more nuanced evaluation of all components of the deformity. At present, using the Refined Classification the recommendation for treatment of a IIB type deformity is incorporation of a lateral column lengthening procedure.[4] The rationale for this is to decrease the amount of abduction/talar head uncovering that is seen through the talonavicular joint by lengthening the structures on the lateral side of the foot. Although good results are frequently obtained with this treatment approach, the recommended surgical procedure applies a 2-dimensional answer to a 3-dimensional problem. The 3-dimensionality of this problem was highlighted by the Seattle group in the use of the "dorsolateral peritalar subluxation" descriptor.[29] The incorporation of WBCT coupled with 3-dimensional rendering of images may allow for a more effective 3-dimensional correction.

SUMMARY

To answer the question whether we should be staging PCFD differently is both no and yes. The work group that has been put together has identified most of the components that need to be addressed. The inclusion of a system that deliberately and lucidly addresses each component of the deformity is necessary. However, there does need to be expansion of the overall framework. Should we include pediatric pathologic conditions for which treatment may be different despite sharing all the same characteristics of those who have developed the deformity as an adult? One question that remains relates to the cause of the deformity in different patient populations: Is the bony morphology of the foot in individuals who have been flat-footed their entire life but only develop symptoms in adulthood different from those individuals who develop PCFD late in life? Perhaps the shape of the talus, navicular, and calcaneus (as well as other bones of the foot) of the former group are substantially different from those of the latter group as a result of differential loading on their physes. If this is the case, in some patients perhaps both bony and soft tissue deformities are developing concomitantly to eventually lead to the painful flatfoot. It would be logical then to use osteotomies to restore normal bony morphology to support soft tissue corrections that are done in conjunction. In some ways this would be coming full circle because we commonly use medializing calcaneal osteotomies to help protect the soft tissue reconstructions on the medial side of the foot when addressing flexible flatfoot deformities.

A large advancement in comprehensively classifying progressive collapsing foot deformity was made by the PCFD Workgroup. The answer to the question as to whether we should be staging PCFD differently is yes, but not substantially so. The current classification of PCFD needs minor improvements. We have the opportunity to build upon a robust system that our colleagues have provided us; orthopedic foot and ankle surgeons look forward to further improvements.

REFERENCES

1. Schatzker J, McBroom R, Bruce D. The tibial plateau fracture. The Toronto experience 1968–1975. Clin Orthopaedics Relat Res 1979;138:94–104.
2. Jawad MU, Scully SP. In brief: classifications in brief: enneking classification: benign and malignant tumors of the musculoskeletal system. Clin Orthopaedics Relat Res 2010;468(7):2000–2.
3. Salter RB, Harris RW. Injuries Involving the Epiphyseal Plate. J bone Jt Surg 1963; 45(3):587–622.
4. Bluman EM, Title CI, Myerson MS. Posterior tibial tendon rupture: a refined classification system. Foot Ankle Clin 2007;12(2). 233–249, v.
5. Müller ME, Koch P, Nazarian S, et al. The comprehensive classification of fractures of long bones. Berlin, Heidelberg: Springer Berlin Heidelberg; 1990.
6. Myerson MS, Thordarson DB, Johnson JE, et al. Classification and nomenclature: progressive collapsing foot deformity. Foot Ankle Int 2020;41(10):1271–6.
7. Johnson KA, Strom DE. Tibialis posterior tendon dysfunction. Clin Orthop Relat Res 1989;239:196–206.
8. Myerson MS. Adult acquired flatfoot deformity: Treatment of dysfunction of the posterior tibial tendon. Instr Course Lect 1997;46:393–405.
9. Raikin SM, Winters BS, Daniel JN. The RAM classification: a novel, systematic approach to the adult-acquired flatfoot. Foot Ankle Clin 2012;17(2):169–81.
10. Deland J. Adult-acquired flatfoot deformity. J Am Acad Orthop Surg 2008;16(7): 399–406.
11. C Schon L, de Cesar Netto C, Day J, et al. Consensus for the indication of a medializing displacement calcaneal osteotomy in the treatment of progressive collapsing foot deformity. Foot Ankle Int 2020;41(10):1282–5.

12. de Cesar Netto C, Myerson MS, Day J, et al. Consensus for the use of weight-bearing CT in the assessment of progressive collapsing foot deformity. Foot Ankle Int 2020;41(10):1277–82.
13. Deland JT, Ellis SJ, Day J, et al. Indications for deltoid and spring ligament reconstruction in progressive collapsing foot deformity. Foot Ankle Int 2020;41(10):1302–6.
14. Ellis SJ, Johnson JE, Day J, et al. Titrating the amount of bony correction in progressive collapsing foot deformity. Foot Ankle Int 2020;41(10):1292–5.
15. Hintermann B, Deland JT, de Cesar Netto C, et al. Consensus on indications for isolated subtalar joint fusion and naviculocuneiform fusions for progressive collapsing foot deformity. Foot Ankle Int 2020;41(10):1295–8.
16. Johnson JE, Sangeorzan BJ, de Cesar Netto C, et al. Consensus on indications for medial cuneiform opening wedge (cotton) osteotomy in the treatment of progressive collapsing foot deformity. Foot Ankle Int 2020;41(10):1289–91.
17. Sangeorzan BJ, Hintermann B, de Cesar Netto C, et al. Progressive collapsing foot deformity: consensus on goals for operative correction. Foot Ankle Int 2020;41(10):1299–302.
18. Thordarson DB, Schon LC, de Cesar Netto C, et al. Consensus for the indication of lateral column lengthening in the treatment of progressive collapsing foot deformity. Foot Ankle Int 2020;41(10):1286–8.
19. Pinney SJ, Lin SS. Current concept review: acquired adult flatfoot deformity. Foot Ankle Int 2006;27(1):66–75.
20. de Cesar Netto C, Deland JT, Ellis SJ. Guest Editorial: Expert Consensus on Adult-Acquired Flatfoot Deformity. Foot Ankle Int 2020;41(10):1269–71.
21. Jones J, Hunter D. Consensus methods for medical and health services research. BMJ (Clinical Research Ed.) 1995;311(7001):376–80.
22. Apostle KL, Coleman NW, Sangeorzan BJ. Subtalar joint axis in patients with symptomatic peritalar subluxation compared to normal controls. Foot Ankle Int 2014;35(11):1153–8.
23. Dibbern KN, Li S, Vivtcharenko V, et al. Three-Dimensional Distance and Coverage Maps in the Assessment of Peritalar Subluxation in Progressive Collapsing Foot Deformity. Foot Ankle Int 2021. 1071100720983227.
24. Schepers T, van Lieshout EMM, Ginai AZ, et al. Calcaneal fracture classification: a comparative study. J Foot Ankle Surg 2009;48(2):156–62.
25. Epstein N, Chandran S, Chou L. Current concepts review: intra-articular fractures of the calcaneus. Foot Ankle Int 2012;33(1):79–86.
26. de Cesar Netto C, Saito GH, Roney A, et al. Combined weightbearing CT and MRI assessment of flexible progressive collapsing foot deformity. Foot Ankle Surg 2020;S1268-7731(20)30262-9.
27. Sanders R. Intra-articular fractures of the calcaneus: present state of the art. J Orthop Trauma 1992;6(2):252–65.
28. Myerson MS. Primary subtalar arthrodesis for the treatment of comminuted fractures of the calcaneus. Orthop Clin North Am 1995;26(2):215–27.
29. Toolan BC, Sangeorzan BJ, Hansen ST. Complex reconstruction for the treatment of dorsolateral peritalar subluxation of the foot. Early results after distraction arthrodesis of the calcaneocuboid joint in conjunction with stabilization of, and transfer of the flexor digitorum longus tendon to, the midfoot to treat acquired pes planovalgus in adults. J Bone J S Am Vol 1999;81(11):1545–60.

Is Advanced Imaging a Must in the Assessment of Progressive Collapsing Foot Deformity?

Francois Lintz, MD, MSc, FEBOT[a,*], Cesar de Cesar Netto, MD, PhD[b]

KEYWORDS

- Magnetic resonance imaging • Weight-bearing cone-beam CT • 3D biometrics
- Spring ligament • Interosseous talocalcaneal ligament • Progressive foot collapse
- Adult acquired flatfoot deformity

KEY POINTS

- Progressive collapsing foot deformity (PCFD) is a 3-dimensional (3D) disease, hence 3D imaging is a requisite.
- Weight-bearing cone-beam CT is a transformative innovation in the clinical and research exploration of PCFD.
- The middle facet has been identified as the center of rotation of the subtalar joint and its uncoverage percentage as an earlier marker of PCFD.
- The 3D Biometric Foot Ankle Offset has been shown to highly correlate with several known conventional PCFD measurements.
- MRI studies have identified lesions of the Spring ligament as being at least as important as tibialis posterior in the characterization of PCFD.

INTRODUCTION: WHAT DO WE CALL ADVANCED IMAGING AND HOW DOES IT APPLY TO PROGRESSIVE COLLAPSING FOOT DEFORMITY

The term "advanced imaging" is not coined in the literature as an exact definition, yet it suggests technologies that are positioned farther down any real or virtual axis deemed to represent some area of progress or at least positive evolution. One of these axes could be time, or in this case, image definition. To be more scientific, the authors performed a literature search with the following query terms in new-PubMed: "advanced imaging" [ti] AND orthopedics. This returned 35 results where MRI was mentioned in

[a] Department of Foot and Ankle Surgery, Ramsay Healthcare Clinique de l'Union, Boulevard de Ratalens, Saint-Jean, Toulouse 31240, France; [b] Department of Orthopaedics and Rehabilitation, University of Iowa, Iowa City, IA, USA
* Corresponding author.
E-mail address: dr.f.lintz@gmail.com

Foot Ankle Clin N Am 26 (2021) 427–442
https://doi.org/10.1016/j.fcl.2021.05.001

92% of occurrences including all modalities of vascular or articular contrast injections, computed tomography (CT) in 69%, also including all modalities of injections for arthro or vascular CT, ultrasound in 8%, bone scan or scintigraphy in 4%. Other modalities that were mentioned in 12% included dual-energy X-ray absorptiometry scan, dynamic fluoroscopy, biplanar low-dose radiography (EOS),[1] PET, even histology and arthroscopy. Surprisingly, cone-beam weight-bearing CT (WBCT) was not picked up by this simple request. We deem that some explanation to this lies in that cone-beam CT (CBCT) technology is not recent, and dates back to the mid-1990s,[2] taking off first in the dental arena, whereas its clinical use in orthopedics dates back only to the mid-2010s (**Fig. 1**). Scientific publications concerning CBCT and orthopedics are currently growing exponentially (currently 30/y), with roughly half (14/y) concerning the foot and the ankle. It is technologically a conventional, low-dose imaging (it is a radiographic beam source that revolves around an object) that is paving the way for advanced computer sciences techniques, such as deep learning and artificial intelligence. de Cesar Netto and Richter[3] did use the term "advanced" with weight-bearing imaging in a recent publication reporting the use of cone-beam WBCT in hallux valgus in a historic publication reporting the first ever fully automatic 3-dimensional (3D) measurement (of the M1-M2 angle).

Advanced imaging is sometimes criticized for being costly, time-consuming, and unnecessary[4]; however, this is more generally true of any new technology before it becomes mainstream. History has shown numerous examples of both being right or wrong in the end. Other investigators emphasize its ability to reduce costs and improve patient workflow, as well as diagnostic accuracy and radiation exposure.[5,6] As such, ultrasonography, which improves patient workflow by decentralizing imaging solutions in point-of-care specialized units may be considered advanced or at least progressive.[7]

In what concerns progressive collapsing foot deformity (PCFD) or until recently adult acquired flatfoot deformity,[8,9] the literature clearly points out 2 major modalities as advanced imaging systems: MRI, which was greatly commented especially between 2010 and 2015, and cone-beam WBCT, which is increasingly being reported on since 2015. In 2014, Baca and colleagues[10] published a paper on PCFD and advanced imaging, only citing MRI and ultrasound, not CT, which seems to emphasize the fact that for this author, CT without weight bearing, could not be considered advanced imaging for PCFD. This is confirmed by a larger literature search on WBCT and PCFD, which shows that the main areas of interest with CT before 2015 were to perform custom load-simulation protocols for conventional CT, or more complex, costly and time-

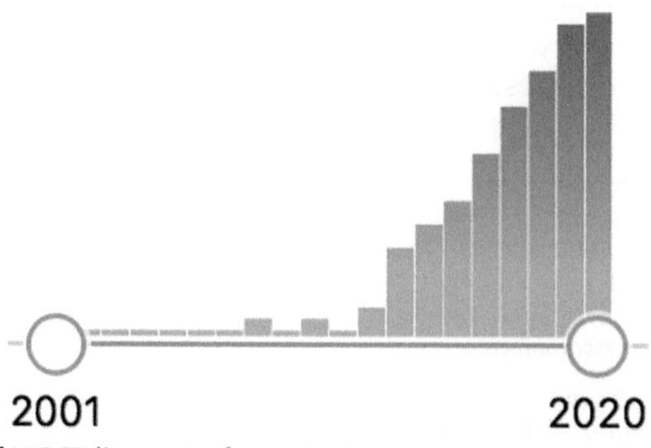

Fig. 1. Evolution of WBCT literature from 2000 to 2020.

consuming computational models such as finite element analysis[11–16] to simulate the effects of load on foot and ankle structures.

In summary, Advanced Imaging in PCFD may be perceived as futuristic, complex, and research oriented, but the evolution of the scientific literature shows us that what truly prevails are technologies that make sense in daily practice through improvement of diagnostic accuracy, clinical outcomes (an indirect consequence of the former), time consumption, and costs. Patient satisfaction influences practitioner choices in terms of clinical decision making and research orientation. In the realm of PCFD, it is clear today that MRI and even more, WBCT are the driving forces. Furthermore, computational models, which were really a trend of research until the mid-2010s are now on the verge of becoming conventional in our everyday practice too. Understanding them is key to remaining at the tip of the arrow.

Discussion: State of the Art Research and its Clinical Relevance: Notable Findings with MRI and Weight-Bearing Computed Tomography in Recent Years

MRI

MRI is nowadays well established in daily clinical practice and largely accessible in developed countries but remains a costly examination. Its ability to visualize bone as well as soft tissue makes it a valuable tool in PCFD as a complex 3D pathology implicating both soft tissue lesions[17,18] and bony alterations, such as impingement syndromes creating bony edema visible on MRI images.[19] Numerous investigators have published research using MRI with a focus on detecting early signs of ongoing foot collapse at a stage in which conservative and joint-sparing measures are still possible before joint sacrificing interventions must be considered.[20–23] The tibialis posterior (TP) (**Fig. 2**) tendon has long been the most investigated structure. Rosenberg and colleagues[24] published the first MRI-based TP classification in 1988, which was then modified by Kong and Van Der Vliet in 2008[25] with excellent intraobserver and interobserver reliability, as demonstrated by Braito and colleagues[26] in 2016, in a study investigating the correlation between MRI and intraoperative findings. The 3-grade classification described by Conti and colleagues[17] had the advantage to be

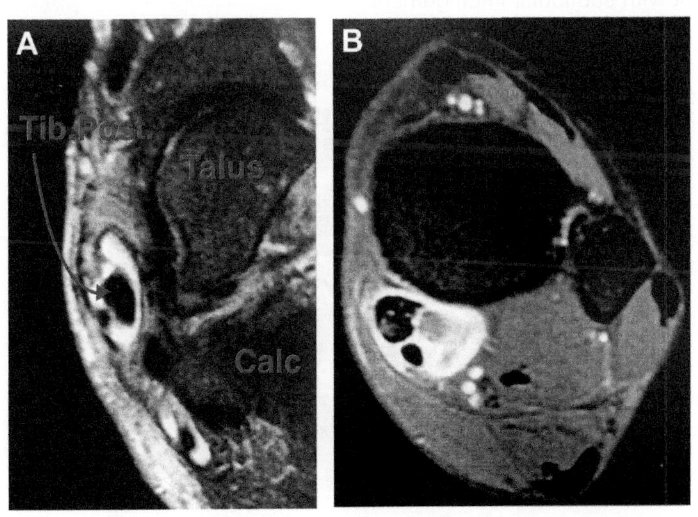

Fig. 2. (*A*) MRI imaging of TP dysfunction Conti Grade 1. (*B*) MRI of TP dysfunction Conti Grade 2.

predictive of postoperative outcomes. In Grade 1, a fine longitudinal split is seen, in grade 2, wider longitudinal splits are seen with gray areas demonstrating degenerative areas. In grade 3, the whole tendon is replaced with degenerative tissue. In this 1992 study, MRI was more sensitive than intraoperative inspection of the TP for intramural degeneration, which is correlated with failure of reconstructive surgery. This emphasizes the functional role of MRI in general and the importance of the "functional" criteria to define imaging technology as "advanced." The capacity for detecting ongoing biological failure of the intrinsic repair mechanisms at the early or later stages of pathology, as illustrated by increased inflammation through water concentration within a seemingly normal tissue, is specific to MRI, and particularly meaningful in PCFD. However, the TP tendon is not always reported as the key feature in PCFD, although we would argue that being a multifactorial process, the search for therapeutic solutions is complex and leads to multiple hypotheses. For example, DeOrio and colleagues[27] showed posterior tibial edema is highly correlated with presence of inflammatory fluid within the TP tendon sheath on MRI findings (sensitivity 86%, specificity 100%), so the investigators did not advocate for systematic use of MRI in the presence of this clinical finding. MRI is also valuable in the differential diagnosis with other causes of medial compartment painful syndromes, such as accessory navicular or tarsal tunnel syndrome.[28] Other investigators have also reported the role of MRI in correlating PCFD with other conditions, particularly to explain associated lateral pain that has long been attributed to sinus tarsi impingement syndrome, where increased signal can be found on the lateral process of the talus and mirroring in the calcaneal floor of the sinus tarsi (**Fig. 3**). In this respect, associated subtalar joint instability and anterior talofibular ligament lesions were reported.[29–31] Another field of research has investigated the spring ligament[18,32,33] (**Fig. 4**) and other structures such as the talocalcaneal interosseus (**Fig. 5**) and deltoid ligament.[34] In a recent publication assessing the combined results of WBCT and MRI assessments in PCFD, the investigators were able to find significant correlations between important WBCT markers of peritalar subluxation (PTS) and MRI findings of soft tissue injury.[19] In particular, degeneration of the TP tendon was associated with sinus tarsi impingement, spring ligament degeneration to subtalar subluxation, and talocalcaneal interosseous ligament involvement with subfibular impingement.

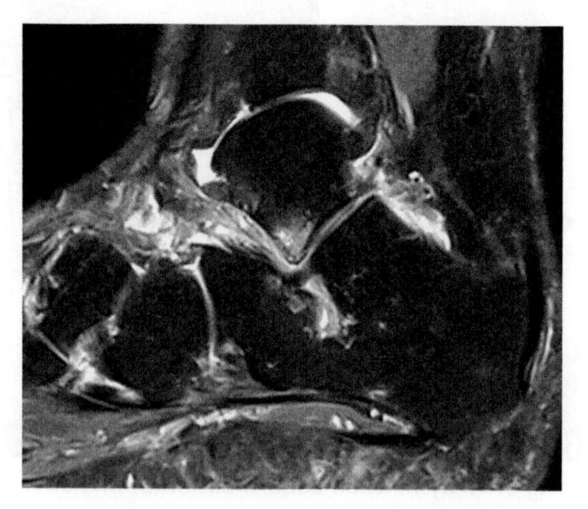

Fig. 3. MRI of STI.

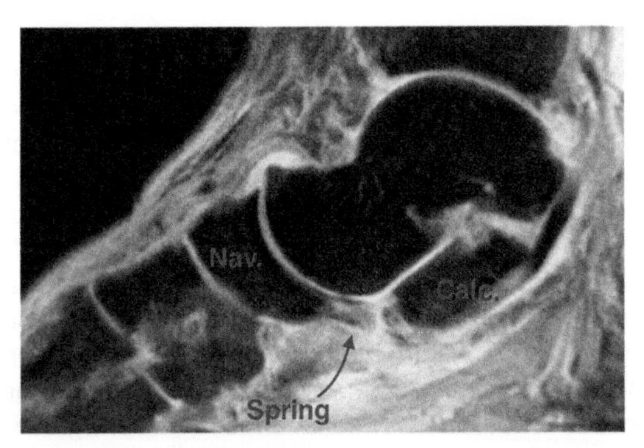

Fig. 4. MRI sagittal view of spring ligament rupture.

In another study correlating clinical signs such as the first metatarsal rise test and the heel rise, Albano and co-authors[35] state that MRI correlated better with clinical signs than histology. Khoury and colleagues[36] stated furthermore that MRI characteristics of severe tendinosis and partial tear may overlap. Shibuya and colleagues[37] had in 2008 found that, based on the Conti classification, and correlating MRI findings with radiographic ones, only severe TP pathology was associated with radiographic findings compatible with PCFD, suggesting that TP is not the only driving force implicated. This was confirmed in 2014 by Williams and colleagues[32] who stated that MRI findings on the spring ligament were possibly at least of equal importance to TP degeneration in patients with moderate to severe PCFD.

In total, MRI is largely used in the context of PCFD and is mostly known for its ability to characterize TP tendon impairment through the Conti classification. However, it should be recognized also for its capacity to investigate exhaustively all deep ligamentous and tendinous structures. In particular, the TP may not be the main driving force and further research on the role of the spring and the interosseous ligaments is warranted. Other roles of MRI should be pointed out with an emphasis on identifying potential differential diagnoses or signs of severity in PCFD such as sinus tarsi and subfibular impingement or subtalar arthritic changes.

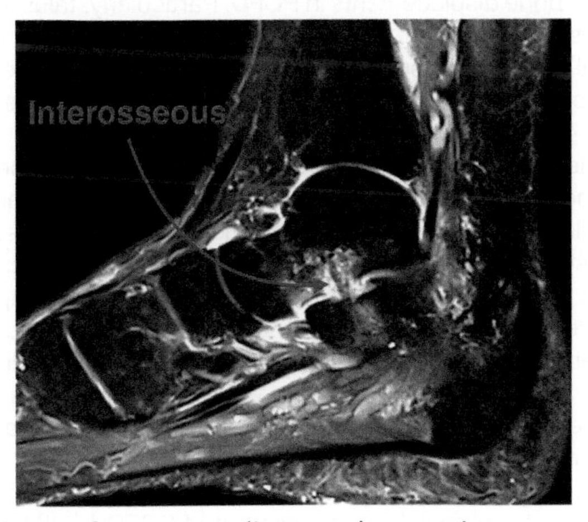

Fig. 5. MRI sagittal view of interosseous ligament degeneration.

Cone-beam weight-bearing computed tomography

Three-dimensional cone-beam WBCT[38,39] is the main paradigm shift of the recent years in orthopedics. In the lower limbs, its weight-bearing imaging capacity is fundamental, even more so in the foot and ankle with its complex and intricate 3D. In this context, PCFD, due to previous research using simulated weight bearing[15,40] showing the importance of load in evaluating this pathology, has been the main area of interest with WBCT. In particular, important work by Ellis and colleagues[41–44] using a large and costly device (Philipps Eleva System) in the context of research, harvested valuable data from 2008 to 2015, before the initiation of WBCT. This research particularly emphasized the importance of weight bearing in PCFD and its superiority to older imaging modalities, being either 3D, but not weight bearing, or weight bearing but not 3D. As Ellis and colleagues[41] cited: "conventional CT is not a surrogate for weight bearing scanning." Recently, de Cesar Netto and colleagues[45] published a landmark paper comparing traditional measurements with and without weight bearing using WBCT. This was a diagnostic level 2 study that demonstrated that in a non–weight-bearing configuration, osseous derangements are underestimated, which has been otherwise constantly reported in the literature[46] also using other image modalities such as MRI.[47] Numerous international review papers[38,39,46] have already reported on the advantages of WBCT compared with the conventional radiograph-CT sequence, including lower radiation dose,[48] easier use, and rapid learning curve whatsoever the experience of the investigating surgeon or radiologist.[49,50] Still, the concentration of literature around few but prolific investigators does reflect the fact that in real life the technology is not yet ubiquitous. In our opinion, this is not due to excessive costs or lack of evidence, but rather to an absence of administrative awareness of the technology and its advantages. The WBCT has already been used as a reference in studies investigating the validity of clinical examination[51,52] or postoperative surgical correction in PCFD[53] and can be considered as the gold standard, considering the evidence today, for 3D measurements. It should not be long before it does become conventional.

Another significant aspect of WBCT imaging, in general, but that applies importantly in PCFD, is the absence of measurement bias as compared with conventional radiography.[38,48,54] It is a mathematical fact that traditional measurements made on weight-bearing radiographs are a sinusoid function of the angle between incident rays and the detector panel. Therefore, what is measured is not the real angle, but only a 2D projection.[55,56] In that sense, WBCT is a paradigm shift. It allows further investigations into the true loaded bone displacements in PCFD. Particularly, talus internal rotation,[44] first tarso-metatarsal joint sagging,[57] and innate valgus of the calcaneus and subtalar joints,[44,58] as well as forefoot supination,[15,40,59] have been studied. Ellis and colleagues[41] also showed better correlation of the real 3D measurements with hindfoot pain.

Hindfoot alignment is the subject for which there has been the most interest in the literature. Switching from a distorted 2D plane and straightforward measurements to a reliable, but complex 3D environment requires a learning curve, research, and clinical validation. The first steps required adaptation of known 2D measurements, such as the hindfoot angle or navicular-to-floor distance to WBCT[45,60] in papers that showed that WBCT provided more reproducibility and better sensitivity. However, achieving these measurements leads to a new kind of bias that could be called "slicing bias," related to the fact that in order to perform a 2D measurement in a 3D environment, one particular slice must be chosen among many possibilities for a single measurement. Concomitantly, novel 3D biometrics making full use of the 3D weight-bearing capacity were introduced and subject to an extensive research effort, demonstrating close to 100% reliability, especially in the context of PCFD.[1,46,61,62] The most stated

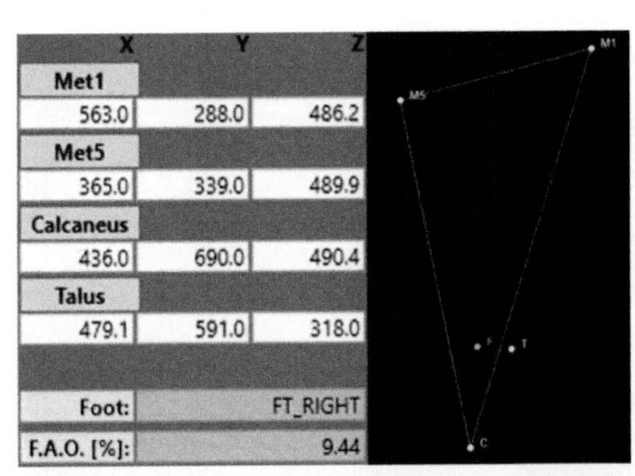

X
Y
Z
Met1
563.0
288.0
486.2
Met5
365.0
339.0
489.9
Calcaneus
436.0
690.0
490.4
Talus
479.1
591.0
318.0
Foot:
FT_RIGHT
F.A.O. [%]:
9.44
M1
M5
T
C

Fig. 6. An example of PCFD measurement of alignment using 3D biometrics. The FAO is 9.44% for a normal value between 0% and 2%) demonstrating severe valgus deformity. The center of the ankle joint is projected outside of the foot triangle, demonstrating fundamental biomechanical imbalance of this particular foot.

measurement has been the Foot Ankle Offset (FAO) described in 2017, which is a semiautomatic, WBCT-based measurement of the coronal rotational torque lever arm generated between the ankle joint and the foot tripod[63,64] (**Fig. 6**). Effectively, a software allows for manual selection of landmark points on the WBCT dataset: the plantarmost or weight-bearing points of the first metatarsal head, fifth metatarsal head (M1 and M5), and the calcaneus (C) define the weight-bearing triangle. The software then calculates the median line of the foot, passing through C and the midpoint of the forefoot (halfway between M1 and M5). A final point (T), describing the center of the ankle joint (uppermost point on the talar dome, halfway between its lateral and medial corners) is manually selected. The program then automatically calculates the distance between T and the median line of the foot (TF). This distance is then divided by the length of the foot line and given as a percentage, so that results are comparable, whatever the length of the foot. The distance corresponds to the offset between the center of the ankle joint (where body weight is applied) and the virtual point where ground reaction force is applied. It therefore accurately represents the torque that acts on the foot and ankle complex during gait, at each step. The whole process takes a few seconds, actually less time than it would take to manually measure any angle. The FAO has demonstrated near perfect intraobserver and interobserver reliability, excellent correlation with on-board pedobarographic data,[65] whereas earlier investigations using 2D measurements had failed to correlate with the pressure sensor data.[66] Three-dimensional biometrics have also allowed progress in understanding the relationship between knee and hindfoot alignment, demonstrating the existence of a pattern in valgus configuration.[1] More recently they also displayed the existence of significant relationship between hindfoot alignment and the development of total ankle replacement periprosthetic cysts.[67] Therefore, it seems reasonable to say that, being the only modality of imaging in functional position, WBCT also answers to the definition of "advanced" imaging, as does MRI.

More generally, WBCT has enabled great progress in the domain of normal and pathologic behavior of the subtalar joint,[42,43,64,68] confirming and helping to develop the concept of subtalar instability.[69] In this area, the middle facet, which was suggested as a key element by Ananthakrisnan and colleagues[70] in 1999 was recognized as a the center of rotation of the subtalar joint[71] and the keystone of subtalar subluxation in PCFD by de Cesar Netto and colleagues in a later publication 2019[62,72]

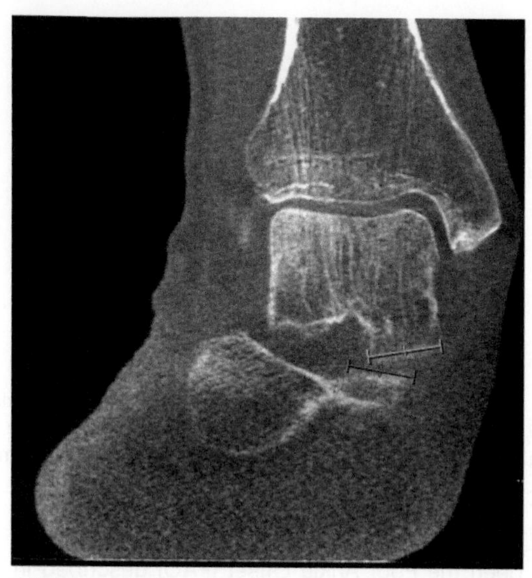

Fig. 7. WBCT coronal imaging and measurement of middle facet subluxation according to de Cesar Netto and colleagues.[62,72]

(**Fig. 7**). The investigators found that middle facet subluxation greater than 18% could be a better predictor of early PTS in PCFD than posterior facet subluxation.[73] It seems clear seeing the consistency and the chronology of these findings that they were only made possible by the advent of WBCT.

Foot and ankle offset was also recently demonstrated to correlate significantly with measurements of forefoot arch angle, talonavicular coverage angle, subtalar horizontal angle, and hindfoot moment arm, explaining approximately 80% of variations of these measurements.[62] The investigators emphasized the possibility of using FAO to provide a relatively simple and easy multiplanar measurement of PCFD. It allowed a global 3D assessment of PCFD using a single measurement, that incorporates 4 of the most commonly conventional PCFD measurements performed in the sagittal, coronal, and axial planes. FAO was also shown to be a great assessment tool of deformity corrections in patients with PCFD after surgical treatment,[61] in a prospective

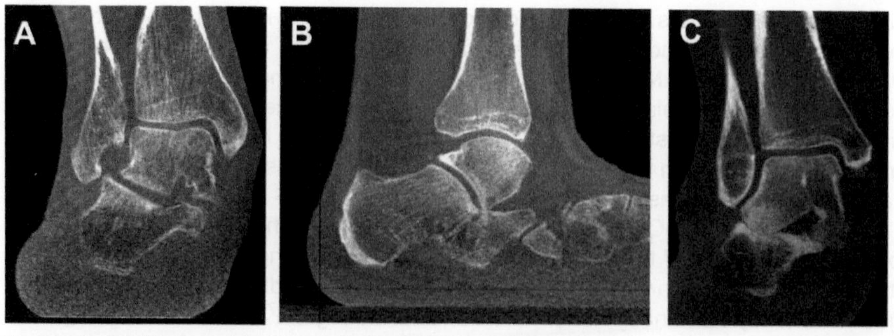

Fig. 8. (*A*) WBCT coronal imaging of subfibular impingement. (*B*) WBCT sagittal imaging of STI. (*C*) WBCT coronal imaging of STI.

comparative study reporting highly significant and sensitive correction of the FAO and improvement of all PROMIS domains.

Subfibular impingement (SFI) and sinus tarsi impingement (STI) (**Fig. 8**), are associated with peritalar instability in PCFD. Jeng and colleagues[74] found that SFI was present in 35% of cases between the fibula and the calcaneus, whereas talocalcaneal impingement was present in 38%. They concluded that, although WBCT confirmed that SFI is a true feature of PCFD, it is less frequent than previously reported. Ellis and colleagues[41] reported that in a series comparing PCFD feet with or without hindfoot pain, SFI was increased in the painful group, but did not reach significance. Eventually, WBCT was able to investigate SFI better than any other imaging modality; however, this is far from being its only indication, as often perceived. On its part, STI has been recently confirmed by many studies and acknowledged in the PCFD consensus papers as a reliable marker on advanced collapse on WBCT.[8]

Computational models: solving the data paradox

The paradigm shift introduced by WBCT leads to a multitude of data we did not have access before in PCFD; however, we are faced with a data paradox. We have been trained and are used to working with a combination of functional 2D distorted datasets (radiographs) and 3D but nonfunctional datasets (conventional CT). Punctual past solutions like simulated horizontal load now seem outdated and unreliable,[39] but also avoidable seeing that WBCT devices are cheaper than conventional CT, growingly available worldwide and resulting in roughly 10 times less radiation exposure. One other factor apart from our training, lies in the fact that interpreting angles and distances in 3D is difficult and mainly implies intuition. Because WBCT potentially provides us constantly with millions of data points, we must rely on computational models to help us make proper measurements and interpret those large quantities of data. The foremost aspect of this matter of fact is the 3D environment is difficult to grasp. Looking at a multiplanar view of a PCFD case, for example, will remain a difficult challenge and we will have to find the correct plane in which to perform a 2D measurement.

However, recent literature is showing that the "gray zone" is losing ground fast. Computational models that were initially dedicated to research are being feverishly automatized by the industry. Among these, many have been already used in PCFD. Segmentation (labeling of individual bones)[53,71] (**Fig. 9**), which is still being performed by hand in many instances, is on the verge of becoming fully automatic,[3] paving the

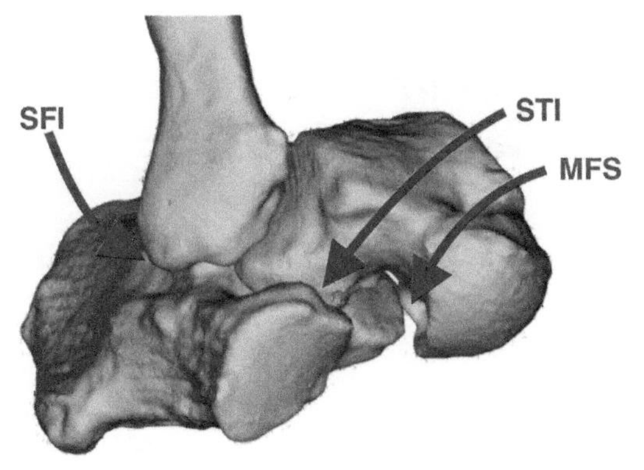

Fig. 9. Segmentation of hindfoot bones from WBCT in a PCFD case, illustrating SFI, STI and MFS.

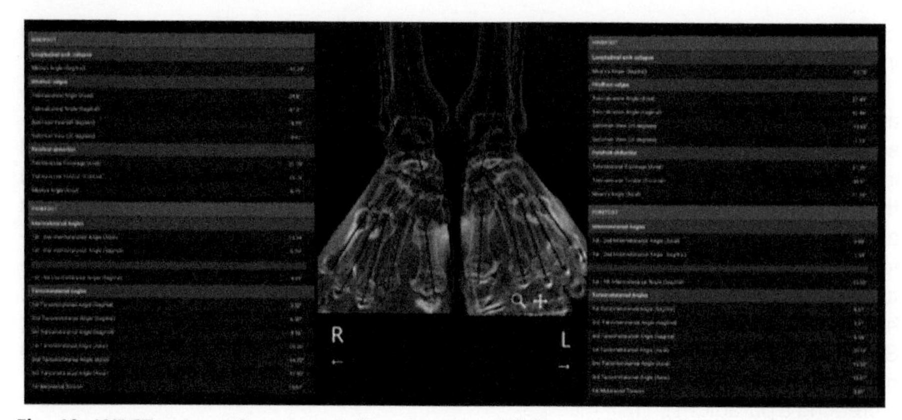

Fig. 10. WBCT automatic segmentation report and fully automatic 3D measurements.

way for automatization of all measurements (**Fig 10**). The use of large, prospectively collected datasets have successfully found mathematical relationships between deformity and pathology[75] using WBCT. Other techniques such as Digital Volume Correlation,[71] which correlates deformity measurements with 3D strain. In other words, minute changes in positioning or density of areas of bone may be detected using this technique and correlated with mechanical or structural changes. Rigid body modeling[76] is another technique, which calculates strain based on 3D displacement of bones. Finally, knowledge of soft tissue resistance is used independently or associated with finite element analysis,[77–79] which has been known for a long time now to simulate forces based on tissue mechanical properties. One of the most promising techniques is distance mapping (DM) (**Fig. 11**), which analyzes the 3D surface interaction maps of joints through color-coded, quantified maps, replacing the traditional eyeball intuitive uniplanar joint space analysis. This has been found to be highly correlated with patient pain.[41,80] A 2019 paper by Kothari and colleagues reported that a

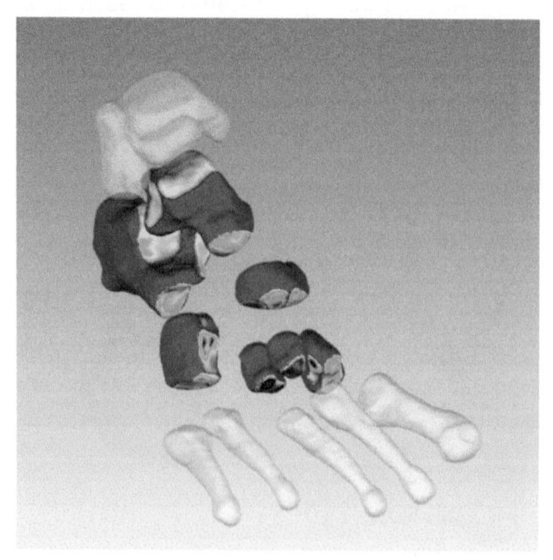

Fig. 11. Exploded view of a mild PCFD case with DM of hindfoot and midfoot joints illustrating joint space narrowing.

joint space width less than 2.0 mm was significantly associated with increased pain in a multicentric series of patients with knee osteoarthritis. The same technique is being used by PCFD authors to investigate the distal syndesmosis[81] or sinus tarsi volumes,[82] finding more precise ways to describe pathologic situations.

Summary: Yes, it Is a Must, and it Will Change the Way We Work

In conclusion, although the term "advanced imaging" is not officially coined in the literature, there seems to be a large consensus on the fact that MRI and WBCT are best fit to represent this category of imaging in PCFD. In the past, MRI has been largely commented as a valuable tool with a focus on correlation with pain and postoperative evolution. It is now commonly integrated in investigation protocols for PCFD. Cone-beam WBCT, on the other hand, is still in its infancy, but already generating a plethora of new knowledge, such as the value of the subtalar middle facet and the FAO. However, it is creating a paradigm shift in that the data produced are too large to be understood intuitively, requiring the help of newly developed computational models, for instance DM. With cone-beam WBCT, we have opened the pandora's box of the digital revolution in the foot and ankle, and PCFD is the gateway into it.

CLINICS CARE POINTS

- MRI and WBCT are the most developed advanced imaging modalities in PCFD.
- MRI is well integrated in diagnostic protocols with an aim to correctly assess ligamentous and tendinous components in PCFD.
- WBCT is gaining traction both in research and in clinical use. It uses advanced computational models to help with the interpretation of datasets. It can already be considered as the Gold Standard and in the process of becoming mainstream.
- WBCT has demonstrated the importance of Middle Facet Subluxation as a very specific early marker of PTS in PCFD and 3D Biometrics such as the Foot Ankle Offset as a reliable measure of hindfoot alignment in general and in PCFD.

DISCLOSURE

F. Lintz and C. de Cesar Netto declare being paid consultants of Curvebeam LLC. They serve on the board of the International Weight Bearing CT Society as Vice President and Treasurer.

REFERENCES

1. Dagneaux L, Dufrenot M, Bernasconi A, et al. Three-dimensional biometrics to correlate hindfoot and knee coronal alignments using modern weightbearing imaging. Foot Ankle Int 2020. https://doi.org/10.1177/1071100720938333.
2. Mozzo P, Procacci C, Tacconi A, et al. A new volumetric CT machine for dental imaging based on the cone-beam technique: preliminary results. Eur Radiol 1998;8:1558–64.
3. de Cesar Netto C, Richter M. Use of advanced weightbearing imaging in evaluation of hallux valgus. Foot Ankle Clin 2020;25:31–45.
4. Natoli RM, Fogel HA, Holt D, et al. Advanced Imaging Lacks Clinical Utility in Treating Geriatric Pelvic Ring Injuries Caused by Low-Energy Trauma. J Orthop Trauma 2017;31:194–9.

5. Rua T, Parkin D, Goh V, et al. The economic evidence for advanced imaging in the diagnosis of suspected scaphoid fractures: systematic review of evidence. J Hand Surg Eur 2018;43:642–51.
6. Fuller CB, Farnsworth CL, Bomar JD, et al. Femoral version: Comparison among advanced imaging methods. J Orthop Res 2018;36:1536–42.
7. Tanaka K, Kudo S. Functional assessment of the spring ligament using ultrasonography in the Japanese population. Foot (Edinb) 2020;44:101665.
8. de Cesar Netto C, Myerson MS, Day J, et al. Consensus for the use of weight-bearing CT in the assessment of progressive collapsing foot deformity. Foot Ankle Int 2020;41:1277–82.
9. Myerson MS, Thordarson DB, Johnson JE, et al. Classification and nomenclature: progressive collapsing foot deformity. Foot Ankle Int 2020;41:1271–6.
10. Baca JM, Zdenek C, Catanzariti AR, et al. Is advanced imaging necessary before surgical repair. Clin Podiatr Med Surg 2014;31:357–62.
11. Er MS, Verim O, Altinel L, et al. Three-dimensional finite element analysis used to compare six different methods of syndesmosis fixation with 3.5- or 4.5-mm titanium screws: a biomechanical study. J Am Podiatr Med Assoc 2013;103:174–80.
12. Wong DW-C, Wang Y, Chen TL-W, et al. Biomechanical consequences of subtalar joint arthroereisis in treating posterior tibial tendon dysfunction: a theoretical analysis using finite element analysis. Comput Methods Biomech Biomed Engin 2017; 20:1525–32.
13. Wong DW-C, Wang Y, Leung AK-L, et al. Finite element simulation on posterior tibial tendinopathy: Load transfer alteration and implications to the onset of pes planus. Clin Biomech (Bristol, Avon) 2018;51:10–6.
14. Xu J, Ma X, Wang D, et al. Comparison of Extraosseous Talotarsal Stabilization Implants in a Stage II Adult-Acquired Flatfoot Model: A Finite Element Analysis. J Foot Ankle Surg 2017;56:1058–64.
15. Zhang Y, Xu J, Wang X, et al. An in vivo study of hindfoot 3D kinetics in stage II posterior tibial tendon dysfunction (PTTD) flatfoot based on weight-bearing CT scan. Bone Joint Res 2013;2:255–63.
16. Wang Z, Imai K, Kido M, et al. A finite element model of flatfoot (Pes Planus) for improving surgical plan. Annu Int Conf IEEE Eng Med Biol Soc 2014;2014:844–7.
17. Conti S, Michelson J, Jahss M. Clinical significance of magnetic resonance imaging in preoperative planning for reconstruction of posterior tibial tendon ruptures. Foot Ankle 1992;13:208–14.
18. Mengiardi B, Pinto C, Zanetti M. Spring Ligament Complex and Posterior Tibial Tendon: MR Anatomy and Findings in Acquired Adult Flatfoot Deformity. Semin Musculoskelet Radiol 2016;20:104–15.
19. de Cesar Netto C, Saito GH, Roney A, et al. Combined weightbearing CT and MRI assessment of flexible progressive collapsing foot deformity. Foot Ankle Surg 2020. https://doi.org/10.1016/j.fas.2020.12.003.
20. C Schon L, de Cesar Netto C, Day J, et al. Consensus for the Indication of a Medializing Displacement Calcaneal Osteotomy in the Treatment of Progressive Collapsing Foot Deformity. Foot Ankle Int 2020;41:1282–5.
21. Hintermann B, Deland JT, de Cesar Netto C, et al. Consensus on Indications for Isolated Subtalar Joint Fusion and Naviculocuneiform Fusions for Progressive Collapsing Foot Deformity. Foot Ankle Int 2020;41:1295–8.
22. Sangeorzan BJ, Hintermann B, de Cesar Netto C, et al. Progressive collapsing foot deformity: consensus on goals for operative correction. Foot Ankle Int 2020;41:1299–302.

23. Thordarson DB, Schon LC, de Cesar Netto C, et al. Consensus for the indication of lateral column lengthening in the treatment of progressive collapsing foot deformity. Foot Ankle Int 2020;41:1286–8.
24. Rosenberg ZS, Cheung Y, Jahss MH, et al. Rupture of posterior tibial tendon: CT and MR imaging with surgical correlation. Radiology 1988;169:229–35.
25. Kong A, Van Der Vliet A. Imaging of tibialis posterior dysfunction. Br J Radiol 2008;81:826–36.
26. Braito M, Wöß M, Henninger B, et al. Comparison of preoperative MRI and intra-operative findings of posterior tibial tendon insufficiency. Springerplus 2016;5:1414.
27. DeOrio JK, Shapiro SA, McNeil RB, et al. Validity of the posterior tibial edema sign in posterior tibial tendon dysfunction. Foot Ankle Int 2011;32:189–92.
28. Chhabra A, Soldatos T, Chalian M, et al. 3-Tesla magnetic resonance imaging evaluation of posterior tibial tendon dysfunction with relevance to clinical staging. J Foot Ankle Surg 2011;50:320–8.
29. Yoon DY, Moon SG, Jung H-G, et al. Differences between subtalar instability and lateral ankle instability focusing on subtalar ligaments based on three dimensional isotropic magnetic resonance imaging. J Comput Assist Tomogr 2018;42:566–73.
30. Kim TH, Moon SG, Jung H-G, et al. Subtalar instability: imaging features of subtalar ligaments on 3D isotropic ankle MRI. BMC Musculoskelet Disord 2017;18:475.
31. Persaud S, Hentges MJ, Catanzariti AR. Occurrence of lateral ankle ligament disease with stage 2 to 3 adult-acquired flatfoot deformity confirmed via magnetic resonance imaging: a retrospective study. J Foot Ankle Surg 2019;58:243–7.
32. Williams G, Widnall J, Evans P, et al. Could failure of the spring ligament complex be the driving force behind the development of the adult flatfoot deformity? J Foot Ankle Surg 2014;53:152–5.
33. Toye LR, Helms CA, Hoffman BD, et al. MRI of spring ligament tears. AJR Am J Roentgenol 2005;184:1475–80.
34. Ormsby N, Jackson G, Evans P, et al. Imaging of the tibionavicular ligament, and its potential role in adult acquired flatfoot deformity. Foot Ankle Int 2018;39:629–35.
35. Albano D, Martinelli N, Bianchi A, et al. Posterior tibial tendon dysfunction: clinical and magnetic resonance imaging findings having histology as reference standard. Eur J Radiol 2018;99:55–61.
36. Khoury NJ, el-Khoury GY, Saltzman CL, et al. MR imaging of posterior tibial tendon dysfunction. AJR Am J Roentgenol 1996;167:675–82.
37. Shibuya N, Ramanujam CL, Garcia GM. Association of tibialis posterior tendon pathology with other radiographic findings in the foot: a case-control study. J Foot Ankle Surg 2008;47:546–53.
38. Lintz F, de Cesar Netto C, Barg A, et al. Weight-bearing cone beam CT scans in the foot and ankle. EFORT Open Rev 2018;3:278–86.
39. Barg A, Bailey T, Richter M, et al. Weightbearing computed tomography of the foot and ankle: emerging technology topical review. Foot Ankle Int 2018;39:376–86.
40. Ferri M, Scharfenberger AV, Goplen G, et al. Weightbearing CT scan of severe flexible pes planus deformities. Foot Ankle Int 2008;29:199–204.
41. Ellis SJ, Deyer T, Williams BR, et al. Assessment of lateral hindfoot pain in acquired flatfoot deformity using weightbearing multiplanar imaging. Foot Ankle Int 2010;31:361–71.

42. Probasco W, Haleem AM, Yu J, et al. Assessment of coronal plane subtalar joint alignment in peritalar subluxation via weight-bearing multiplanar imaging. Foot Ankle Int 2015;36:302–9.
43. Kunas GC, Probasco W, Haleem AM, et al. Evaluation of peritalar subluxation in adult acquired flatfoot deformity using computed tomography and weightbearing multiplanar imaging. Foot Ankle Surg 2018;24:495–500.
44. Cody EA, Williamson ER, Burket JC, et al. Correlation of Talar Anatomy and Subtalar Joint Alignment on Weightbearing Computed Tomography With Radiographic Flatfoot Parameters. Foot Ankle Int 2016;37:874–81.
45. de Cesar Netto C, Schon LC, Thawait GK, et al. Flexible adult acquired flatfoot deformity: comparison between weight-bearing and non-weight-bearing measurements using cone-beam computed tomography. J Bone Joint Surg Am 2017;99:e98.
46. Shakoor D, de Cesar Netto C, Thawait GK, et al. Weight-bearing radiographs and cone-beam computed tomography examinations in adult acquired flatfoot deformity. Foot Ankle Surg 2020. https://doi.org/10.1016/j.fas.2020.04.011.
47. Ikoma K, Ohashi S, Maki M, et al. Diagnostic characteristics of standard radiographs and magnetic resonance imaging of ruptures of the tibialis posterior tendon. J Foot Ankle Surg 2016;55:542–6.
48. Richter M, Lintz F, de Cesar Netto C, et al. Results of more than 11,000 scans with weightbearing CT — Impact on costs, radiation exposure, and procedure time. Foot Ankle Surg 2019. https://doi.org/10.1016/j.fas.2019.05.019.
49. Pilania K, Jankharia B, Monoot P. Role of the weight-bearing cone-beam CT in evaluation of flatfoot deformity. Indian J Radiol Imaging 2019;29:364–71.
50. de Cesar Netto C, Shakoor D, Dein EJ, et al. Influence of investigator experience on reliability of adult acquired flatfoot deformity measurements using weightbearing computed tomography. Foot Ankle Surg 2019;25:495–502.
51. Patel S, Bernasconi A, Thornton J, et al. Relationship between foot posture index and weight bearing computed tomography 3D biometrics to define foot alignment. Gait Posture 2020;80:143–7.
52. de Cesar Netto C, Shakoor D, Roberts L, et al. Hindfoot alignment of adult acquired flatfoot deformity: A comparison of clinical assessment and weightbearing cone beam CT examinations. Foot Ankle Surg 2019;25:790–7.
53. Burssens A, Barg A, van Ovost E, et al. The hind- and midfoot alignment computed after a medializing calcaneal osteotomy using a 3D weightbearing CT. Int J Comput Assist Radiol Surg 2019;14:1439–47.
54. Baverel L, Brilhault J, Odri G, et al. Influence of lower limb rotation on hindfoot alignment using a conventional two-dimensional radiographic technique. Foot Ankle Surg 2017;23:44–9.
55. Lintz F, Barg A, de Cesar Netto C, et al. Comments on the paper: "Impact of the rotational position of the hindfoot on measurements assessing the integrity of the distal tibio-fibular syndesmosis". Foot Ankle Surg 2020. https://doi.org/10.1016/j.fas.2020.04.003.
56. Richter M, Seidl B, Zech S, et al. PedCAT for 3D-imaging in standing position allows for more accurate bone position (angle) measurement than radiographs or CT. Foot Ankle Surg 2014;20:201–7.
57. Kido M, Ikoma K, Imai K, et al. Load response of the medial longitudinal arch in patients with flatfoot deformity: in vivo 3D study. Clin Biomech (Bristol, Avon) 2013;28:568–73.
58. Colin F, Horn Lang T, Zwicky L, et al. Subtalar joint configuration on weightbearing CT scan. Foot Ankle Int 2014;35:1057–62.

59. Yoshioka N, Ikoma K, Kido M, et al. Weight-bearing three-dimensional computed tomography analysis of the forefoot in patients with flatfoot deformity. J Orthop Sci 2016;21:154–8.
60. Burssens A, Peeters J, Buedts K, et al. Measuring hindfoot alignment in weight bearing CT: A novel clinical relevant measurement method. Foot Ankle Surg 2016;22:233–8.
61. Day J, de Cesar Netto C, Nishikawa DRC, et al. Three-dimensional biometric weightbearing CT evaluation of the operative treatment of adult-acquired flatfoot deformity. Foot Ankle Int 2020. https://doi.org/10.1177/1071100720925423.
62. de Cesar Netto C, Bang K, Mansur NS, et al. Multiplanar semiautomatic assessment of foot and ankle offset in adult acquired flatfoot deformity. Foot Ankle Int 2020;41:839–48.
63. Lintz F, Welck M, Bernasconi A, et al. 3D biometrics for hindfoot alignment using weightbearing CT. Foot Ankle Int 2017;38:684–9.
64. Zhang JZ, Lintz F, Bernasconi A, et al. 3D biometrics for hindfoot alignment using weightbearing computed tomography. Foot Ankle Int 2019;40:720–6.
65. Richter M, Lintz F, Zech S, et al. Combination of PedCAT weightbearing CT with pedography assessment of the relationship between anatomy-based foot center and force/pressure-based center of gravity. Foot Ankle Int 2018;39:361–8.
66. Richter M, Lintz F, Zech S, et al. Combination of PedCAT weightbearing CT with pedography assessment of the relationship between anatomy-based foot center and force/pressure-based center of gravity. Foot Ankle Int 2018;39:361–8.
67. Lintz F, Mast J, Bernasconi A, et al. 3D, weightbearing topographical study of periprosthetic cysts and alignment in total ankle replacement. Foot Ankle Int 2020;41:1–9.
68. Krähenbühl N, Burssens A, Davidson NP, et al. Can weightbearing computed tomography scans be used to diagnose subtalar joint instability? A cadaver study. J Orthop Res 2019;37:2457–65.
69. Krähenbühl N, Weinberg MW, Davidson NP, et al. Currently used imaging options cannot accurately predict subtalar joint instability. Knee Surg Sports Traumatol Arthrosc 2019;27:2818–30.
70. Ananthakrisnan D, Ching R, Tencer A, et al. Subluxation of the talocalcaneal joint in adults who have symptomatic flatfoot. J Bone Joint Surg Am 1999;81(8):1147–54.
71. Peña Fernández M, Hoxha D, Chan O, et al. Centre of rotation of the human subtalar joint using weight-bearing clinical computed tomography. Sci Rep 2020;10:1035.
72. de Cesar Netto C, Godoy-Santos AL, Saito GH, et al. Subluxation of the middle facet of the subtalar joint as a marker of peritalar subluxation in adult acquired flatfoot deformity: a case-control study. J Bone Joint Surg Am 2019;101:1838–44.
73. de Cesar Netto C, Silva T, Li S, et al. Assessment of posterior and middle facet subluxation of the subtalar joint in progressive flatfoot deformity. Foot Ankle Int 2020. https://doi.org/10.1177/1071100720936603.
74. Jeng CL, Rutherford T, Hull MG, et al. Assessment of Bony Subfibular Impingement in Flatfoot Patients Using Weight-Bearing CT Scans. Foot Ankle Int 2019 Feb;40(2):152–8.
75. Lintz F, Bernasconi A, Baschet L, et al. Relationship between chronic lateral ankle instability and hindfoot varus using weight-bearing cone beam computed tomography. Foot Ankle Int 2019;40:1175–81.

76. Spratley EM, Matheis EA, Hayes CW, et al. Effects of degree of surgical correction for flatfoot deformity in patient-specific computational models. Ann Biomed Eng 2015;43:1947–56.
77. Cifuentes-De la Portilla C, Larrainzar-Garijo R, Bayod J. Analysis of biomechanical stresses caused by hindfoot joint arthrodesis in the treatment of adult acquired flatfoot deformity: A finite element study. Foot Ankle Surg 2020;26:412–20.
78. Xu D, Wang Y, Jiang C, et al. Strain distribution in the anterior inferior tibiofibular ligament, posterior inferior tibiofibular ligament, and interosseous membrane using digital image correlation. Foot Ankle Int 2018;39:618–28.
79. Iaquinto JM, Wayne JS. Effects of surgical correction for the treatment of adult acquired flatfoot deformity: a computational investigation. J Orthop Res 2011;29: 1047–54.
80. Kothari MD, Rabe KG, Anderson DD, et al. The relationship of three-dimensional joint space width on weight bearing CT with pain and physical function. J Orthop Res 2019. https://doi.org/10.1002/jor.24566.
81. Bhimani R, Ashkani-Esfahani S, Lubberts B, et al. Utility of volumetric measurement via weight-bearing computed tomography scan to diagnose syndesmotic instability. Foot Ankle Int 2020;41:859–65. https://doi.org/10.1177/1071100720917682.
82. Malicky ES, Crary JL, Houghton MJ, et al. Talocalcaneal and subfibular impingement in symptomatic flatfoot in adults. J Bone Joint Surg Am 2002;84:2005–9.

Progressive Collapsing Foot Deformity. Is There Really a Johnson and Strom Stage I?

Manuel Monteagudo, MD*, Pilar Martínez-de-Albornoz, MD

KEYWORDS

• Adult acquired flatfoot • Progressive collapsing flatfoot • Deformity • Stage I
• Tibialis tendon • Tenosynovitis • Gastrocnemius

KEY POINTS

- Johnson and Strom Stage I Progressive Collapsing Foot Deformity (PCFD) patients may have pain and swelling along the course of the posterior tibial tendon, but there is preserved function and no hindfoot deformity.
- A group of experts have proposed a new PCFD classification scheme based on the flexibility and the type and location of deformity only, and therefore does not include Johnson and Strom stage I disease.
- Diagnosis of Johnson and Strom stage I is clinical, and magnetic resonance imaging is the gold standard image study.
- Pathomechanics explains the overloading of the tendon that may be worsened by a tight gastrocnemius. Systemic inflammatory disease may be responsible for a Johnson and Strom stage I condition without underlying mechanical abnormalities.
- Conservative treatment with medial heel wedged orthoses is effective in most patients. Surgical treatment usually consists of open/endoscopic tenosynovectomy. In cases of complete posterior tibialis tendon rupture, flexor digitorum longus to posterior tibialis tendon transfer or tendon reconstruction may be considered.
- Patients with a higher risk of progression—inflammatory conditions, excessive laxity, obese—may benefit from a "prophylactic" medializing calcaneal osteotomy.

 **Video content accompanies this article at http://www.foot.theclinics.com.**

INTRODUCTION

A group of experts have recently questioned the term *adult-acquired flatfoot deformity* (AAFD) and advocated for the use of the term *progressive collapsing flatfoot deformity* (PCFD) to define the final pathway for a variety of conditions. According to these

Orthopaedic Foot and Ankle Unit, Orthopaedic and Trauma Department, Hospital Universitario Quirónsalud Madrid, Calle Diego de Velazquez 1, Pozuelo de Alarcon, Madrid 28223, Spain
* Corresponding author.
E-mail address: mmontyr@yahoo.com

Foot Ankle Clin N Am 26 (2021) 443–463
https://doi.org/10.1016/j.fcl.2021.05.002

authors, PCFD would be a multifactorial disorder, and the prior terminology for the symptomatic flatfoot underappreciated the severity and complexity of a collapsing foot.[1] Around 30% of flatfeet are not symptomatic, do not affect daily activities, and therefore need no treatment.[2] Prevalence of painful PCFD is approximately 3.3% in the UK, 2.7% in the United States, and 3.7% to 8% in China.[3] Not many primary care physicians (nor even orthopedic surgeons) get their patients to walk in their clinics. Therefore, many PCFD cases may be undiagnosed. And the more subtle the PCFD is, the more cases that will end up with no specific diagnosis or the wrong diagnosis. That scenario specifically applies to early stages of the disease in the Johnson and Strom classification when PCFD is not evident on a quick conventional orthopedic examination. This staging of PCFD consider phase I to be the initiation of a progressive condition that finally comprises flattening and arthritic changes of the midfoot, hindfoot, and ankle. Johnson and Strom stage I disease presents with tenderness and tenosynovitis of the tibialis posterior tendon without deformity. An ideal classification system not only should provide a reproducible description but also should be easily applied to guide treatment and predict outcomes. However, the “in situ” stage I flatfoot without deformity does not always progress toward stage II, and stage I management is sometimes controversial. Stage I remains a rare stage for presentation at our clinics. So many questions arise: Is there really a Johnson and Strom stage I? Do we all share the same standards to define a Johnson and Strom stage I? Are all “stage I” patients equal in terms of pain, progression, and management? How should we treat those patients? The aim of the present article is to present the most updated diagnostic and therapeutic approaches to Johnson and Strom stage I PCFD based on the most specific literature and our own experience.

HISTORY OF POSTERIOR TIBIALIS TENDON DYSFUNCTION

In 1936, Kulowski was the first to publish on a case of tenosynovitis of the sheath of the posterior tibial tendon (PTT).[4] In 1950, Lipscomb reported on a large series of cases.[5] Lapidus and Seidenstein[6] studied two cases of tenosynovitis, stating *“nonspecific chronic tenosynovitis must be considered a rarity, particularly at the ankle.”* These early reports were mainly focused on the state of the tendon, and no deformities were reported. In 1955, A.W. Fowler published seven cases of tenosynovectomies with relief of both pain and function.[7] In 1967, Langenskiöldn operated on six cases of tenosynovitis debriding the granulation tissue with great pain relief.[8] In 1953, Key registered the first case of a posterior tibial partial rupture treated with excision of the torn component and debridement of the residual thickened tendon.[9]

In the 1960s, focus was on “spontaneous” posterior tibialis tendon ruptures in rheumatoids and patients with systemic disease, but no direct correlation was made between degeneration with rupture of the tendon and deformity. Surgical procedures acted on the tendon alone, and results were poor.[10] In the 1970s, Goldner and colleagues[11] transferred the flexor hallucis longus to the diseased PTT and performed a plicature of the spring ligament in 9 patients. The authors believed that a contracted gastrocnemius–soleus complex contributed to the deformity and had to be addressed at the time of surgery.

In the 1980s, focus changed toward deformity and the search for etiology, pathophysiology correlating soft tissue damage and progressive arch collapse, and successful treatment options. Mann and Specht[12] used the flexor digitorum longus tendon instead of the flexor hallucis longus to maintain flexion strength in the hallux. In 1989, Johnson and Strom[13] classified PTT dysfunction into three categories which helped to provide a framework to understand the different types of presentations of the progressive condition.

Staging

Staging in orthopedics is the process of determining the extent to which a condition has developed by growing and spreading to other joint segments. The seminal classification of PTT dysfunction was formulated in 1989 by Johnson and Strom[13] and divided the deformity into three stages (**Table 1**). This classification assumed a progressive course from tenosynovitis with no deformity to a fixed flatfoot with degenerative arthritis and instability. Stage I of the disease includes tenderness, tenosynovitis (with or without tendinopathy), and absence of deformity.

Mueller[14] classified PTT dysfunction into four etiologic categories depending on the cause of tendon damage or rupture (**Table 2**) with no significant differences being made with respect to stage I. Myerson later added a fourth stage to define the extension of the deformity to the tibiotalar joint.[15] In 2007, Bluman and colleagues[16] modified all stages to subdivide them into different categories (**Table 3**). This modified classification has been widely used for its added value to serve as a guide for the indication/type of surgical procedure. Stage I was subdivided into three different categories including slight valgus deformity (less valgus than in stage II).

Raikin and colleagues[17] developed a new classification considering the involvement of the midfoot. The so-called RAM (Rearfoot, Ankle, Midfoot) classification subdivided stage I into IA (tenosynovitis of PTT with neutral midfoot and ankle alignment) and IB (tendinopathy with mild flexible midfoot supination with mild hindfoot valgus [around 5°]). Recently, the spring (plantar calcaneonavicular) ligament has gained popularity as one of the structures that would suffer damage at the beginning of the arch collapse, and some authors have set up a classification with the spring ligament as the reference (**Table 4**).[18] Stage I in this scenario would present with spring ligament laxity/failure and tendinopathy but normal tendon length and no deformity.

Another clinical classification, reported by Richter in 2013, divided the disease into four stages depending on the function of the posterior tibialis tendon independently

Table 1
Clinical stages and surgical interventions in adult pes plano valgus according to the classical classification by Johnson and Strom

Stage	Clinical Findings	Surgical Options
I	Medial foot and ankle pain, swelling, mild weakness, tendon length is normal. No deformity (pre-existing relative flatfoot often present)	Decompression of tendon synovectomy ± FDL transfer open debridement
II	Moderate flexible deformity (minimal abduction through talonavicular joint, <30% talonavicular uncoverage). Medial or lateral pain or both. The "too many toes sign" and single limb heel rise are present. The tendon is elongated and functionally incompetent	FDL transfer and medial displacement calcaneal osteotomy. Spring ligament repair. Cobb procedure. Achilles tendon lengthening. Gastrocnemius recession (open or endoscopic). Arthroereisis
III	Fixed deformity (involving the triple-joint complex). Lateral pain at the calcaneal-fibular contact	Isolated hindfoot fusions (eg, subtalar fusion) or medial column fusion. Double or triple fusion.

Surgical options include the most reported in the literature.

Abbreviations: FDL, flexor digitorum longus.

From Johnson KA, Strom DE. Tibialis posterior tendon dysfunction. Clin Orthop Relat Res. 1989;239:196-206.

Table 2
Mueller classification according to the type of damage to the PTT

Type I	Direct: injury to the tendon resulting in dysfunction of the tibialis posterior tendon
Type II	Pathologic rupture: for example, tendon degeneration associated with rheumatoid arthritis
Type III	Idiopathic rupture: etiology unknown
Type IV	Functional rupture: the tibialis posterior tendon is intact but not functioning well

Abbreviations: PTT, posterior tibialis tendon.
From Mueller TJ. Acquired flatfoot secondary to tibialis posterior dysfunction: biomechanical aspects. J Foot Surg. 1991 Jan-Feb;30(1):2-11.

from the stiffness of the joints (**Table 5**).[19] In Richter's idea, there is a difference between the PTT insufficiency and flexibility of the deformity. Indeed, it is not uncommon to find a collapsed foot that is not stiff and viceversa. Stage I would correspond to the possibility of a single leg heel rise, with the heel moving to varus during heel rise.

Recently, a group of experts have questioned the term AAFD and recommended the use of the term PCFD.[1] These authors believe that the historical nomenclature for the AAFD is confusing, with different names and many focused on the rupture of the PTT. But most of these deformities are not associated with PTT rupture. Degeneration of the PTT would be the consequence of a PCFD in a small group of patients. The use of the terms *progressive* and *collapsing* would give a better idea of the worsening and evolving nature of the complexity of this 3D deformity.[20] This expert consensus group agreed to propose a new classification scheme based on the flexibility, and the type and location of deformity only, and therefore does not include Johnson and Strom stage I disease. They question whether the original stage I ought to be included in the description of PCFD as they argue it is a stable process associated with minor tendon inflammation and/or degeneration.[20] In their group, the most important finding of conventional stage I disease was the presence of PTT pain (5/9%, 56%), followed by gastrocnemius tightness and mild hindfoot valgus (2/9%, 22%). Some experts believed there was no valid description of stage I disease, and only 56% (5/9) felt that there was some indication for surgery in this stage. Surgeries indicated were a gastrocnemius recession, PTT debridement, and calcaneus osteotomy (5/9%, 56%), followed by a medial cuneiform osteotomy, PTT tenosynovectomy, and arthroereisis (1/9%, 11%). For the new classification, the new stage I would refer to a flexible deformity and stage II to a rigid deformity, and they further add letters depending on the deformities present (**Table 6**).

Unlike the controversy in defining more advance stages and the new PCFD classification, the characteristics of conventional stage I disease are not quite different when analyzing all classifications available. If we study clinical findings and image studies, stage I might be defined as follows:

- Pain and swelling occur along the course of the tendon and are defined as tenosynovitis or tendinosis.
- Tendon length is preserved and motor strength unchanged.
- The heel inverts on single toe rise, and there is no loss of strength.
- Repetitive toe raises may reproduce symptomatic pain.

Table 3
Johnson and Strom classification as modified by Bluman/Myerson

Stage	Substage	Characteristics	Treatment
I	IA	Inflammatory disease: PTT rupture that results from a systemic disease such as rheumatoid arthritis and the other inflammatory arthritides. Hindfoot and foot alignment is normal.	Conservative or tenosynovectomy or tendon reconstruction.
	IB	Partial PTT tear with normal hindfoot anatomy.	Conservative or tenosynovectomy or tendon reconstruction.
	IC	Partial PTT tear with subtle hindfoot valgus (deviation of 5° or less).	Conservative, tenosynovectomy and medial translational osteotomy of the calcaneus.
II	IIA1	Flexible hindfoot valgus flexible forefoot varus ± pain along PTT.	Orthotics, MDCO + FDL transfer ± Achilles tendon lengthening.
	IIA2	Flexible hindfoot valgus Fixed forefoot varus ± pain along PTT.	MDCO + FDL transfer + Cotton osteotomy
	IIB	Flexible hindfoot valgus Forefoot abduction	MDCO + FDL transfer + lateral column lengthening
	IIC	Flexible hindfoot valgus Fixed forefoot varus Medial column instability First ray dorsiflexion with hindfoot correction Sinus tarsi pain	MDCO + FDL transfer + Cotton osteotomy + medial column fusion
III	IIIA	Rigid hindfoot valgus Sinus tarsi pain	Double or triple arthrodesis
	IIIB	Rigid hindfoot valgus Sinus tarsi pain Forefoot abduction	Remodeling double or triple arthrodesis
IV	IVA	Hindfoot valgus and flexible ankle valgus without significant ankle arthritis.	Subtalar, double, or triple arthrodesis with deltoid reconstruction.
	IVB	Hindfoot valgus with rigid ankle valgus or flexible deformity with significant ankle arthritis	Triple arthrodesis with total ankle replacement or pantalar (tibiotalocalcaneal + talonavicular) fusion

Abbreviations: FDL, flexor digitorum longus; MDCO, Medial displacement calcaneal osteotomy; PTT, posterior tibialis tendon.
From Bluman EM, Title CI, Myerson MS. Posterior tibial tendon rupture: a refined classification system. Foot Ankle Clin. 2007;8(3):637-45.

- There is no deformity; hindfoot valgus is absent, too-many toes sign is also absent, and arch height remains unchanged.
- Dynamic subtle hindfoot valgus (around 5°) may be observed on visual gait analysis in the third rocker of gait in a subset of patients.
- Radiographs are normal. Magnetic resonance imaging (MRI) will demonstrate edema around the tendon and occasional intrasubstance degeneration. Exuberant tenosynovitis may be a hallmark of an inflammatory or rheumatic etiology.
- Systemic diseases cause a more aggressive condition than mechanical backgrounds.

DIAGNOSIS

Clinical Examination

Diagnosis is made clinically. Clinical examination should start with a visual gait analysis with the patient barefoot and both knees and ankles visible. It is particularly important to rule out proximal deformities because PCFD may be secondary to compensation of a varus knee. With the patient seated and feet hanging from the examination couch, palpation reveals pain mainly in the medial soft tissues around the ankle. Tibialis posterior tendon may be swollen and painful in different segments or all the way from the retromalleolar region down to its insertion in the navicular (**Fig. 1**). In Johnson and Strom

Table 4
RAM classification of AAFD according to rearfoot (R), ankle (A), or midfoot (M) involvement

Stage	Rearfoot	Ankle	Midfoot
IA	Tenosynovitis of PTT	Neutral alignment	Neutral alignment
IB	PTT tendonitis without deformity	Mild valgus (5°)	Mild flexible midfoot supination
IIA	Flexible planovalgus (<40% talar uncoverage, <30° Meary angle, incongruency angle 20° to 45°)	Valgus with deltoid insufficiency (no arthritis)	Midfoot supination without radiographic instability
IIB	Flexible planovalgus (>40% talar uncoverage, >30° Meary angle, incongruency angle >45°)	Valgus with deltoid insufficiency with tibiotalar arthritis	Midfoot supination with midfoot instability—no arthritis
IIIA	Fixed/arthritic planovalgus (<40% talar uncoverage, <30° Meary angle, incongruency angle 20° to 45°)	Valgus secondary to bone loss in the lateral tibial plafond (deltoid normal)	Arthritic changes isolated to medial column (navicular-medial cuneiform or first TMT joints)
IIIB	Fixed/arthritic planovalgus (>40% talar uncoverage, >30° Meary angle, incongruency angle >45°)—not correctable through triple arthrodesis	Valgus secondary to bone loss in the lateral tibial plafond and with deltoid insufficiency	Medial and middle column midfoot arthritic changes (usually with supination and/or abduction of the midfoot)

Abbreviations: AAFD, adult acquired flatfoot deformity; PTT, posterior tibialis tendon; RAM, Rearfoot, Ankle, Midfoot; TMT, Tarsometatarsal.

From Raikin SM, Winters BS, Daniel JN. The RAM classification: a novel, systematic approach to the adult-acquired flatfoot. Foot Ankle Clin. 2012 Jun;17(2):169-81.

Table 5
Clinical stages/deformity of pes plano valgus centered on the spring ligament

Stage	Deformity
0	Spring ligament laxity but no tendinopathy or planovalgus
1	Spring ligament laxity/failure with tendinopathy but normal tendon length and no deformity
2	Spring ligament failure with tendon lengthening and flexible planovalgus deformity
3	Spring ligament failure with tendon lengthening, and fixed planovalgus deformity

From Pasapula C, Cutts S. Modern Theory of the Development of Adult Acquired Flat Foot and an Updated Spring Ligament Classification System. Clin Res Foot Ankle. 2017;5:247. doi: 10.4172/2329-910X.1000247.

stage I, medial structures—spring ligament, deltoid, and the flexor tendons of the toes (hallucis longus and digitorum)—will have minor or no pain. With further progression of the condition, tenderness initially present may diminish and instead patients complain of fatigue and pain with a reduction in walking distance.

Dynamic examination should include a heel raise test—monopodal and bipodal—to address the presence of a hindfoot valgus and PTT function and power to invert the subtalar joint. Johnson and Strom stage I should not present with valgus deformity or with a very subtle tilting. Gastrocnemius tightness should be assessed using the Silfverskiöld's test. Examination of the gastroc-soleus complex for contracture should be made with the subtalar joint in the reduced position and the foot supinated to eliminate dorsiflexion through the midtarsal joints. In Johnson and Strom stage I of the condition, the hindfoot is supple and easily reducible when evaluating subtalar motion. Weakness of supination may be encountered on manual testing of the muscle (inversion strength of the hindfoot by plantar flexed ankle).

Imaging Studies

Weight-bearing radiographs with anteroposterior and lateral views of the foot and anteroposterior view of the ankle may aid in excluding an underlying tarsal coalition (C-sign, a talar beak, or an anteater sign) and other deformities secondary to trauma and other congenital conditions. Weight-bearing conventional radiographic evaluation is mandatory to understand the type of collapse and classify the type of PCFD.[20]

Table 6
Classification of AAFD according to PTT function

Stage	PTT Function
I	Single leg heel-rise possible, heel moves to varus during heel-rise.
II	Single leg heel-rise possible, heel moves to neutral during heel-rise.
III	Single leg heel-rise possible, heel stays in valgus during heel-rise.
IV	Single leg heel-rise is not possible.

Abbreviations: AAFD, Adult Acquired Flatfoot Deformity; PTT, posterior tibialis tendon.

From Richter M, Zech S. Lengthening osteotomy of the calcaneus and flexor digitorum longus tendon transfer in flexible flatfoot deformity improves talo-1st metatarsal-Index, clinical outcome and pedographic parameter. Foot Ankle Surg 2013; 19:56-61.

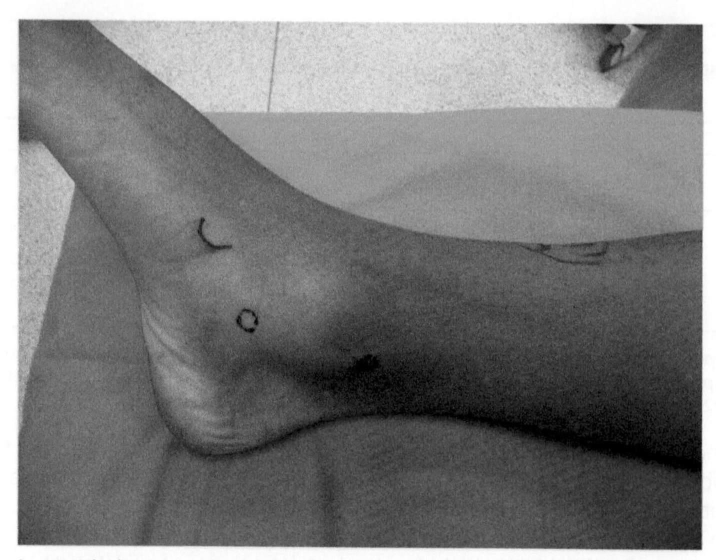

Fig. 1. Patient with rheumatoid arthritis and stage I posterior tibial tendon dysfunction presenting with retromalleolar swelling. Circles delimitate the more tender segment of the tendon.

Ultrasound is useful for the assessment of the integrity of the tendon, visualization of tendon fibers, dynamic properties, and tenderness to sonopalpation. Associated hypervascularity on color Doppler and thickening of the peritendinous tissues may suggest tendinopathy. Partial or total ruptures may also be diagnosed. Some authors suggest that ultrasound may be superior to MRI on evaluating tendon integrity based on speed, convenience, cost, and its dynamic nature. Still, an experienced sonographer is necessary to interpret the images.[21,22]

MRI is considered the gold standard for the study of PTT disorders. In Johnson and Strom stage I, focus is made on the state of posterior tibialis tendon that runs behind the medial malleolus and changes its orientation almost 90° around the tip of the malleolus to finally insert in the navicular. That abrupt change of orientation is responsible for signal abnormalities in the MRI that result in many false-positive and false-negative interpretations of partial and/or complete ruptures. MRI findings have a poor correlation with surgical findings.[23] Longitudinal tears of the PTT that can be identified on MRI are sometimes difficult to reveal on open surgery. Some authors have demonstrated that in the presence of inflammation near the tendon, MRI may falsely indicate a high-grade rupture of the PTT.[21,22] Exogenous origin of inflammation caused changes in the MRI signal in the PTT that resemble those seen in ruptures. Identification of tenosynovial fluid on MRI may help in the differential diagnosis of Johnson and Strom stage I disease.[24] Other medial soft tissue structures, different from PTT, have been found to be more severely degenerated than the PTT.[2,25] Therefore, findings in MRI should not guide surgical planning. Computerized tomography (CT) and weight-bearing CT scan help to better define arthritic changes and the state of neighboring joints, helping by better characterizing the PCFD.[26] Furthermore, the assessment of PCFD at very early stages may benefit from the use of weight-bearing CT as it may demonstrate sinus tarsi impingement, subluxation of the subtalar joint at the posterior and/or middle facet, and most importantly when deformity is still not too evident, the increased valgus inclination of the posterior facet of the subtalar joint.[27]

Other Studies

PTT injuries may result from a systemic disease—rheumatoid arthritis and the other inflammatory arthritis—so laboratory studies may help with the diagnosis and etiology at early stages of this condition. Diagnostic injections may also help in some cases. Neurophysiological studies and genetic studies may reveal conditions affecting the strength of the PTT.[28]

PATHOMECHANICS

Proper function of PTT may be impaired by direct or indirect trauma, systemic inflammatory diseases, PCFD, or iatrogenic causes. PTT courses posterior to the medial malleolus within the flexor retinaculum, just slightly posterior to the ankle joint axis. Then it continues inferior to the medial malleolus and passes medial and plantar to the subtalar joint axis and plantar to the oblique midtarsal joint axis.[29]

We will refer to the "rockers" from gait analysis to better understand the pathomechanics of Johnson and Strom stage I flatfoot deformity.[30] The contact pattern between the foot and the ground varies during the stance phase. The tibia keeps on rotating forward throughout stance. A rocking point for the tibia to rotate is needed all along the stance phase to achieve simultaneously both continuous progression and stability. During the *first rocker*, the tibia internally rotates and is brought "up and over" the talus and on the heel, which is the only part of the sole of the foot contacting the ground. As soon as the forefoot contacts the ground, the tibia can no longer rotate on the heel and starts rotating onto the talus. Contraction of the anterior compartment muscles controls this motion. Eccentric contraction of the PTT, and the intrinsic muscles of the foot together with the passive tightening of the plantar fascia (via windlass effect), allows for the maintenance of the medial longitudinal arch. Posterior tibial muscle/tendon is physiologically stretched during the first rocker of gait to allow subtalar pronation. The foot-ground contact pattern during the *second (ankle) rocker* is plantigrade. During the second rocker of gait, PTT helps to center the talus over the navicular. The last milliseconds of the second rocker signal the triceps surae to fire. By then, the ankle should ideally be in maximum dorsiflexion and the knee in full extension with the gastrocnemius in full stretch. If the calf becomes too tight, thus limiting its ultimate available length, the rotation of the ankle is hindered and stopped too early. Yet, the body continues to progress forward over the planted foot, which will produce increased leveraged forces in the foot and ankle.[31] Ground reaction forces that are unavoidable provide the balance of this equation. The tighter the calf becomes, the higher and earlier the leveraged forces that result.[32] Compensatory mechanisms to avoid damage to the foot and ankle are the adoption of a "bouncy gait" and/or subtalar pronation.[33] The latter would invariably translate moments acting throughout the sagittal plane into moments acting in the transverse plane thus potentially damaging PTT. Owing to the triceps surae, the *third rocker* or propulsive phase allows for the body center of mass to elevate, increasing potential energy. PTT actively external rotates the tibia/leg and induces foot supination. The ankle undergoes progressive plantarflexion, and the longitudinal axis of the foot is placed vertically on the ground. Because of the anatomic location of the tendon in relation to the axis of the ankle, subtalar and midtarsal joints, contraction of the posterior tibial muscle causes a plantarflexion moment across the ankle joint axis, a supination moment across the subtalar, and a supination moment across the oblique midtarsal joint. During the third rocker, the foot behaves similar to a wheelbarrow, which is balanced by the peroneal tendons and the PTT. PTT allows for the dynamic locking of the medial column of the foot during the third rocker creating a rigid lever, with the calcaneus firmly seating into the cuboid and the talus into the navicular.[34]

The PTT is a "gliding tendon" as it changes direction by curving around the medial malleolus. Fibrocartilage found within connective tissue is due to repetitive stimulus of intermittent compressive and shear forces. The fibrocartilaginous region of PTT is located around the medial malleolus and is more vulnerable to repetitive microtrauma. It is in this region where most ruptures occur.[34] Degeneration may arise because of the poor repair response of the hypovascular fibrocartilaginous tissue. This portion of the tendon rubs back and forth between the underlying malleolus and the overlying flexor digitorum longus. The sliding properties of PTT may be altered because of synovitis, an irregular medial malleolus, longitudinal or transverse splits, elongation because of continuous overpronation, or a combination of several disorders. All these entities may lead to fibrous tissue formation between the tendon and the surrounding synovial sheath.[35] Secondarily, neoinnervation after neovascularization may be a cause of pain in PTT tendinopathy.

IS THERE REALLY A JOHNSON AND STROM STAGE I?

We may affirm that there is indeed a Johnson and Strom stage I because it is present in most classification systems regardless the focus of each of them. Most classifications agree with the description of stage I as an initial inflammatory phase characterized by swelling and pain around the medial malleolus, tenosynovitis, with no changes in tendon length and no hindfoot deformity.[36] The "too many toes" sign is not present, and the patient is able to perform a single heel raise with some discomfort but clear evidence of hindfoot inversion. Image studies reveal synovitis and/or partial tears on MRI, but the overall continuity of the tendon is maintained. It is important to notice that classic stage I may or may not be accompanied by systemic inflammatory disease, and it has been associated with seronegative disorders, such as ankylosing spondylitis, psoriasis, and Reiter syndrome.

If we assume there is a Johnson and Strom stage I of the condition, next question would be, are all Johnson and Strom stage I cases equal? There are a variety of different patients that would fit into the Johnson and Strom stage I of the disease. It seems that inflammatory conditions affect the tendon differently than mechanical conditions. Some authors suggest that PTT ruptures are common in rheumatoid patients, but other authors found no strong relationship between rheumatoid arthritis and structural damage to the tendon.[37,38] Bluman and Myerson added three subsections to this stage I (see **Table 3**),[16] with different treatment proposals, from tenosynovectomy in stage IA to even consider a bony procedure in stage IC. It is our impression that Johnson and Strom stage I PCFD may behave and progress differently in patients with underlying mechanical causes compared with in those with inflammatory initiation of the condition. Patients with generalized laxity and obesity show a more rapid progression of the disease. Most of these patients without a primary mechanical background might be considered as an early Johnson and Strom stage II rather than a late Johnson and Strom stage I of the disease in terms of management. Our threshold to perform a "prophylactic" medializing calcaneal osteotomy in those patients has been lower over the last years.

The authors however disagree with the classical theory of initial damage of the PTT leading to progressive deformity. We have long believed that conventional symptomatic PCFD was due to mechanical causes—malalignment with loss of compensatory mechanisms leading to soft-tissue damage—so that the PTT is the victim rather than the cause of the condition known as AAFD or PCFD. And our belief is supported by different publications.[2,25] Indeed, in the last 12 years, we have skipped any medial soft-tissue reconstruction in flexible deformities relying on our bony procedures and found no differences on a 10-year follow-up (Manuel Monteagudo, unpublished data, 2021). In this context, should classical Johnson and Strom stage I continue to exist? Some experts believe it should be eliminated from a comprehensive classification.[20] We modestly believe there still might be a place for Johnson and Strom stage I when considering patients with subtle valgus deformity (not evident on weight-bearing x-rays but evident on weight-bearing CT), with pain and swelling in the medial peritalar soft tissues (PTT, spring, deltoid), and with risk factors for progression of the condition (obesity, generalized laxity, inflammatory disease, gastrocnemius tightness). Might that scenario fit as a "stage 0" in future revisions of the new classification of PCFD?

HOW SHOULD WE TREAT THOSE PATIENTS?

Conservative management is recommended as the initial treatment in all patients presenting with a Johnson and Strom stage I PCFD. Most patients will respond well to conservative measures which, in the opinion of the authors, should always be tried before surgery is indicated.

Conservative

The goal of nonoperative treatment is to alleviate pain and restore function while preventing progression toward stage II of the disease. Resting or relieving the tension on the PTT may be done in a graduated fashion. The patient should be encouraged to lose weight, wear supportive shoes, and modify loading activities. A review of conservative interventions for mobile PCFD in adults selected four studies that met the inclusion criteria to minimize biases.[39] One of the studies suggested that, after 4 weeks of use, orthoses may result in a significant improvement in mediolateral sway and may result in improved, although nonsignificant, general foot-related quality of life.[40] Another study suggests that their effect on plantar pressure distribution may facilitate better function regardless the orthoses are custom or prefabricated devices.[41] But another study failed to find any significant effect on prefabricated orthoses on pain, injury incidence, foot health, or quality of life in a group of air force recruits.[42] The fourth study suggests that exercising the intrinsic foot muscles may enhance the effect of orthoses.[43]

Rest: Whenever tenosynovitis is present, the first level of rest involves the use of a below-the-knee walking cast or walker boot for around 4 to 6 weeks, along with oral nonsteroidal anti-inflammatory drugs.[44] Blake and colleagues[45] emphasize that protected weight-bearing encourages tendon repair by organizing new collagen along the direction of stress. After immobilization, a semi-rigid stirrup brace or lace-up sport brace crossing the ankle joint should be used to limit excursion of the PTT.

Medication: Steroids can create local microvascular attenuation, further compromising healing of the diseased PTT. Johnson and Strom[13] felt that steroid injections were contraindicated because of accelerated tendon weakening. In fact, Holmes and Mann[38] reported that in an age-stratified population, 28% of the younger patients and 17% of the older patients with rupture of the PTT had a history of multiple steroid injections or a history of oral corticosteroid use.

Rehabilitation: The role of physiotherapy is controversial. Combining orthotic management with a concentrated, aggressive exercise program has support in lessening PTT symptoms, as noted by Alvarez and colleagues[46] The authors evaluated 47 consecutive patients with stage 1 or 2 PTT dysfunction. An above-ankle articulated device (70%) or orthotic (30%) was used in combination with a home program of strengthening and stretching therapy over a 4-month interval. Eighty-nine percent were satisfied after the conclusion of treatment (although only 83% had successful subjective and objective outcomes). A recent randomized, controlled trial found significant benefit of combining the use of ankle-foot orthoses with eccentric and concentric progressive resistive exercises.[47] Therapeutic strengthening exercises, along with stretching of the gastrocsoleus complex and iliopsoas, could improve important clinical outcomes, such as muscle activity, and dynamic balance in flatfeet.[48]

Footwear: Footwear modifications include extra-depth shoes, soft leather uppers to accommodate insoles, a high toe box, and a cushioned, rocker bottom to reduce ground reaction forces acting on the PTT. Rocker bottom soles assist in toe-off during the transition from the second to the third rockers of gait.[49,50] In athletes with PCFD Johnson and Strom stage I, care should be taken to wear a running shoe with a flared heel and not run more than 650 km (around 400 miles) on any one pair of shoes.[51] Midfoot cushioning significantly dissipates after that distance, resulting in less arch support, less ability to control pronation, and increased tension on the PTT.

Orthoses: Orthotic and brace management has been a large focus of attention in conservative management of PCFD at any stage of the condition.[52] Orthoses are generally the most effective conservative intervention in the management of PCFD. The aim of orthoses in Johnson and Strom stage I dysfunction is to support the medial arch while preventing the subtalar tilting into pronation and lessening the strain across the PTT. The ideal orthotic for PCFD should have a supinatory wedge in the heel area with around 10 to 12 mm of height medially to create an antipronatory effect during the first milliseconds of the first rocker (just after heel strike) (**Fig. 2**).[53,54] Longitudinal medial arch support should not be more elevated than the supinatory wedge, otherwise it would create a shearing effect around the talonavicular region over the painful and sore medial soft tissues. There is a variety of other orthotic options if the conventional fails to alleviate pain, but they are usually bulkier, and compliance is difficult.[55] The University of California Biomechanics Laboratory, the Arizona brace, Airlift-type brace, and the ankle-foot orthosis are usually recommended in more advanced stages of PCFD, although may have an impact in the occasional Johnson and Strom stage I patient.[56,57]

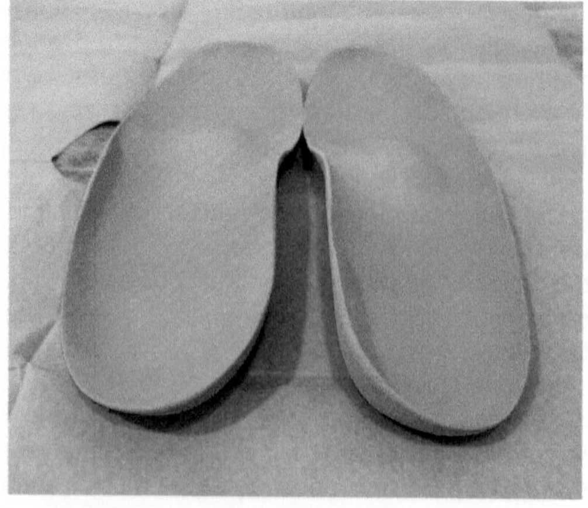

Fig. 2. Orthoses with a pronatory medial heel wedge and longitudinal arch support allows for the unloading of the posterior tibial tendon.

While there may be some benefit associated with the conservative interventions described in the previous studies, there is insufficient evidence from randomized controlled trials to determine which conservative treatment is the most appropriate for the management of Johnson and Strom stage I PCFD. For most (mechanical) cases, conservative interventions should be continued for 4 to 6 months, and if they fail, then surgical treatment may be warranted. The only circumstance to consider operative intervention sooner is in patients afflicted with seronegative spondyloarthropathy and PTT tenosynovitis. Myerson[58] suggests that failure of conservative care over a 6-week period should prompt surgical tenosynovectomy to prevent potential tendon rupture.

Surgical

Rarely surgical treatment is necessary in Johnson and Strom stage I PCFD. When needed, most surgical interventions depend on the state of the PTT. Open tendon debridement, tenosynovectomy, and repair of longitudinal tears are the most common procedures for stage I cases.[59] Intraoperative findings in conventional open debridement and tenosynovectomy include tenosynovitis, often with granulation tissue, increased tenosynovial fluid, and an interstitial longitudinal rupture, usually between the medial malleolar tip and the navicular insertion of the tendon. Conventional surgical treatment involves opening the tendon sheath from at least the medial malleolus to the navicular insertion. If hypertrophied, the tendon is debrided and debulked sharply via a longitudinal incision in the tendon itself. Postoperatively, immobilization is recommended for 3 weeks, followed by rigid bracing for another 3 weeks. After immobilization, supportive shoewear with a custom-made arch support is recommended for 3 months.[58]

Open surgery is frequently needed to establish a diagnosis and treatment but is not free of complications such as adhesions and painful scars. Over the last decade, tendoscopy has become a useful tool to diagnose and treat tendon disorders by providing a close and dynamic anatomic assessment of the PTT (**Fig. 3**) (Video 1). It was first performed by Wertheimer in 1994,[60] although it was van Dijk and colleagues who described the procedure in detail.[61] Most indications for open surgery of the PTT

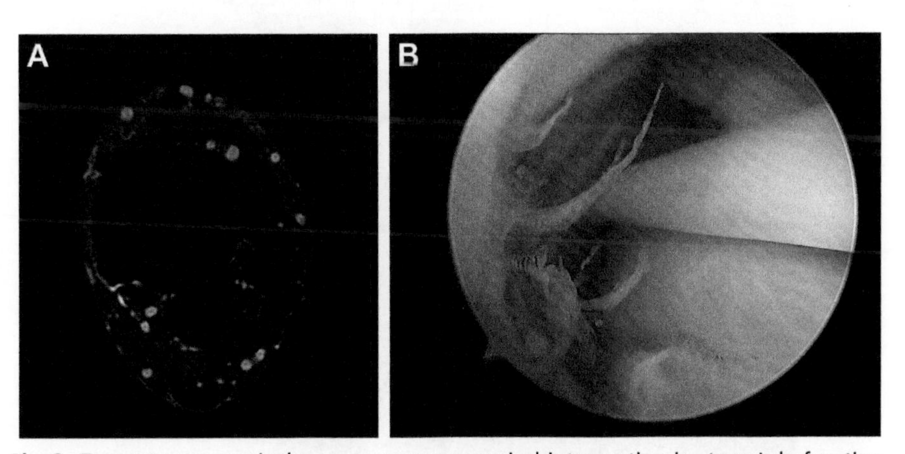

Fig. 3. Tenosynovectomy is the more common surgical intervention in stage I dysfunction. (*A*) MRI showing an irregular posterior tibialis tendon with a rounded structure that might simulate a partial tear. (*B*) Tendoscopy finally revealed a synovial plica with synovitis. Motorized synovectomy was performed with the help of a shaver (Video 1).

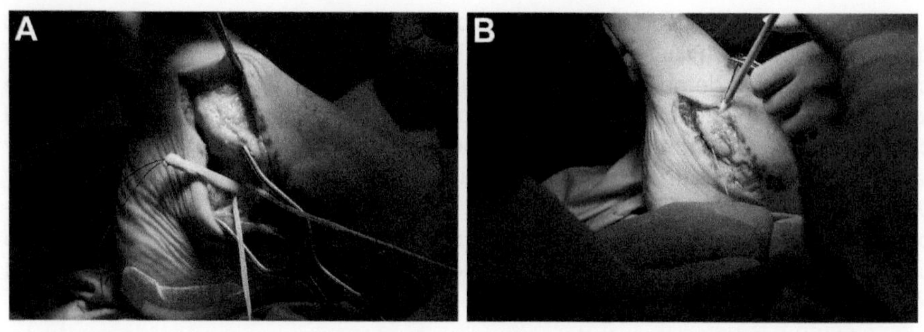

Fig. 4. Patient with advanced degenerative changes of the posterior tibialis tendon. (*A*) Flexor digitorum longus tendon is prepared to be transferred. (*B*) Fixation of the transfer into the navicular using an interference screw.

are now covered by tendoscopy with less morbidity and faster return to daily activities including sport.[62] Timing of tenosynovectomy is influenced by the suspected cause of the condition. Patients with florid tenosynovitis resulting from conditions such as the seronegative spondyloarthropathies benefit from an early tenosynovectomy after a 6-week trial of conservative care.[63]

Although a very uncommon scenario in classic Johnson and Strom stage I, when severe substance damage in the tendon is present, flexor digitorum longus transfer is considered to reinforce the dysfunctional tendon (**Fig. 4**). A free donor tendon (autograft or allograft) may also be an option for reconstruction.[64] In older patients presenting with a Johnson and Strom stage I disease but advanced degeneration of the tendon, some authors consider side-to-side tenodesis of the flexor digitorum longus tendon to the PTT.[65–67] Deciding between reconstruction versus transfer largely depends on the muscle quality (liposubstitution).[68] Gastrocnemius recession should be indicated if the patient has gastrocnemius-dependent equinus on Silfverskiöld

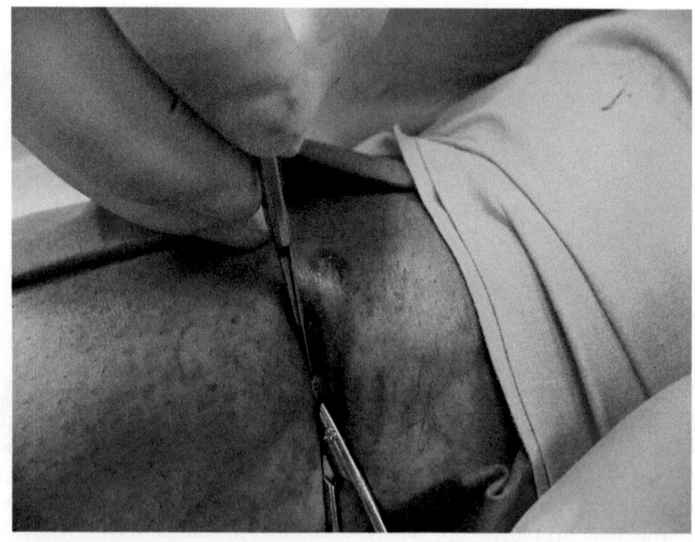

Fig. 5. Proximal medial gastrocnemius release in a patient with stage I dysfunction.

test, to diminish pronatory moments acting on the subtalar joint at the end of the second rocker of gait (**Fig. 5**) (Video 2).[69]

Bluman and colleagues[16] suggested PCFD Bluman's stage IA should be treated with open debridement and tenosynovectomy. Bluman's IB care should begin with a conservative treatment consisting of anti-inflammatory medications and immobilization in a cast, walking boot, or custom brace before considering tenosynovectomy. Bluman's IC care should also begin with conservative treatment, but subtle valgus deformity and a more incipient rupture may be managed by a medial translational osteotomy of the calcaneus. Raikin and colleagues[17] suggested similar management when considering stages R-Ia and R-Ib. Although bone work is rarely needed in Raikin's stage I, in patients with extreme laxity, with obesity, or with degenerative or inflammatory disease, consideration should be given to a medial sliding calcaneal osteotomy.

It is our impression that Johnson and Strom stage I PCFD may behave and progress differently in patients with an underlying mechanical condition (subtalar valgus tilt) than in patients with inflammatory/rheumatoid trigger of the condition. Patients with generalized laxity, and/or with obesity, and/or gastrocnemius tightness may progress to a classical stage II of the disease. In most of these latter patients, Johnson and Strom stage I might be considered as an early Johnson and Strom stage II, and treatment should possibly be adjusted to the conventional Johnson and Strom stage II including a "prophylactic" medializing calcaneal osteotomy (**Fig. 6**) (Video 3). A 10 mm of medial shift is usually enough to change valgus/pronation moments across the subtalar joint into varus/supination moments.[69] A posterior tibialis tendoscopy may be associated to evaluate and treat potential synovitis, plicae, or partial rupture that might continue to be painful despite the unloading effect of the osteotomy. Some authors find arthroereisis of the subtalar joint to be useful for deformity correction in early stages of PCFD by blocking subtalar pronation with a sinus tarsi implant.[70] It has the potential advantage of the minimally invasive approach, but it reduces subtalar motion, and it is not difficult to overcorrect into a varus hindfoot (poorly tolerated and a very unusual complication of a calcaneal osteotomy).

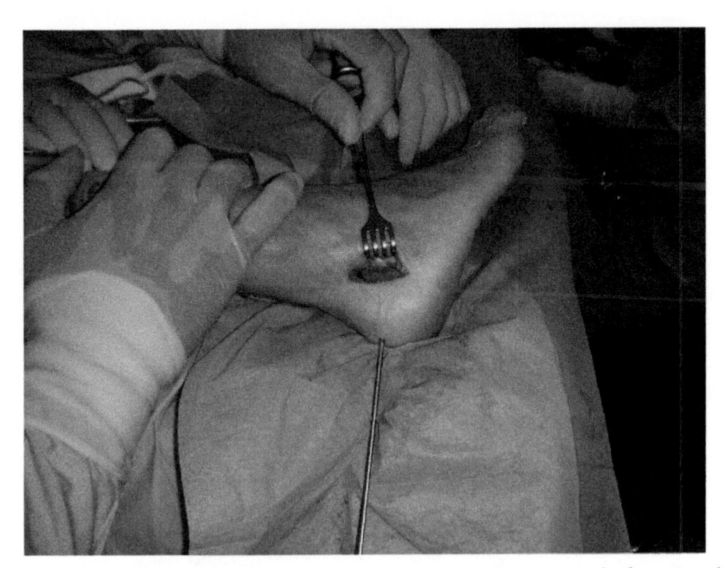

Fig. 6. Medializing calcaneal osteotomy in a patient with stage I dysfunction but with obesity and inflammatory background.

RESULTS AND OUTCOMES

Funk and colleagues[71] looked at tenosynovectomy with and without repair of a split tendon tear and found 89% of patients with absent or minor pain. Teasdall and Johnson[72] reported 74% success after tenosynovectomy but believed debridement alone should be reserved for patients without a progressive deformity. Tendoscopic tenolysis has shown consistent results in Johnson and Strom stage I of the condition in different studies.[61,73] Crates and Richardson[74] evaluated seven patients with Johnson and Strom stage I dysfunction who underwent tenosynovectomy with three requiring simultaneous repairs of a split tear or fissure. Six out of seven patients were pain free. McCormack and colleagues[75] reviewed eight competitive athletes with Johnson and Strom stage I disease who underwent tenosynovectomy at an average age of 22 years. All could return to sports, and seven continued to participate at their sport without incident. The authors recommend early intervention in this subset of patients with stage I disease after an aggressive trial of conservative care. Bulstra and colleagues[76] published their series of 33 patients who underwent tendoscopy with good results for pathologic vincula and rheumatoid arthritis, but poor results for adhesiolysis. Chow and colleagues[77] reported on a series of 6 patients with synovectomy in PCFD Johnson and Strom stage I with no complications and no progression to stage II.

Further research is needed in this area to have a more evidence-based approach to PCFD Johnson and Strom stage I. Future knowledge of factors that can predispose the tendon to attenuation and degeneration may allow for a more specific intervention. Polymorphisms at genes involved in collagen degradation and remodeling may play a role, although these factors are still being investigated.[78] The relative effect of many of these factors is still not well understood.

After reviewing the most updated diagnostic, and therapeutic approaches to Johnson and Strom stage I PCFD based on the most specific literature and considering our

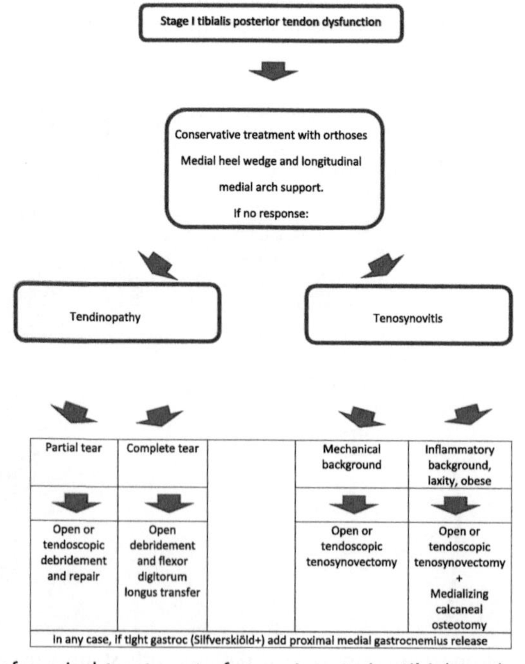

Fig. 7. Algorithm of surgical treatment of stage I posterior tibial tendon dysfunction.

own experience in over 20 years of dealing with PCFD patients, an algorithm of treatment is proposed (**Fig. 7**).

SUMMARY

Is There Really a Stage I?

On one hand, our answer would be, yes, there is. According to most classifications, stage I of PCFD would correspond to the initial condition of some PCFD with PTT pain and swelling but no evident hindfoot deformity. Tenosynovitis and partial tears of the PTT are common findings both on MRI and surgery.

But on another hand, our answer would be no, there is not. The authors disagree with the classical theory of initial damage of the PTT leading to progressive deformity. We have always believed that conventional symptomatic PCFD was due to mechanical causes—malalignment with loss of compensatory mechanisms leading to medial soft-tissue damage—therefore the PTT being the victim rather than the villain/cause of the condition known as AAFD or PCFD.

In this controversial context, should classical stage I continue to exist? Some experts believe it should be eliminated from a comprehensive classification.[20] We modestly believe there might still be a place for Johnson and Strom stage I when considering patients with subtle valgus deformity (not evident on weight-bearing x-rays but evident on weight-bearing CT), with pain and swelling in the medial peritalar soft tissues (PTT, spring, deltoid), and with risk factors for progression of the condition (obesity, generalized laxity, inflammatory disease, gastrocnemius tightness).

How should we treat those patients? Most patients respond well to conservative orthotic treatment with medial heel wedged and longitudinal arch support. When surgery is needed, “inflammatory cases” usually respond well to open/endoscopic tenosynovectomy, whereas “mechanical cases” usually need tendon debridement of partial tears with/without reinforcement with flexor digitorum longus tendon. Gastrocnemius proximal release unloads posterior tibialis tendon in patients with tight gastrocnemius. In a subset of patients with special risk of progression—systemic disease, laxity, obesity—a medializing calcaneal osteotomy will unload the diseased tendon while possibly preventing progression to stage II.

CLINICS CARE POINTS

- Diagnosis of Johnson and Strom stage I is clinical by checking there is preserved function with no hindfoot deformity..
- Pathomechanics include overloading of the posterior tibial tendon worsened by a tight gastrocnemius. But rule out systemic inflammatory disease if no mechanical abnormalities are found.
- Most patients respond well to medial heel wedged orthoses. Those who fail to orthoses may benefit from endoscopic tenosynovectomy. Very rarely a tendon transfer is needed at this initial stage.
- A "prophylactic" medializing calcaneal osteotomy may be considered in those patients with risk factors for progression (inflammatory, obese, excessive laxity).

DISCLOSURE

The authors have nothing to disclose.

SUPPLEMENTARY DATA

Supplementary data related to this article can be found online at https://doi.org/10.1016/j.fcl.2021.05.002.

REFERENCES

1. de Cesar Netto C, Deland JT, Ellis SJ. Guest Editorial: Expert Consensus on Adult-Acquired Flatfoot Deformity. Foot Ankle Int 2020;41(10):1269–71.
2. Deland JT, de Asla RJ, Sung IH, et al. Posterior tibial tendon insufficiency: which ligaments are involved? Foot Ankle Int 2005;26(6):427–35.
3. Kohls-Gatzoulis J, Angel JC, Singh D, et al. Tibialis posterior dysfunction: a common and treatable cause of adult acquired flatfoot. BMJ 2004;329(7478):1328–33.
4. Kulowski J. Tenovaginitis (tenosynovitis). J Mo Med Assoc 1936;35:135–7.
5. Lipscomb PR. Tendons. I. Non-suppurative tenosynovitis and para tendinitis. Instr Course Lect 1950;7:254–61.
6. Lapidus PW, Seidenstein H. Chronic non-specific tenosynovitis with effusion about ankle. J Bone Joint Surg 1950;32-A:175–7.
7. Fowler AW. Tibialis posterior syndrome. J Bone Joint Surg 1955;37-B:520.
8. Langenskiöld A. Chronic Non-Specific Tenosynovitis of the Tibialis Posterior Tendon. Acta Orthop Scand 1967;38(1–4):301–5.
9. Key JA. Partial rupture of the tendon of the posterior tibial muscle. J Bone Joint Surg 1953;35-A:1006–8.
10. Kettlekamp DB, Alexander HH. Spontaneous rupture of the posterior tibial tendon. J Bone Joint Surg Am 1969;51:759–64.
11. Goldner JL, Keats PK, Bassett FH III, et al. Progressive talipes equinovalgus due to trauma or degeneration of the posterior tibial tendon and medial plantar ligaments. Orthop Clin North Am 1974;5(1):39–51.
12. Mann RA, Specht LH. Posterior tibial tendon ruptures: Analysis of eight cases. J Foot Ankle 1982;2:350–3.
13. Johnson KA, Strom DE. Tibialis posterior tendon dysfunction. Clin Orthop Relat Res 1989;239:196–206.
14. Mueller TJ. Acquired flatfoot secondary to tibialis posterior dysfunction: biomechanical aspects. J Foot Surg 1991;30(1):2–11.
15. Myerson MS. Adult acquired flatfoot deformity: treatment of dysfunction of the posterior tibial tendon. Instr Course Lect 1997;46:393–405.
16. Bluman EM, Title CI, Myerson MS. Posterior tibial tendon rupture: a refined classification system. Foot Ankle Clin 2007;8(3):637–45.
17. Raikin SM, Winters BS, Daniel JN. The RAM classification: a novel, systematic approach to the adult-acquired flatfoot. Foot Ankle Clin 2012;17(2):169–81.
18. Pasapula C, Cutts S. Modern theory of the development of adult acquired flat foot and an updated spring ligament classification system. Clin Res Foot Ankle 2017;5:247.
19. Richter M, Zech S. Lengthening osteotomy of the calcaneus and flexor digitorum longus tendon transfer in flexible flatfoot deformity improves talo-1st metatarsal-Index, clinical outcome and pedographic parameter. Foot Ankle Surg 2013;19:56–61.
20. Myerson MS, Thordarson DB, Johnson JE, et al. Classification and Nomenclature: Progressive Collapsing Foot Deformity. Foot Ankle Int 2020;41(10):1271–6.
21. Wake J, Martin K. Posterior tibial tendon endoscopic debridement for stage i and ii posterior tibial tendon dysfunction. Arthrosc Tech 2017;6(5):e2019–22.

22. Chen YJ, Liang SC. Diagnostic efficacy of ultrasonography in stage I posterior tibial tendon dysfunction: sonographic-surgical correlation. J Ultrasound Med 1997;16(6):417–23.
23. Lesiak AC, Michelson JD. Posterior tibial tendon dysfunction: Imperfect specificity of magnetic resonance imaging. Foot Ankle Surg 2020;26(2):224–7.
24. Gonzalez FM, Harmouche E, Robertson DD, et al. Tenosynovial fluid as an indication of early posterior tibial tendon dysfunction in patients with normal tendon appearance. Skeletal Radiol 2019;48(9):1377–83.
25. de Cesar Netto C, Saito GH, Roney A, et al. Combined weightbearing CT and MRI assessment of flexible progressive collapsing foot deformity. Foot Ankle Surg 2020. https://doi.org/10.1016/j.fas.2020.12.003.
26. de Cesar Netto C, Shakoor D, Dein EJ, et al. Influence of investigator experience on reliability of adult acquired flatfoot deformity measurements using weightbearing computed tomography. Foot Ankle Surg 2019;25(4):495–502.
27. de Cesar Netto C, Myerson MS, Day J, et al. Consensus for the use of weightbearing CT in the assessment of progressive collapsing foot deformity. Foot Ankle Int 2020;41(10):1277–82.
28. Blasimann A, Eichelberger P, Brülhart Y, et al. Non-surgical treatment of pain associated with posterior tibial tendon dysfunction: study protocol for a randomised clinical trial. J Foot Ankle Res 2015;8:37.
29. Pohl MB, Rabbito M, Ferber R. The role of tibialis posterior fatigue on foot kinematics during walking. J Foot Ankle Res 2010;3:6.
30. Perry J, Schoneberger B. Gait analysis: normal and pathological function. Thorofare (NJ): Slack Inc; 1992.
31. Rabbito M, Pohl MB, Humble N, et al. Biomechanical and clinical factors related to stage I posterior tibial tendon dysfunction. J Orthop Sports Phys Ther 2011;41(10):776–84.
32. Arangio G, Rogman A, Reed JF 3rd. Hindfoot alignment valgus moment arm increases in adult flatfoot with Achilles tendon contracture. Foot Ankle Int 2009;30(11):1078–82.
33. Maceira E, Monteagudo M. Subtalar anatomy and mechanics. Foot Ankle Clin 2015;20(2):195–221.
34. Imhauser CW, Siegler S, Abidi NA, et al. The effect of posterior tibialis tendon dysfunction on the plantar pressure characteristics and the kinematics of the arch and the hindfoot. Clin Biomech (Bristol, Avon) 2004;19(2):161–9.
35. Benjamin M, Qin S, Ralphs JR. Fibrocartilage associated with human tendons and their pulleys. J Anat 1995;187:625–33.
36. Abousayed MM, Tartaglione JP, Rosenbaum AJ, et al. Classifications in brief: johnson and strom classification of adult-acquired flatfoot deformity. Clin Orthop Relat Res 2016;474(2):588–93.
37. Anzel SH, Covey KW, Weiner AD, et al. Disruption of muscles and tendons; an analysis of 1,014 cases. Surgery 1959;45(3):406–14.
38. Holmes GB, Mann RA Jr. Possible epidemiological factors associated with rupture of the posterior tibial tendon. Foot Ankle 1992;13:70–9.
39. Ashford RL, Mathieson I, Rome K. Conservative interventions for mobile pes planus in adults: a systematic review. Rev Int de Cienc Podol 2016;10(2):42–61.
40. Rome K, Brown CL. Randomized clinical trial into the impact of rigid foot orthoses on balance parameters in excessively pronated feet. Clin Rehabil 2004;18(6):624–30.

41. Redmond AC, Landorf KB, Keenan AM. Contoured, prefabricated foot orthoses demonstrate comparable mechanical properties to contoured, customised foot orthoses: a plantar pressure study. J Foot Ankle Res 2009;2:20.
42. Esterman A, Pilotto L. Foot shape and its effect on functioning in Royal Australian Air Force recruits. Part 1: Prospective cohort study. Mil Med 2005;170(7):623–8.
43. Jung DY, Koh EK, Kwon OY. Effect of foot orthoses and short-foot exercise on the cross-sectional area of the abductor hallucis muscle in subjects with pes planus: a randomized controlled trial. J Back Musculoskelet Rehabil 2011;24(4):225–31.
44. Hockenbury RT, Sammarco GJ. Medial sliding osteotomy with flexor hallucis longus transfer for the treatment of posterior tibial tendon insufficiency. Foot Ankle Clin 2001;6:569–81.
45. Blake RL, Anderson K, Ferguson H. Posterior tibial tendinitis. A literature review with case reports. J Am Podiatr Med Assoc 1994;84(3):141–9.
46. Alvarez RG, Marini A, Schmitt C, et al. Stage I and II posterior tibial tendon dysfunction treated by a structured nonoperative management protocol: an orthosis and exercise program. Foot Ankle Int 2006;27(1):2–8.
47. Kulig K, Reischl SF, Pomrantz AB, et al. Nonsurgical management of posterior tibial tendon dysfunction with orthoses and resistive exercise: a randomized controlled trial. Phys Ther 2009;89(1):26–37.
48. Alam F, Raza S, Moiz JA, et al. Effects of selective strengthening of tibialis posterior and stretching of iliopsoas on navicular drop, dynamic balance, and lower limb muscle activity in pronated feet: A randomized clinical trial. Phys Sportsmed 2019;47(3):301–11.
49. Tan JM, Auhl M, Menz HB, et al. The effect of Masai Barefoot Technology (MBT) footwear on lower limb biomechanics: A systematic review. Gait Posture 2016;43: 76–86.
50. Giza E, Cush G, Schon LC. The flexible flatfoot in the adult. Foot Ankle Clin 2007; 12(2):251–71.
51. Conti SF. Posterior tibial tendon problems in athletes. Clin Podiatr Med Surg 1999; 763:557–77.
52. Imhauser CW, Abidi NA, Frankel DZ, et al. Biomechanical evaluation of the efficacy of external stabilizers in the conservative treatment of acquired flatfoot deformity. Foot Ankle Int 2002;23(8):727–37.
53. Pascual-Huerta J, Ropa JM, Kirby KA, et al. Effect of 7 degree varus and valgus rearfoot wedging on rearfoot kinematics and kinetic during the stance phase of walking. J Am Podiatr Med Assoc 2009;99(5):415–21.
54. Kirby KA, Green DR. Evaluation and Nonoperative Management of Pes Valgus. In: DeValentine SJ, editor. Foot and ankle disorders in children. New York: Churchill-Livingstone; 1992. p. 295–327.
55. Richie D. Biomechanics and orthotic treatment of the adult acquired flatfoot. Clin Podiatr Med Surg 2020;37(1):71–89.
56. Havenhill TG, Toolan BC, Draganich LF. Effects of a UCBL orthosis and a calcaneal osteotomy on tibiotalar contact characteristics in a cadaver flatfoot model. Foot Ankle Int 2005;26(8):607–13.
57. Augustin JF, Lin SS, Berberian WS, et al. Nonoperative treatment of adult acquired flat foot with the Arizona brace. Foot Ankle Clin 2003;8(3):491–502.
58. Myerson MS. Correction of the flatfoot deformity in the adult. In: Reconstructive foot and ankle surgery: management of complications. 2nd edition. Philadelphia: Elsevier (Saunders); 2010. p. 201–20.
59. Vulcano E, Deland JT, Ellis SJ. Approach and treatment of the adult acquired flatfoot deformity. Curr Rev Musculoskelet Med 2013;6(4):294–303.

60. Wertheimer SJ. The role of endoscopy in treatment of stenosing posterior tibial tenosynovitis. J Foot Ankle Surg 1995;34:15–22.
61. van Dijk CN, Knort N, Scholten PE. Tendoscopy of the posterior tibial tendon. J Arthroscopic Rel Surg 1997;13(6):692–8.
62. Monteagudo M, Maceira E. Posterior tibial tendoscopy. Foot Ankle Clin 2015; 20(1):1–13.
63. Myerson MS, Solomon G, Shereff M. Posterior tibial tendon dysfunction: its association with seronegative inflammatory disease. Foot Ankle 1989;9(5):219–25.
64. Dominick DR, Catanzariti AR. Posterior Tibial Tendon Allograft Reconstruction for Stage II Adult Acquired Flatfoot: A Case Series. J Foot Ankle Surg 2020;59(4): 821–5.
65. Conti MS, Garfinkel JH, Ellis SJ. Outcomes of reconstruction of the flexible adult-acquired flatfoot deformity. Orthop Clin North Am 2020;51(1):109–20.
66. Jahss MH. Spontaneous rupture of the tibialis posterior tendon: clinical findings, tenographic studies, and a new technique of repair. Foot Ankle 1982;3(3):158–66.
67. Arronow MS. Tendon transfer options in managing the adult flexible flatfoot. Foot Ankle Clin 2012;17:205–26.
68. Kuo KN, Wu KW, Krzak JJ, et al. Tendon transfers around the foot: when and where. Foot Ankle Clin 2015;20(4):601–17.
69. Arangio GA, Salathe EP. Medial displacement calcaneal osteotomy reduces the excess forces in the medial longitudinal arch of the flat foot. Clin Biomech (Bristol, Avon) 2001;16:535–9.
70. Viladot R, Pons M, Alvarez F, et al. Subtalar arthroereisis for posterior tibial tendon dysfunction: a preliminary report. Foot Ankle Int 2003;24(8):600–6.
71. Funk DA, Cass JR, Johnson KA. Acquired adult flat foot secondary to posterior tibial-tendon pathology. J Bone Joint Surg Am 1986;68(1):95–102.
72. Teasdall RD, Johnson KA. Surgical treatment of stage I posterior tibial tendon dysfunction. Foot Ankle Int 1994;15(12):646–8.
73. Khazen G, Khazen C. Tendoscopy in stage I posterior tibial tendon dysfunction. Foot Ankle Clin 2012;17(3):399–406.
74. Crates JM, Richardson EG. Treatment of stage I posterior tibial tendon dysfunction with medial soft tissue procedures. Clin Orthop Relat Res 1999;(365):46–9.
75. McCormack AP, Varner KE, Marymont JV. Surgical treatment for posterior tibial tendonitis in young competitive athletes. Foot Ankle Int 2003;24(7):535–8.
76. Bulstra GH, Olsthoom PGM, van Dijk CN. Tendoscopy of the posterior tibial tendon. Foot Ankle Clin 2006;11(2):421–7.
77. Chow HT, Chan KB, Lui TH. Tendoscopic debridement for stage I posterior tibial tendon dysfunction. Knee Surg Sports Traumatol Arthrosc 2005;13:695–8.
78. Vaughn NH, Stepanyan H, Gallo RA, et al. Genetic factors in tendon injury: a systematic review of the literature. Orthop J Sports Med 2017;5(8). 2325967117724416.

Tendon Transfer versus Allograft Reconstruction in Progressive Collapsing Foot Deformity

Michael J. Kelly, MD, Nicholas D. Casscells, MD*

KEYWORDS

- Posterior tibial tendon • Progressive collapsing foot deformity • Flatfoot
- Posterior tibial tendon dysfunction • Tendon transfer • Allograft

KEY POINTS

- The posterior tibial tendon muscle belly must be functional and non-atrophied for an allograft reconstruction.
- If the posterior tibial tendon muscle belly is scarred and not "springy" when assess intraoperatively, an FDL transfer should be performed.
- The foot deformity must be corrected at the time of reconstruction.

The posterior tibial tendon (PTT) is the principal dynamic stabilizer of the medial longitudinal arch of the foot.[1] Attenuation of the PTT, seen with diabetes, obesity, corticosteroid use, and pre-existing developmental progressive collapsing foot deformity, contributes to an inability to support the arch.[1] This disease process, formerly adult acquired flatfoot deformity, is now known as progressive collapsing foot deformity (PCFD).[2] The basic goal of surgically reconstructing PCFD is to restore the foot's medial longitudinal arch, often through a combination of bony and soft tissue procedures. The PTT, thus, is a common surgical target. How exactly to restore its function, however, has recently been called into question.[3]

Before 2015, tendon transfer would have been the obvious answer, and for most foot and ankle surgeons, it probably still is. Transfer of the flexor digitorum longus (FDL) to the primary insertion site of the PTT on the navicular (most often in combination with calcaneal osteotomies and other procedures) has produced excellent results.[4] Transfers of the flexor hallucis longus (FHL) or a portion of the tibialis anterior tendon have also been described but have their respective drawbacks.[5,6] Restoring the critical function of the PTT with a completely separate, healthy myotendinous

Department of Orthopaedic Surgery, MedStar Georgetown University Hospital, 3800 Reservoir Road, Ground Floor PHC, Washington, DC 20007, USA
* Corresponding author.
E-mail address: ncasscells@gmail.com

Foot Ankle Clin N Am 26 (2021) 465–471
https://doi.org/10.1016/j.fcl.2021.06.008
1083-7515/21/Published by Elsevier Inc.

unit, which itself has a native function deemed sacrificable, has undoubtedly provided reliable outcomes. However, tendon transfer surgery, especially about the foot and ankle, has its limitations, namely, the size and strength differences between the FDL and PTT.[7,8] Asking the FDL to perform the duties of the much stouter PTT can be a bit of a stretch, and some would argue that the FDL acts more as a cable supporting the arch of the foot than as a dynamic inverter.

Dissatisfaction with the transfer inspired Myerson and Shariff[9] to describe an allograft tendon reconstruction as a means of managing flexible PCFD. The premise of this technique is rooted in the limitations of tendon transfers, exemplified in 2 landmark studies, by Silver and colleagues[10] and Jeng and colleagues,[11] which helped define the discrepancies in size and power of the myotendinous units affecting foot and ankle motion. By analyzing the cross-sectional area of the individual tendons and the strength of the tendons' respective muscle bellies by quantifying muscle volume on MRI, these studies demonstrated significant discrepancies between the strength of the PTT and the other historically transferred myotendinous units of the leg.[12] For the purposes of this discussion, the FDL has 28% the strength of the PTT; the FHL, although stronger, still pales in comparison with the PTT, only able to garner 50% of its strength.[9]

The principles of tendon transfers were established more than 100 years ago, and are still referenced today, albeit with some updates.[13] The most important of these when considering PCFD reconstruction is the expected loss of one grade of muscle strength upon transferring a muscle-tendon unit. This premise, not surprisingly, has brought some to ask: if the patient has a degenerative posterior tibial tendon, but a mobile and nonatrophied tibialis posterior muscle belly, why are we transferring another, weaker muscle-tendon unit—that we can expect to weaken even further—and expecting it to do the job? Thus, the growing (albeit small) trend is away from tendon transfer, and toward allograft tendon reconstruction.

Allograft tendon reconstruction has been described as a method that addresses several of the limitations of tendon transfers in flat foot reconstruction.[12] Allograft effectively salvages the tibialis posterior muscle belly and its inherent strength designed to support the medial arch, while avoiding reliance on a smaller-diameter and diminished-strength transferred tendon to shoulder this responsibility.[9] Allografts are readily accessible and are available in various calibers and lengths. In addition, using allograft tendon has the potential to decrease operative time, as the procedure avoids additional surgical incisions and dissections required to harvest autogenous tendon (which also decreases soft tissue manipulation and donor site morbidity).[13]

To perform the technique, first the diseased posterior tibial tendon is resected off of the medial pole of the navicular through a standard medial approach as seen in **Fig. 1**.

The springiness of the PTT must be assessed. If the PTT tendon and/or muscle belly is proximally scarred, the allograft reconstruction must be abandoned in favor of the FDL transfer. **Fig. 2** demonstrates adequate springiness of the native PTT.

An incision is then made proximally to expose the posterior tibial tendon at the medial border of the tibia at the musculotendinous junction. The PTT tendon is then pulled proximally through the tarsal tunnel. An allograft semitendinosus can be used because it generally has plenty of length and has a width comparable to the PTT. The allograft can be secured to the musculotendinous junction using a pulvertaft weave technique and then passed through the tarsal tunnel behind the medial malleolus using a Kelly clamp. Once in the distal surgical field, the allograft can be secured and tensioned in inversion using a bone tunnel and biotenodesis screw in the medial pole of the navicular. Conversely, as performed in the included images, the allograft can first be secured to the medial pole of the navicular as seen in **Fig. 3**.

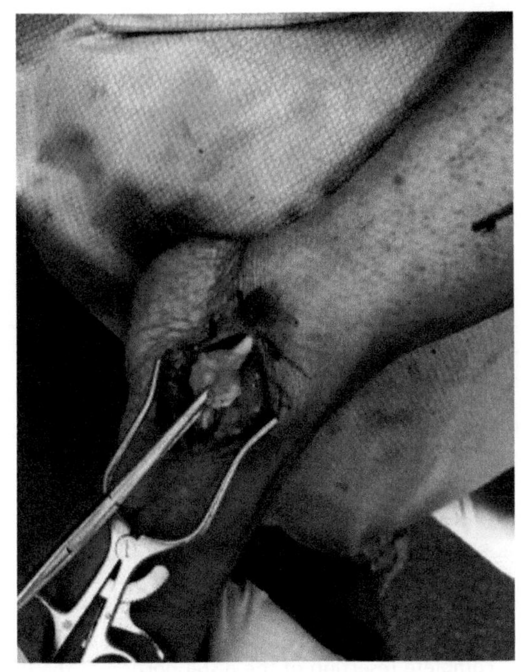

Fig. 1. Medial approach to the PTT with appreciable tendinopathy.

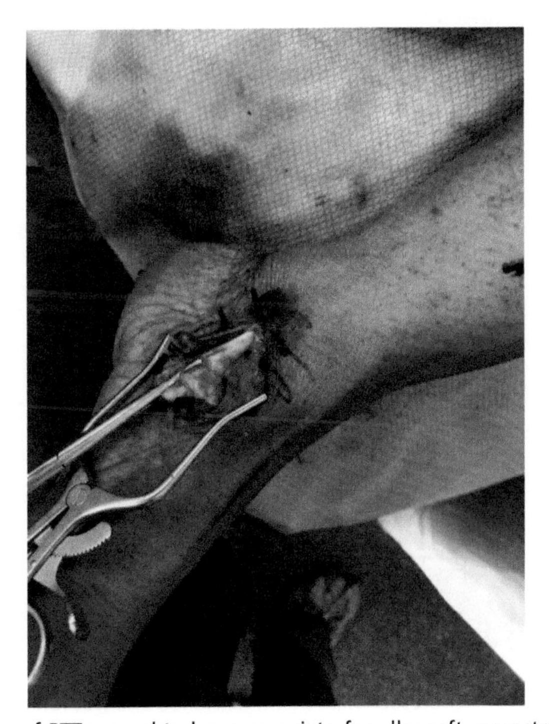

Fig. 2. Springiness of PTT proved to be appropriate for allograft reconstruction.

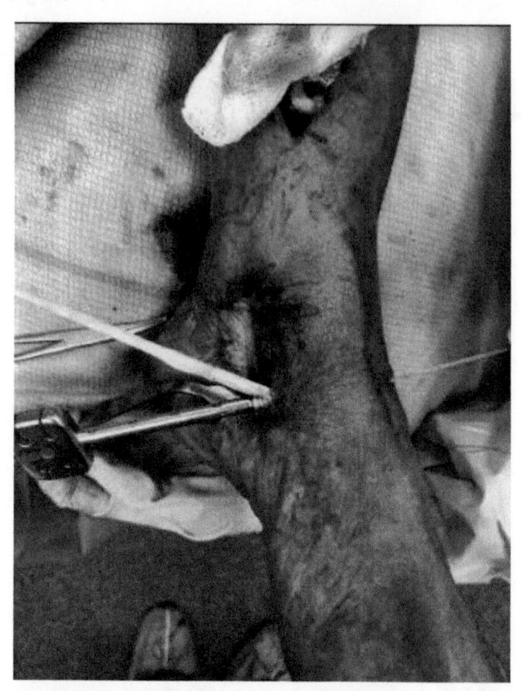

Fig. 3. Biotenodesis fixation of allograft tendon into the native PTT insertion site on the medial midfoot, after complete resection of the distal portion of the PTT's tendinopathy.

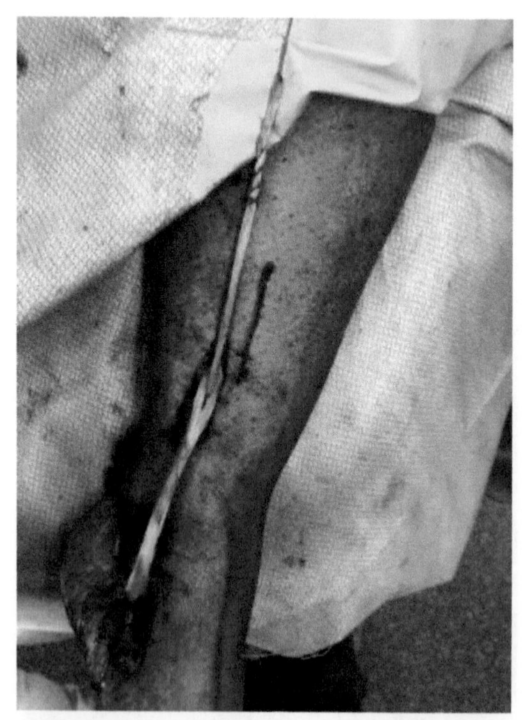

Fig. 4. Semitendinosus allograft seen here being tensioned and weaved through the musculotendinous junction of the PTT.

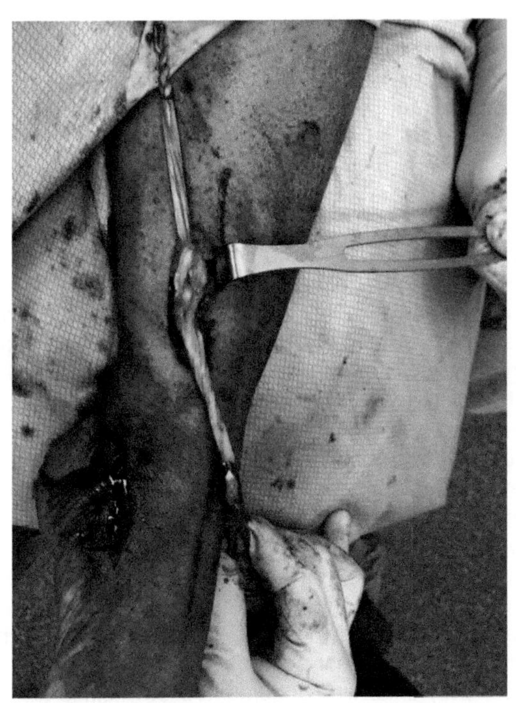

Fig. 5. Completed pulvertaft weave between the allograft and the native PTT at the musculotendinous junction.

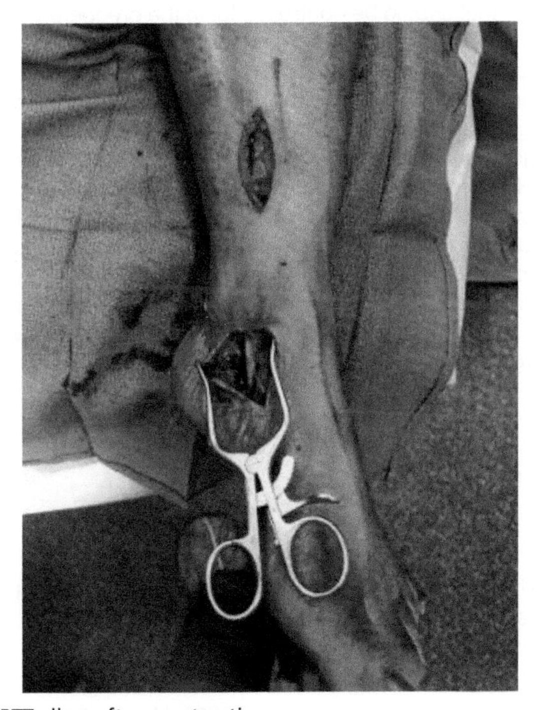

Fig. 6. Complete PTT allograft reconstruction.

The allograft is passed proximally through the tarsal tunnel, tensioned, and secured to the myotendinous junction of the native PTT as seen in **Figs. 4** and **5**.

The tendon edges can be trimmed, and the bulk of the pulvertaft weave nicely tucks in behind the tibia. **Fig. 6** demonstrates the completed allograft reconstruction.

This technique is predicated on patient selection. Not all those with PCFD are considered good candidates, and tendon transfer surgery will likely never become obsolete in the flatfoot population. Myserson and Shariff[9] recommend obtaining a preoperative MRI of the leg to evaluate for fatty atrophy of the tibialis posterior muscle belly. The other requirement for this technique is an intraoperative assessment of the mobility or springiness of the PTT; this helps to exclude scarred and immobile myotendinous units, which would not be good candidates for use of an allograft cable.[9,12] The recommendation in these patients is to pursue standard tendon transfer.[9]

Although certainly an interesting phenomenon, at this time there remains little published evidence to support its use. Myerson and colleagues have published review articles and technique papers, none of which present patient outcomes.[9,12,13] This technique is, however, referenced in 2 recent articles in the foot and ankle literature. Torres and colleagues[14] report on 15 patients undergoing allograft reconstruction of multiple different tendons, only one being the PTT; on average, their patients did quite well. More recently, Dominick and Catanzariti[3] published a case series of 4 patients, all undergoing PTT reconstruction, noting very reasonable outcomes. Specifically, all 4 patients demonstrated grade 5 muscle strength and were able to perform a single-limb heel rise at final follow-up 1 year postoperatively.[3]

However, there certainly exist well-documented downsides and limitations to the use of allograft tendons. Allografts come at additional cost; yet this cost may be offset by shorter time in the operating room, as noted previously. Availability of allografts may remain a concern for some surgeons in their respective practices, although this is certainly a variable that should be controlled for in the preoperative planning stages. Additional risks include viral transmission and host rejection, lack of incorporation and rerupture, and infection.[13] Finally, as outlined previously, there are limitations to which patients this technique will benefit, and thus, tendon transfer should remain an indelible tool for all surgeons undertaking flatfoot reconstructions.

As of now, the gold standard for restoring the PTT in PCFD likely remains the FDL tendon transfer. However, there certainly should and likely will be much future research into allograft reconstruction, due to the theoretic benefits that this technique affords in the appropriate patient. First, we must see more studies into this technique's safety and efficacy; only after this can we expect comparisons of this procedure with tendon transfer. In addition, radiographic studies working toward a Goutallier-equivalent grading system for fatty atrophy of the leg musculature would likely aid in stratification of surgical patients in the preoperative planning stage.[15]

DISCLOSURE

The authors have nothing to disclose.

REFERENCES

1. Flores DV, Mejía Gómez C, Fernández Hernando M, et al. Adult acquired flatfoot deformity: anatomy, biomechanics, staging, and imaging findings. Radiographics 2019;39(5):1437–60.
2. de Cesar Netto C, Deland JT, Ellis SJ. Guest editorial: expert consensus on adult-acquired flatfoot deformity. Foot Ankle Int 2020;41(10):1269–71.

3. Dominick DR, Catanzariti AR. Posterior tibial tendon allograft reconstruction for stage II adult acquired flatfoot: a case series. J Foot Ankle Surg 2020;59(4): 821–5.
4. Conti MS, Garfinkel JH, Ellis SJ. Outcomes of reconstruction of the flexible adult-acquired flatfoot deformity. Orthop Clin North Am 2020;51(1):109–20.
5. Backus JD, McCormick JJ. Tendon transfers in the treatment of the adult flatfoot. Foot Ankle Clin 2014;19(1):29–48.
6. Helal B. Cobb repair for tibialis posterior tendon rupture. J Foot Surg 1990;29(4): 349–52.
7. Ibano D, Cortese MC, Duarte A, et al. Predictive role of ankle MRI for tendon graft choice and surgical reconstruction. Radiol Med 2020;125:763–9.
8. Briggs LC, Otis JC, Deland JT, et al. Lower extremity tendon strengths - implications for posterior tibial tendon reconstruction. Presented at the 45th Annual Meeting, Orthopaedic Research Society, February 1999.
9. Myerson M, Shariff R. Managing the adult flexible flatfoot deformity. An evolution of thinking. Medicina Fluminensis 2015;51(1):91–102.
10. Silver RL, de la Garza J, Rang M. The myth of muscle balance. A study of relative strengths and excursions of normal muscles about the foot and ankle. J Bone Joint Surg Br 1985;67:432–7.
11. Jeng CL, Thawait GK, Kwon JY, et al. Relative strengths of the calf muscles based on MRI volume measurements. Foot Ankle Int 2012;33:394–9.
12. Geaney LE, Myerson MS. Management of posterior tibial tendon rupture with allograft reconstruction, osteotomy, and peroneus brevis to longus transfer. Tech Foot Ankle Surg 2015;14:112–9.
13. Aiyer A, Smyth N, Avila A, et al. Evolution of tendon transfer to allograft reconstruction in foot and ankle surgery. Tech Foot Ankle Surg 2017;16(3):108–16.
14. Torres NO, Cisterna C, Ortiz C, et al. Allograft Reconstruction for Irreparable Foot and Ankle Tendon Ruptures. Med Res Arch 2018;6(12). https://doi.org/10.18103/mra.v6i12.1884.
15. Goutallier D, Postel JM, Bernageau J, et al. Fatty muscle degeneration in cuff ruptures. Pre- and postoperative evaluation by CT scan. Clin Orthop Relat Res 1994;(304):78–83.

Calcaneal Osteotomies in the Treatment of Progressive Collapsing Foot Deformity. What are the Restrictions for the Holy Grail?

Carsten Schlickewei, MD[a], Alexej Barg, MD[a,b,c,*]

KEYWORDS

- Progressive collapsing foot deformity • Posterior tibial tendon dysfunction
- Adult acquired flatfoot deformity • Medial displacement calcaneal osteotomy
- Clinical/radiographic outcomes • Complications

KEY POINTS

- Progressive collapsing foot deformity is a common disabling process.
- Progressive collapsing foot deformity is complex with several components, including abduction forefoot deformity, foot pronation/supination, and heel valgus deformity.
- Medial displacement calcaneal osteotomy is a reliable surgical procedure to realign the heel position; however, often, further surgical steps are necessary to fully correct the underlying deformity.

Video content accompanies this article at http://www.foot.theclinics.com.

INTRODUCTION

The progressive collapsing foot deformity (PCFD) is a complex deformity consisting of several components with variable degree of severity: (1) abduction deformity of the midfoot mostly due to lateral deviation at the talonavicular joint; (2) peritalar subluxation resulting in foot and hindfoot deviation in all three major planes with subtalar joint eversion, talus plantarflexion, and forefoot abduction; (3) forefoot varus with the first ray elevated above the fifth metatarsal; and (4) hindfoot valgus.[1] The complexity of the PCFD was recognized a long time ago, as published by Whitman in 1889 in the

[a] Department of Orthopaedics, Trauma and Reconstructive Surgery, University of Hamburg, Martinistr. 52, Hamburg 20246, Germany; [b] Department of Orthopaedics, University of Utah, 590 Wakara Way, Salt Lake City, UT 84108, USA; [c] Department of Trauma and Orthopaedic Surgery, BG Hospital Hamburg, Bergedorfer Str. 10, Hamburg 21033, Germany
* Corresponding author. Department of Orthopaedics, Trauma and Reconstructive Surgery, University of Hamburg, Martinistr. 52, Hamburg 20246, Germany.
E-mail address: al.barg@uke.de

Foot Ankle Clin N Am 26 (2021) 473–505
https://doi.org/10.1016/j.fcl.2021.05.003

very first issue of the Journal of Bone and Joint Surgery (back then known as "Transactions of the American Orthopedic Association").[2] The recently published consensus on flatfoot deformity recommended replacing the term "adult-acquired flatfoot deformity" with "progressive collapsing foot deformity".[1,3]

In patients with flexible PCFD, joint-preserving procedures are indicated to address the underlying deformity. The calcaneal osteotomies are the major tool to address the inframalleolar valgus malalignment of the heel.[4–6] The medial displacement calcaneal osteotomy (MDCO) was first described by Gleich in 1893[7] and initially modified by Obalinski in 1895.[8] Since then, the MDCO has been established as a reliable surgical method to restore the hindfoot axis.[4,5,9–11]

Several Foot and Ankle Clinics publications addressed the role of the MDCO in the past.[4,11–18] This review article aims to provide an updated comprehensive understanding of the biomechanics of the MDCO, indications and contraindications, detailed description of surgical technique, and systematic literature review of publication reporting clinical and radiographic outcomes after the MDCO.

BIOMECHANICS OF MEDIAL DISPLACEMENT CALCANEAL OSTEOTOMY

In 1998, Michelson and colleagues[19] investigated ankle kinematics, including ankle motion using a cadaveric model of 1-cm MDCO. At maximal dorsiflexion, a significant increase of internal rotation by 76% was observed. However, there were no significant differences at maximal plantar flexion.[19]

Thordarson and colleagues[20] demonstrated in a cadaveric study that the division of the plantar fascia does not have any effect on the corrective potency of the MDCO. Horton and colleagues[21] demonstrated that the 1-cm MDCO resulted in an average of 1.2 ± 0.5 mm (range, .6–2.2 mm) loosening of the plantar fascia. Adding of the lateral lengthening osteotomy strengthened the observed effect with measured values of 2.7 ± 1.9 mm (range, 1.1–6.6 mm).[21] This may explain why the symptoms of plantar fasciitis often resolve after the MDCO without a plantar fascia release. Hadfield and colleagues[22] analyzed the effect of the 1-cm MDCO on Achilles tendon length and plantar foot pressures in 14 cadaveric specimens. The length of the Achilles tendon remained the same after the osteotomy. The MDCO resulted in a significant decrease in average pressure underneath the first and second metatarsals while the pressure under the medial and lateral aspects of the heel substantially increased. The results of this study support the suggestion that the MDCO often results in a substantial inversion of the forefoot.[22] The same researcher group analyzed the effect of superior translation of tuber calcanei on the same parameters, including Achilles tendon length and plantar foot pressures.[23] It has been demonstrated that the addition of 5-mm superior translation may result in a substantial offloading of the medial forefoot and may help to avoid the increase of lateral forefoot and heel pressures as observed in the previous study.[22,23]

In 1999, Otis and colleagues[24] analyzed the length of the spring ligament under a load of 100 N in 9 cadaveric specimens. The length of the spring ligament was comparable before versus after the MDCO.[24] In 2001, Arangio and Salathé[25] used a 3D biomechanical multisegmental model to analyze the effect of MDCO on the excess forces in the medial longitudinal arch. It has been demonstrated that the MDCO with 10 mm of displacement results in a substantial shift of the excess forces toward the lateral side and hereby decreases the load on the medial arch.[25] In 2011, Iaquinto and Wayne[26] created a computational model mimicking stage II PCFD. Under PCFD conditions, 80% increase of plantar fascia strain was observed. Then a 1-cm MDCO was simulated, resulting in a significant drop of plantar fascia strain to 87% of normal value. Furthermore, the calcaneocuboid contact load was analyzed. The joint contact load increased 16% from normal to PCFD conditions. The MDCO almost normalized the load with only 1% over the standard load.[26] Similar results were observed in the later study by the same researcher group.[27]

In 2001, Davitt and colleagues[28] measured pressure in tibiotalar and subtalar joints in a cadaver study while performing medial and lateral displacement calcaneal osteotomies. After the 1-cm MDCO, the average center of force shifted medially by 1.0 mm; however, the observed changes were not statistically significant. In the subtalar joint, the pressure distribution shifted slightly medially (5.9%, $P = .06$) and more anteriorly (9.6%, $P = .02$).[28] Patrick and colleagues[29] analyzed subtalar joint force, contact area, and peak contact pressure before and after 1-cm MDCO in 4 cadaveric specimens. After the MDCO, there was a slight decrease of subtalar joint force from 211.4 N (range, 88.3–341.7 N) to 168.8 N (range, 52.0–307.1 N), a decrease of contact area from 3.5 cm^2 (range, 3.3–4.5 cm^2) to 3.1 cm^2 (range, 1.4–4.4 cm^2), and a decrease of peak contact pressure from 1810 kPa (range, 848–2475 kPa) to 1276 kPa (range, 1074–2511 kPa). However, all observed changes were not statistically significant. Similar to the study by Davitt and colleagues,[28] in this study, a slight anteromedial shift of the subtalar joint center of pressure was measured.[29] Steffensmeier and colleagues[30] demonstrated in a cadaveric study that the 1-cm MDCO results in a shift of the pressure center in the tibiotalar joint of 1.58 mm medially. The differences in the contact area, mean contact stress, and maximum stress in the tibiotalar joint were not statistically significant after osteotomy.[30]

Nyska and colleagues[31] established an experimental cadaveric PCFD model by releasing the posterior tibial tendon (PTT), spring ligament, and plantar fascia. Applying axial load with a range between 700 and 1400 N and concomitant Achilles tendon loading substantially aggravated the PCFD as confirmed radiographically. Adding of 1-cm MDCO before the loading reduced the arch-flattening effect of the Achilles tendon.[31]

Marks and colleagues[32] analyzed gait parameters as well as radiographic alignment in 14 patients with MDCO and six patients with lateral lengthening osteotomy of the calcaneus. In both groups, a significant improvement of all gait parameters was observed. The MDCO group demonstrated improved first ray plantarflexion, while the lateral lengthening group presented with a better heel inversion.[32]

INDICATIONS FOR MEDIAL DISPLACEMENT CALCANEAL OSTEOTOMY

The main indication for MDCO is the substantial inframalleolar valgus deformity of the hindfoot in patients with flexible PCFD.[4–6,9,11–16,18,33,34] The MDCO can be performed as an isolated procedure or in combination with other surgical steps. The isolated MDCO should be performed only in patients with isolated hindfoot valgus without substantial additional deformities—that means with an appropriate talonavicular joint coverage (at least 60%) and absence of substantial midfoot abduction and forefoot varus (supination).[5] The substantial midfoot abduction in combination with mild valgus heel malalignment can be reliably addressed by lateral lengthening osteotomy of the calcaneus (**Fig. 1**).[35,36] In patients with substantial inframalleolar valgus deformity and midfoot abduction deformity, a double osteotomy of the calcaneus is indicated—the MDCO followed by lengthening osteotomy of the calcaneus (**Fig. 2**).[37–42] In patients with rigid PCFD, the MDCO is indicated to address the residual valgus heel deformity after a subtalar arthrodesis.[4]

The contraindications for the MDCO include isolated forefoot deformity,[4] patients with flat midfoot/forefoot and concomitant varus alignment of the heel (also known

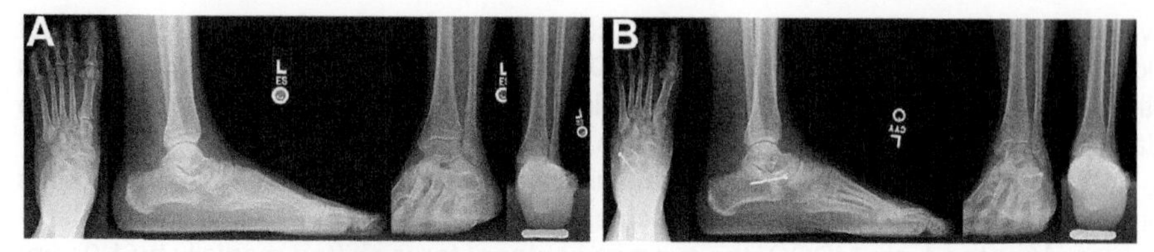

Fig. 1. (*A*) Preoperative weightbearing radiographs of a 40-year-old female demonstrate moderate pes planovalgus et abductus deformity with the pronounced forefoot abductus as seen on anteroposterior view of the foot. (*B*) At 1-year follow-up, a substantial improvement of underlying deformity after the lateral lengthening of the calcaneus was observed on weightbearing radiographs.

as pes planovarus deformity),[43] substantial degeneration of the subtalar joint, and/or limited and painful subtalar joint range of motion.[44–47] Recently, subluxation of the middle facet of the subtalar joint on weightbearing computed tomography (WBCT) has been identified as a reliable radiographic marker of peritalar instability in patients with PCFD.[48,49] Future clinical studies are needed to assess the prognostic value of this marker in patients who underwent joint-preserving realignment surgery to address the underlying PCFD.

SURGICAL TECHNIQUE GREENFIELD

Preoperative Planning

Detailed radiographic assessment, including weightbearing radiographs, routinely belongs to preoperative planning. In the previous issue of *Foot and Ankle Clinics*, we described the imaging of peritalar instability in patients with PCFD, including conventional radiographs, WBCT, and magnetic resonance imaging (MRI) in greater detail.[50]

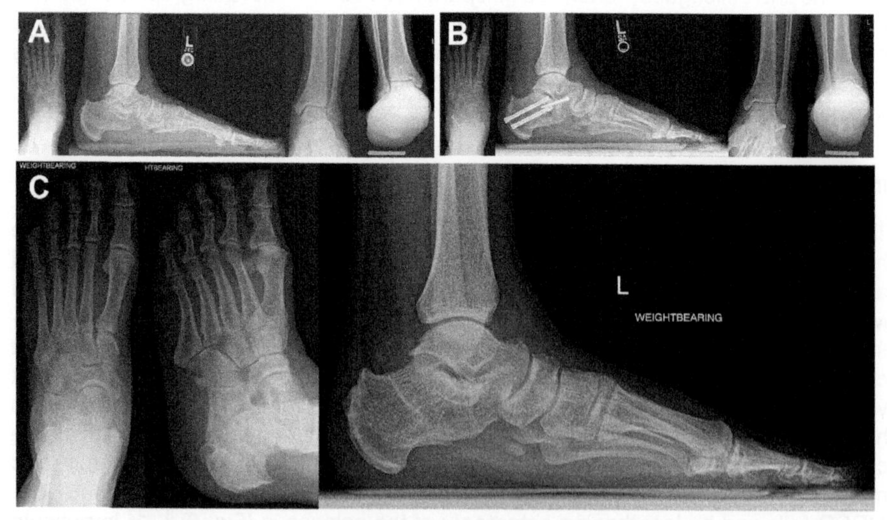

Fig. 2. (*A*) Preoperative weightbearing radiographs of a 41-year-old male demonstrate severe pes planovalgus deformity. (*B*) At 1-year follow-up, a neutral hindfoot and midfoot alignment after the double osteotomy was observed on weightbearing radiographs. (*C*) Removal of hardware was performed due to discomfort causes by the cranial screw at the tuber calcanei.

The hindfoot alignment view and measurement of the calcaneal moment arm is the gold standard for assessment of the inframalleolar hindfoot alignment.[51] Chan and colleagues[38] analyzed 30 patients who underwent surgical correction of PCFD. They found a strong linear correlation between the amount of osteotomy shift and postoperative improvement of the calcaneal moment arm with an adjusted R^2 value of 0.93. The final regression model indicated that each millimeter of medial shifting might reliably result in a 1.52-mm valgization of the calcaneal moment arm.[38] However, the preoperative assessment of the calcaneal moment arm measured using conventional weightbearing hindfoot alignment view should be interpreted carefully. First, there is a magnification factor of about 40%, as revealed in an internal pilot study. Second, in a study comparing hindfoot alignment in a retrospective cohort study with 375 consecutive patients assessed with conventional weightbearing radiographs versus WBCT, we found that conventional imaging may overestimate on average 3.9 mm of varus alignment compared with WBCT (**Fig. 3**).[52]

Preparation and Patient Positioning

- General or regional anesthesia can be used for surgery.
- The patient is placed in a supine position with the feet on the edge of the table. The ipsilateral back of the patient is lifted for a better approach to the lateral aspect of the calcaneus. The bump can be removed intraoperatively if needed for surgical steps on the medial side.
- Esmarch exsanguination and a thigh tourniquet can be applied unless contraindicated. The total tourniquet time of 2 hours should not be exceeded.
- Preoperative antibiotic prophylaxis is generally performed with intravenous cefazolin unless contraindicated.

Surgical Approach

- The anatomic landmarks include on the lateral side distal fibula with the tip of the lateral malleolus, course of palpable peroneal tendons with the base of the fifth metatarsal, and palpable plantar edge of the calcaneus (**Fig. 4**).
- The anatomic landmarks include on the medial side (if medial soft-tissue reconstruction is needed) medial malleolus, course of the palpable PTT, and tuberosity of the navicular bone (**Fig. 5**).
- A standard oblique lateral approach to the lateral calcaneus is made. The incision is made posterior to the palpable peroneal sheath. For alternative osteotomy

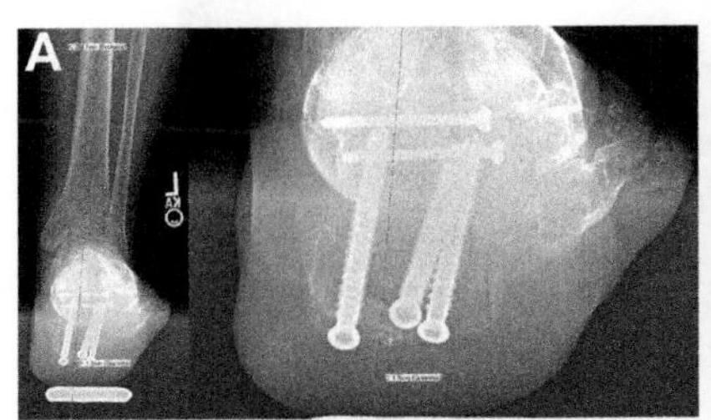

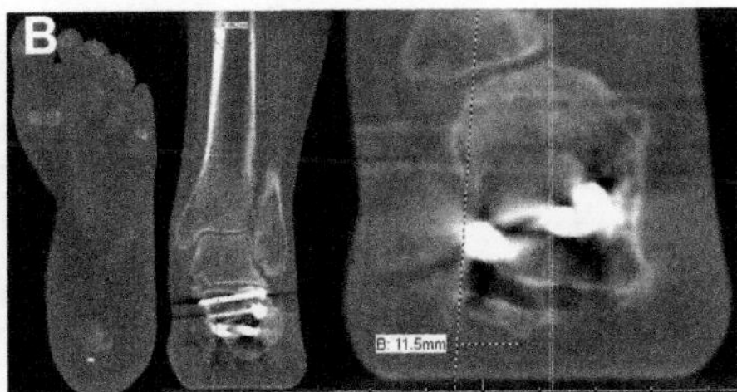

Fig. 3. A 62-year-old female patient who underwent open reduction and internal fixation of the calcaneus fracture. (*A*) Conventional weightbearing hindfoot alignment view demonstrates 1.3 mm (0.9 mm adjusted) of valgus. (*B*) weightbearing computed tomography was used to identify the lowest point of calcaneus contacting the ground (*left*), then identification of the long axis of the tibia (*middle*), resulting in the calcaneal moment arm of 11.5 mm of valgus (*right*).

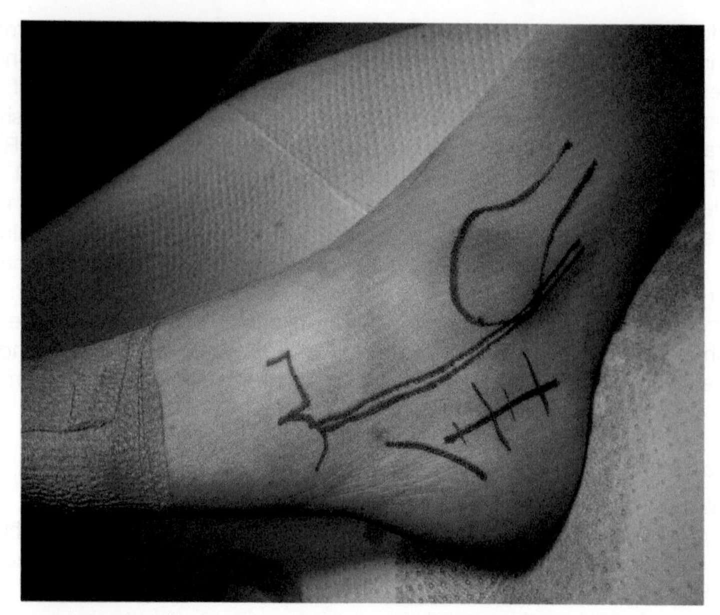

Fig. 4. Anatomic landmarks for the surgical approach on the lateral side (for details please see Surgical Approach).

techniques, the incision can be modified with a less oblique course.[4] The sural nerve is not routinely visualized in this approach; however, the deep dissection is performed very carefully using tenotomy scissors to avoid iatrogenic injury of descending nerve branches (**Fig. 6**). Deep dissection continues until the lateral wall of the calcaneus is exposed.

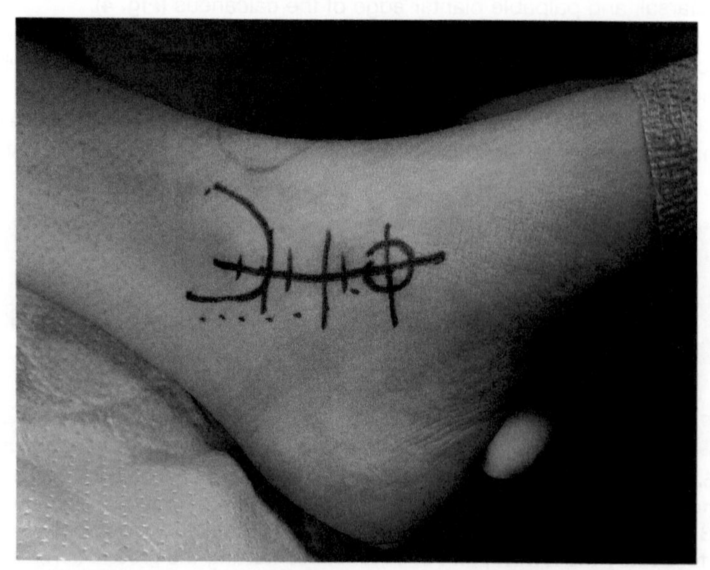

Fig. 5. Anatomic landmarks for the surgical approach on the medial side (for details please see Surgical Approach).

- The sural nerve runs superficially between the lateral malleolus and the Achilles tendon and curves around the lateral malleolus more distally.[53] The tip of the lateral malleolus is an important landmark to plan the lateral incision and to avoid the injury of the sural nerve. The main horizontal, vertical, and 45°-oblique distances between the tip of the lateral malleolus and the sural nerve are 13.5 ± 3.4 mm (8.3–20.0 mm), 13.1 ± 4.1 mm (5.0–19.7 mm), and 12.6 ± 3.0 mm (7.0–18.3 mm), respectively, as demonstrated in a cadaveric dissection study with 20 specimens.[54]

Osteotomy Technique

- Once the lateral calcaneus wall is exposed, the periosteum is longitudinally excised along the planned osteotomy plane. Two Hohmann retractors are placed on the cranial and plantar aspects of the calcaneus along the planned osteotomy plane, which is confirmed clinically and radiographically (**Fig. 7**).
- Talusan and colleagues[55] suggested the landmark line runs from the posterosuperior aspect of the calcaneal tuberosity to the plantar fascia origin (**Fig. 8**). In their anatomic study with 40 specimens, the safe zone for osteotomy plane to avoid medial structures injuries was determined to be within the area of 11.2 ± 2.7 mm anterior to the aforementioned landmark line.[55]
- The osteotomy is performed using a narrow fan-blade oscillating saw from lateral to medial with permanent water irrigation. It is important to pay extra attention to osteotomy completion at the medial cortex. An osteotome should be used instead of an oscillating saw to avoid injury of the medial neurovascular structures (**Fig. 9**). Surgeons with limited experience with this surgery may complete the osteotomy under fluoroscopy to avoid excessive instrument protrusion on the medial side.
- Greene and colleagues[56] performed an anatomic study with 22 specimens and analyzed the medial neurovascular structures in relation to the MDCO. Following

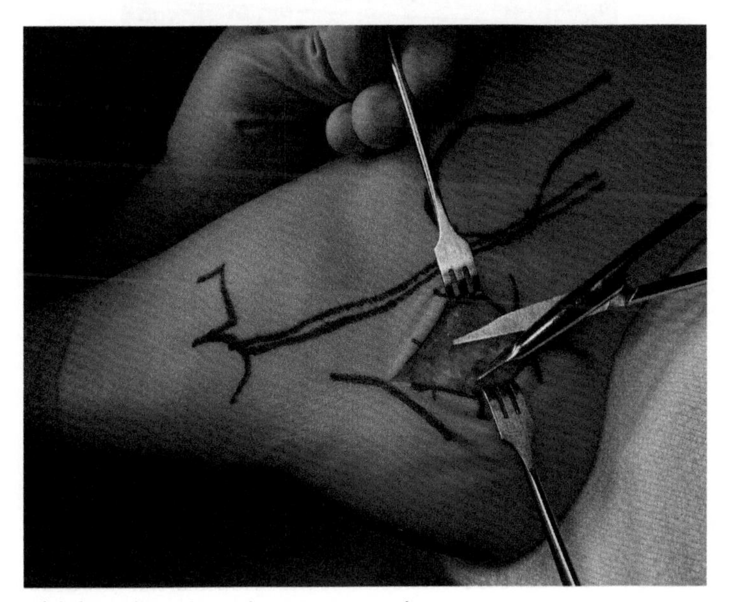

Fig. 6. Careful deep dissection using tenotomy scissors.

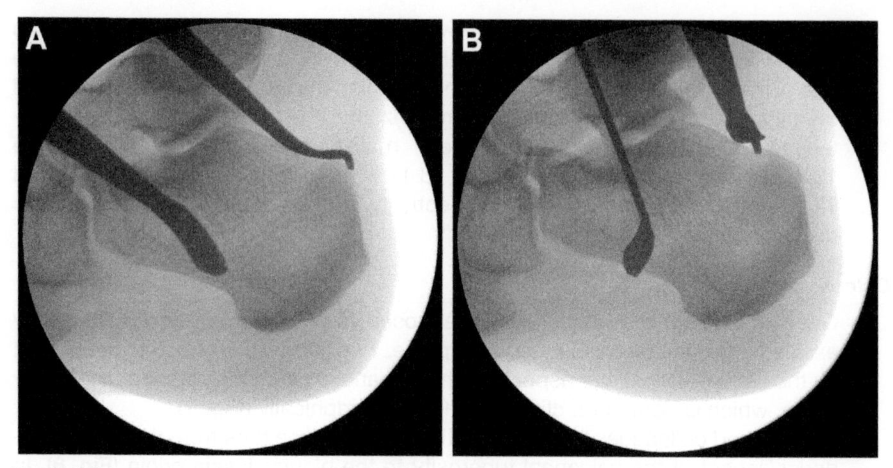

Fig. 7. (*A*) Incorrect placement of both Hohmann retractors; the upper one is too posterior, and the inferior one is not placed exactly on the plantar aspect of the calcaneus. (*B*) Correct placement of both Hohman retractors along planned osteotomy plane.

distances and rates of positions along the osteotomy were observed: medial plantar nerve, 15.4 ± 3.3 mm and 38%; lateral plantar nerve, 7.4 ± 4.4 mm and 51%; posterior tibial artery, 5.7 ± 4.7 mm and 24%, respectively.[56]

- A smooth laminar spreader is inserted into the osteotomy gap. The lamina spreader is used to mobilize the osteotomy resulting in distraction at the osteotomy site and elongating the surrounding soft tissues (**Fig. 10**, Video 1).
- The calcaneus tuberosity is shifted according to the preoperative planning (Video 2). The ankle is held in a plantarflexed position to relax the gastrocsoleus

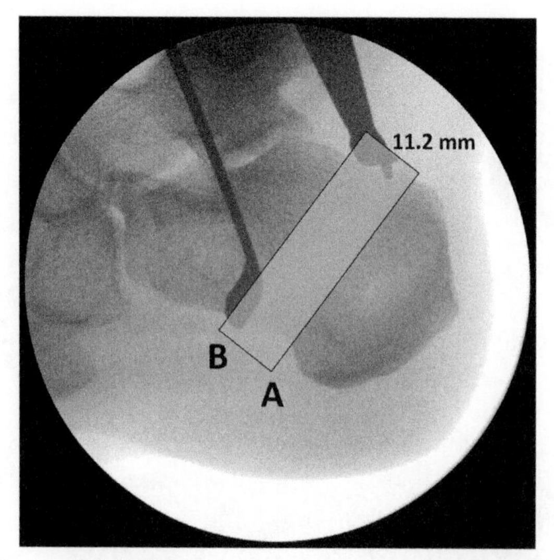

Fig. 8. Safe zone for medial displacement osteotomy plane. Line A runs from the posterosuperior aspect of the calcaneal tuberosity to the plantar fascia origin. Line B is drawn parallel to the line A. The safe zone is the shaded area with the distance between both lines of 11.2 mm.

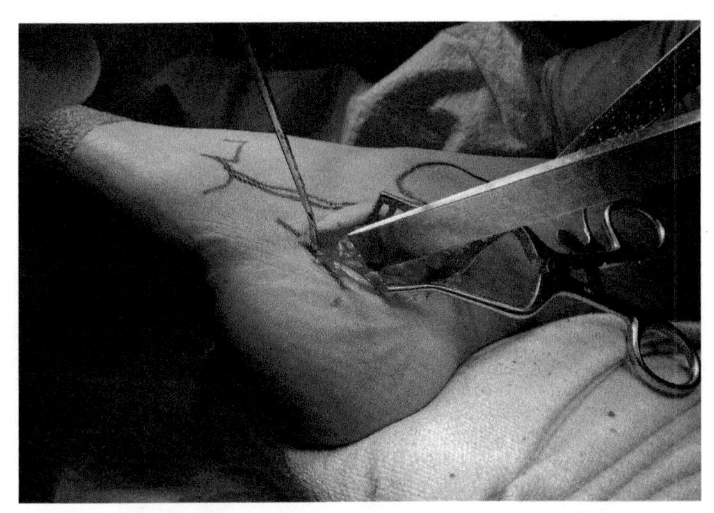

Fig. 9. Osteotome is used to complete the calcaneal osteotomy on the medial side.

complex allowing free mobilization of the tuber calcanei. After the desired correction is achieved, the ankle should be dorsiflexed, so the shifted tuber calcanei are locked in the position by the natural tension of the gastrocsoleus musculature. The clinical alignment is checked from posterior (**Fig. 11**).

- In general, the typical range of medial shifting of the tuber calcanei is between 7 and 15 mm.[5] While lateral displacement calcaneal osteotomy has been demonstrated to increase the risk of tarsal tunnel syndrome, the medial shifting of calcaneus does not have this effect, as demonstrated in a cadaver study.[57] As expected, a significant improvement of the 3D hindfoot angle was observed, and the improvement linearly correlated with the amount of medial translation of the tuberosity. In addition, in the midfoot, substantial improvement of navicular height and rotation as well as the Meary angle were achieved.[58]
- Deland and colleagues[59] described a modification of the MDCO by inserting an 8-mm wedge on the lateral side into the distracted osteotomy. The correction potency was significantly higher than that with the standard MDCO as measured on the lateral radiographs with talar first-metatarsal angle of $5.5° \pm 4.2°$ versus $2.7° \pm 5.7°$ and arch height from medial cuneiform of 4.5 ± 3.1 mm versus 1.6 ± 0.9 mm, as well as on the anteroposterior radiographs with talar first-metatarsal angle of $3.3° \pm 3.4°$ versus $2.1° \pm 2.5°$ and calcaneal pitch of

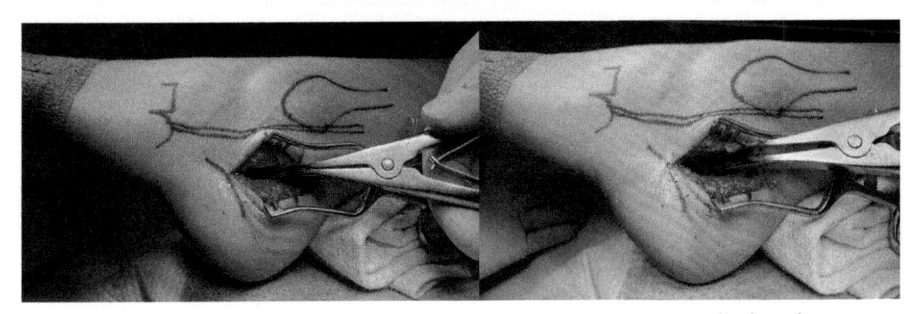

Fig. 10. A smooth laminar spreader is used to mobilize the osteotomy (Video 1).

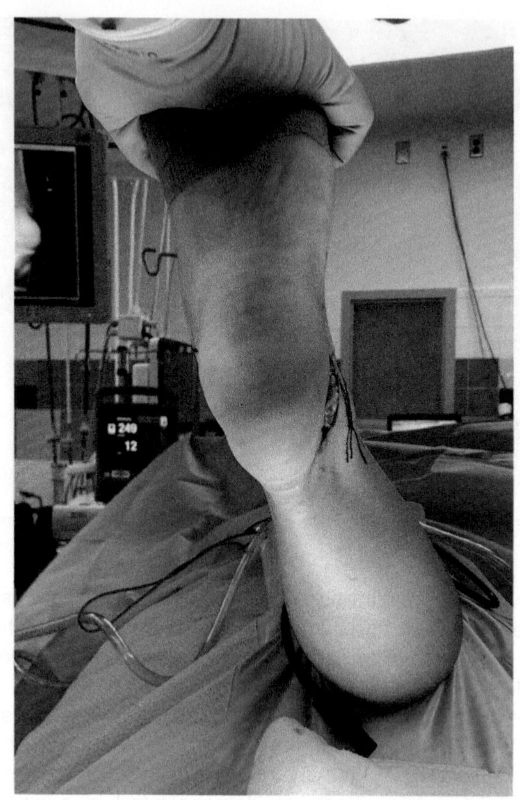

Fig. 11. The clinical alignment after medial shifting of tuber calcanei is checked visually from posterior.

8.4° ± 3.4° versus 1.8° ± 2.0°. However, this was a cadaveric study, and up to date, there are no clinical studies confirming the superiority of this modification.[59]

- The osteotomy is preliminary stabilized with a Kirschner-wire (K-wire) brought through a stab incision (**Fig. 12**). The position of the K-wire, as well as the amount of correction, is checked using fluoroscopy (**Fig. 13**). The position of the K-wire should be checked not only in the lateral plane but also in the axial plane to ensure the position of the K-wire inside the calcaneus (**Fig. 14**).
- We routinely use two-screw fixation (for example, 7.0 cannulated headless screws) (**Figs. 15** and **16**); however, it has been demonstrated that the single-screw fixation may achieve comparable outcomes as double-screw fixation.[60] We prefer to avoid too plantar insertion of calcaneal screws, which may results in hardware/incision irritation while walking.
- Lucas and colleagues[61] investigated screw size and insertion technique in a retrospective study including 149 patients. Thirty patients in this cohort underwent the removal of hardware. The patients with smaller screws (4.0 or 4.5 mm) used for fixation had a lower rate of removal of hardware than patients with larger screws (6.5 or 7.0 mm) with 9% versus 25%, respectively ($P = .032$). The superior and inferior insertion of screws resulted in a comparable rate of screw removal in both groups.[61]
- The alternative fixation of the osteotomy is the lateral plate. Konan and colleagues[62] compared the mechanical stability of MDCO fixation using a single

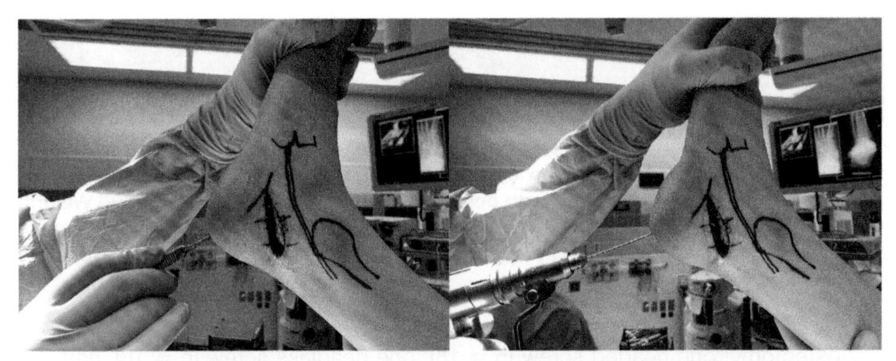

Fig. 12. Preliminary stabilization of the calcaneal osteotomy using a Kirschner-wire through a posterior stab incision.

compression screw versus locking step-plate in eight matched pairs of cadaveric specimens. A 10-mm MDCO was performed, and specimens were loaded up to 4500 N to failure. The median failure force was 1779 N (range, 1099–2312 N) and 826 N (range, 288–1607 N) in the plate and screw groups, respectively. However, it remains unclear whether the observed difference is clinically relevant or not.[62] Saxena and Patel[63] performed a retrospective comparative study including 17 patients with single-screw fixation versus 14 patients with locking plate fixation. The clinical and radiographic outcomes were comparable in both subcohorts. The rate of symptomatic hardware requiring secondary surgery was slightly higher in patients with plate fixation than that in those with screw fixation with 3/17 (21.4%) and 1/14 (5.9%), respectively.[63] Recently, Haggerty and colleagues[64] reported results of a retrospective consecutive case series of 46 patients who underwent MDCO fixed with a lateral plate. The union rate was 100%, and no complications, including the need for removal of hardware, were observed in this patient cohort.[64]

- Abbasian and colleagues[65] performed a retrospective comparative study in a patient cohort who underwent three different fixation types of the calcaneal

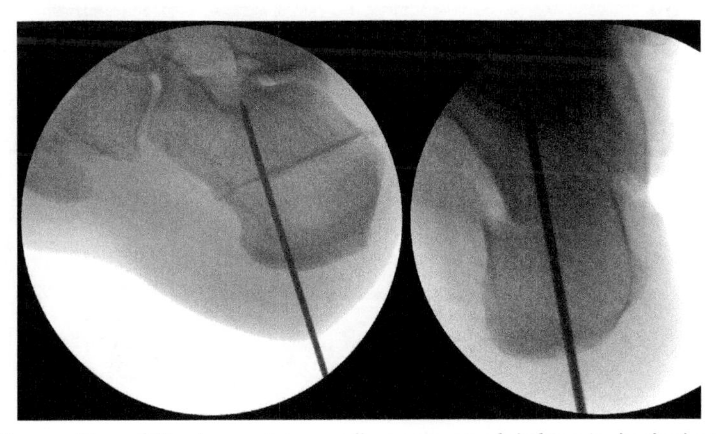

Fig. 13. The position of Kirschner-wire as well as amount of shifting is checked using fluoroscopy in both planes.

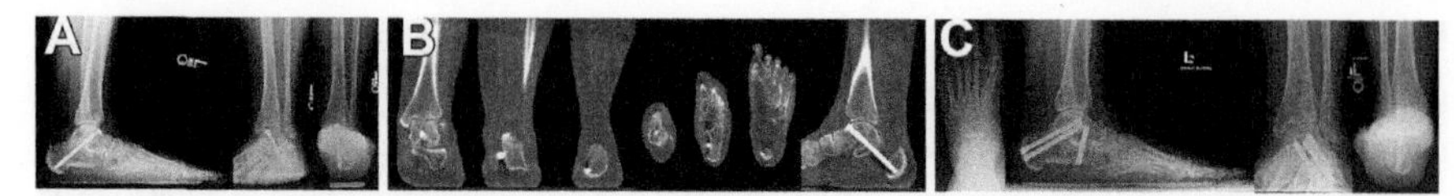

Fig. 14. Erroneous position of the calcaneus fixation screw. (*A*) Weightbearing radiographs of a 32-year-old female patient who underwent subtalar fusion with one screw fixation (performed outside). She presented with persisting pain at 14-month follow-up. (*B*) Weightbearing computed tomography confirmed complete nonunion of the subtalar joint and the erroneous position of the screw. (*C*) Weightbearing radiographs at 6-month follow-up after revision surgery.

osteotomy: one headed screw (n = 18), one headless screw (n = 18), and one lateral plate (n = 32). Three patients had wound healing problems; all three patients had lateral plate fixation. The overall union rate was 97%: both patients with nonunion had lateral plate fixation; however, symptoms were quite low in both patients. The hardware removal rate was 8/17, 2/18, and 2/32 in groups with headed screw, headless screw, and lateral plate, respectively, demonstrating a statistically significant difference ($P = .003$).[65] The favorite use of headless screws versus headed screws was confirmed in a retrospective study by Kunzler and colleagues.[66]

- In patients with substantial abductus deformity, we recommend performing a double calcaneal osteotomy (see **Fig. 2**), including lateral lengthening osteotomy of the calcaneus as described by Hintermann.[67] In patients where a double osteotomy of the calcaneus is indicated, the bicortical structural autograft for lateral lengthening osteotomy can be harvested from the calcaneus itself using the approach for the MDCO as described by Desai.[68]
- In patients with preoperative pain along the PTT and/or radiographic confirmation of degeneration of the PTT and/or spring ligament, we recommend medial soft-tissue reconstruction, which may include debridement of PTT, flexor digitorum longus (FDL)/PTT tendon transfer in patients with substantial (at least 30%) degeneration of PTT, excision of the accessory navicular bone, and/or anatomic reconstruction of the spring ligament (**Figs. 17** and **18**). In the current literature,

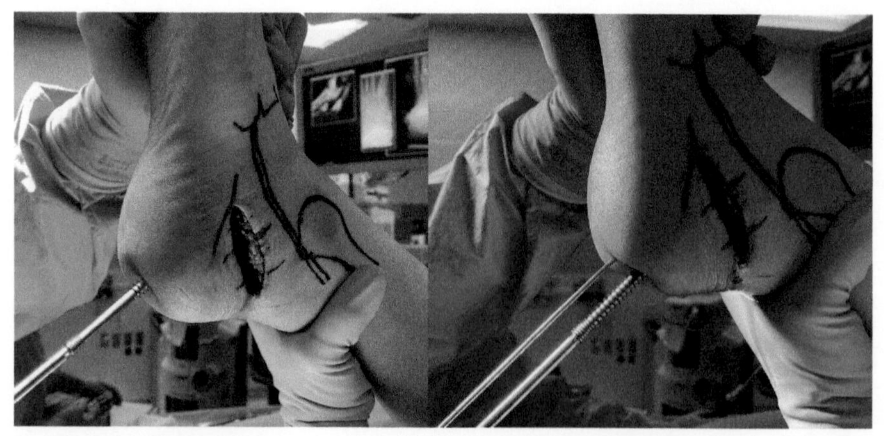

Fig. 15. Screw fixation of the osteotomy over previously positioned Kirschner-wires through a posterior stab incision.

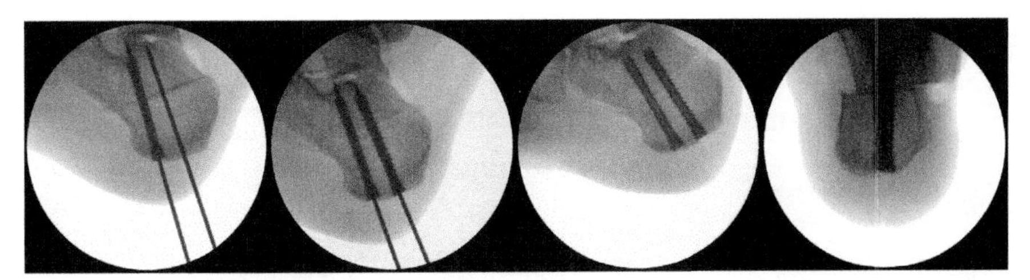

Fig. 16. Radiographic check confirming appropriate position of both screws.

there is still debate whether the diseased PTT should be resected or not.[69] Rosenfeld and colleagues[70] analyzed outcomes of 8 patients who underwent the MDCO with FDL tendon transfer with (4 patients) versus without (4 patients) resection of PTT. The clinical and radiographic outcome was comparable in both groups. However, MRI at the mean 13.4 months postoperatively (range, 11.6–17.7 months) demonstrated substantial atrophy and fatty replacement of posterior tibial muscle.[70] The FDL/PTT tendon transfer is a common procedure with the aim to improve the function of the posterior tibial muscle. However, it should not be performed routinely without a clear indication, especially in younger and sportive active patients, as it has been demonstrated that this procedure may results in impaired function of the lesser toes during the stance phase.[71]

- The calcaneal wall step is smoothened using a bone tamp (**Fig. 19**). The wound closure is completed with subcutaneous and skin sutures.

Percutaneous Minimally Invasive Medial Displacement Calcaneal Osteotomy

In the last decade, there are an increasing number of publications describing the percutaneous minimally invasive method to perform the MDCO.[72–75]

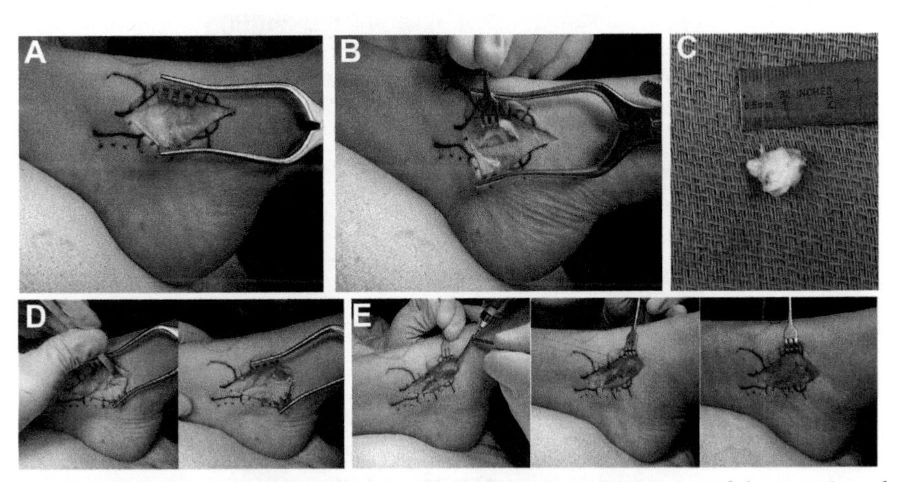

Fig. 17. (*A*) Medial approach to the posterior tibial tendon. (*B*) Exposure of the insertion of the posterior tibial tendon. (*C*) Excision of the accessory navicular bone. (*D*) Partial resection of the medial aspect of the navicular bone. (*E*) Refixation of the distal tibial tendon using transosseous sutures.

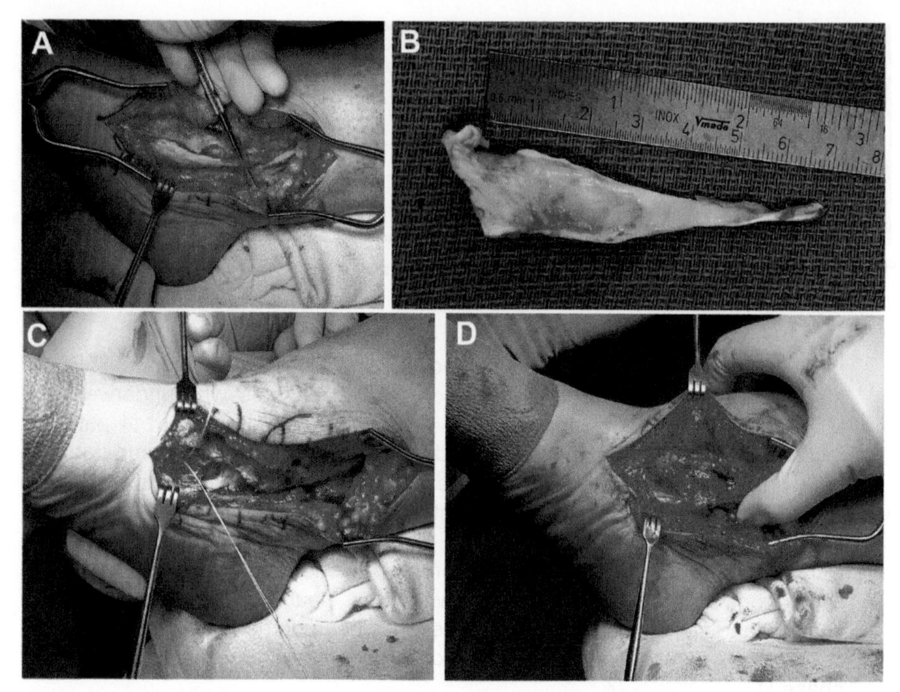

Fig. 18. (*A*) Severe degeneration of the distal posterior tibial tendon with subtotal rupture retromalleolarly. (*B*) Complete resection of the distal part of the posterior tibial tendon. (*C*) Placement of an anchor into the medial aspect of the navicular bone. (*D*) Reconstruction of the posterior tibial tendon using the allograft (anterior tibial tendon).

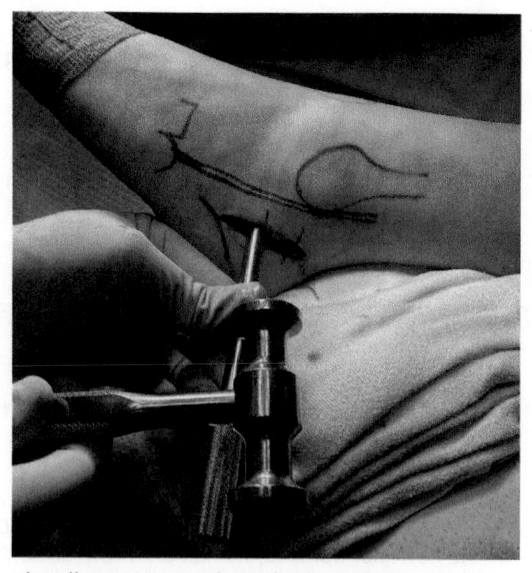

Fig. 19. The calcaneal wall step is smoothened using a bone tamp.

- DiDomenico and colleagues[76] used 20 fresh below-the-knee cadaveric specimens to assess the medial and lateral neurovascular structures after the percutaneous MDCO. The osteotomy was performed using a Gigli saw using four stab incisions. In all 20 specimens, the sural nerve, medial plantar nerve, lateral plantar nerve, and posterior tibial neurovascular bundle remained intact.[76]
- Durston and colleagues[77] used 13 fresh below-the-knee cadaveric specimens to assess the safety of using a Shannon burr for osteotomy competition. The osteotomies were performed by 11 consultant orthopedic surgeons, who did not have any experience with this surgical technique before, and two demonstrators. No significant neurovascular injury was observed in any of the specimens. In two specimens, very small proximal branches of the sural nerve were transected. In all 13 specimens, the path of the osteotomy was within 13 mm of the medial neurovascular bundle, and in 4 of 13 specimens, the bundle was found over the osteotomy plane. However, the calcaneal insertion of the medial head of the quadratus plantae muscle seems to have protecting function of the medial neurovascular bundle.[77]
- Gutteck and colleagues[78] performed a cadaveric biomechanical comparison of straight versus chevron-like osteotomy using a Shannon burr. Both types of osteotomies were stabilized using one 6.5-mm cancellous screw. The stiffness was comparable in both groups at all force levels between 100 and 500 N. However, the failure rate was higher in the group with the straight osteotomy (5 of 9, 4 and 1 at cyclic testing with 500 and 600 N, respectively) than in the group with V-osteotomy (2 of 9, 1 in each cyclic testing with 500 and 600 N).[78]
- Jowett and colleagues[79] analyzed the distance from the exit points of the osteotomy on the medial and lateral side to the tibial and sural nerves. The mean shift of the tuberosity was 16.7 ± 3.4 mm with a range between 12 and 21 mm. For the superomedial exit point of the osteotomy, the mean distance to the bifurcation of the tibial nerve was 7.3 ± 3.6 mm (range, 4–12 mm). In all specimens, the distance between the lateral plantar nerve and the inferomedial exit point of the osteotomy was at least 10 mm. For the superolateral exit point, the mean distance to the sural nerve was 6.2 ± 4.8 mm (range, 0–14 mm). In the same article, the authors shared their clinical experience with 35 procedures. No complications, including neurovascular injuries, were reported. In all patients, the osseous union of the osteotomy was confirmed clinically and radiographically; however, one patient had a delayed union with 9 months. In 34 of 35 patients, an appropriate correction of the PCFD was achieved, while one patient presented with overcorrection treated successfully with orthotics. Four patients underwent removal of hardware due to discomfort.[79]
- Kheir and colleagues[80] retrospectively reported short-term results of 30 patients who underwent minimally invasive MDCO. No complications were observed with a radiological and clinical union rate of 100%. All patients had a neutral hindfoot alignment postoperatively. One patient had heel pain which was resolved by the removal of hardware.[80]
- Mourkus and Prem[81] presented their results of combining the traditional open lateral lengthening osteotomy of the calcaneus with minimally invasive MDCO. Fifteen patients with an age range between 9 and 19 years were followed up for an average of 30 weeks. No complications were reported. At short-term follow-up, a significant improvement of radiographic parameters was observed.[81]
- Coleman and colleagues[82] reported short-term results of 160 consecutive patients with 1989 minimally invasive MDCO procedures in their retrospective

study. Osteotomy healing complications were observed in 7% of all cases, including four patients with delayed union and nine patients with nonunion. Interestingly, 12 of these 13 complications occurred within a 12-month time period in 2017: in this time period, the overall complication rate was 28% (12 out of 43 patients). This case cluster could not be explicitly explained; however, heat osteonecrosis from using the burr has been discussed. Other complications included mild wound dehiscence (3%), superficial infection (2%), transient (6%) and persistent (2%) nerve symptoms, and removal of hardware (2%).[82]
- Catani and colleagues[83] analyzed the functional outcomes, including pain assessment in 20 patients before the minimally invasive MDCO and then at 6 months and 1 year postoperatively. The pain level dropped significantly from 8.0 ± 1.4 to 1.1 ± 1.1 at 6 months follow-up. The further pain decrease was also observed at 1-year follow-up with 0.8 ± 0.7.[83]

COMPLICATIONS

- Injury to the lateral neurovascular structures (especially sural nerve).
- Injury to the medial neurovascular structures (tibial nerve and/or artery).
- Wound healing problems.
- Thromboembolic complications.
- Delayed union or nonunion at the osteotomy site (**Fig. 20**).
- Undercorrection of PCFD (**Fig. 21**).
- Progression of the PCFD and/or degenerative changes of the subtalar joint requiring revision surgery (**Fig. 22**).
- Symptomatic hardware (see **Fig. 2**).

LITERATURE REVIEW

Kou and colleagues[40] performed a prospective study including 24 patients who underwent surgical correction of the PCFD (**Table 1**). All patients have been evaluated at 6, 12, and 24 months postoperatively. Several clinical parameters improved significantly at 6 months follow-up. However, results continued to improve in the following 6 months, with an improved plateau reaching by the second follow-up year. The results of this study support the suggestion that the patients should be informed that the maximal postoperative improvement should not be expected before 1-year follow-up.[40]

Burssens and colleagues[58] used WBCT to analyze the preoperative and postoperative midfoot and hindfoot alignment in their prospective study, including 18 patients who underwent MDCO. The WBCT was performed at 3 months follow-up. This is the

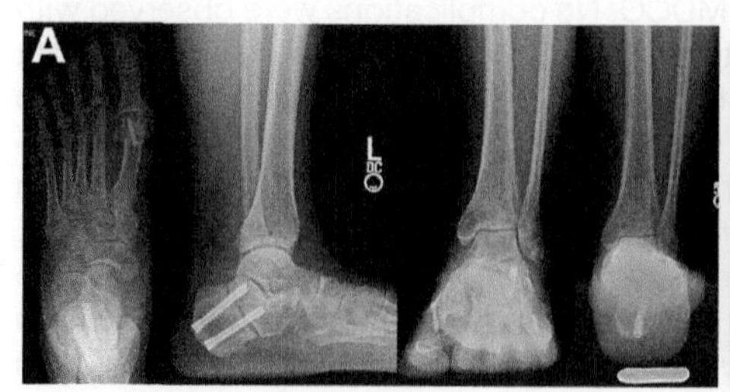

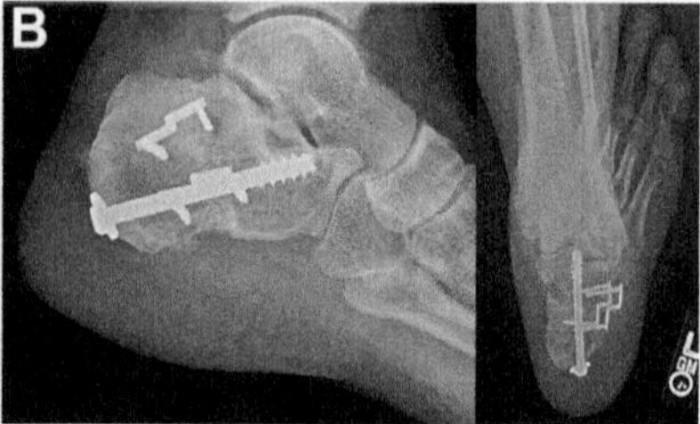

Fig. 20. (*A*) A 50-year-old female patient with a symptomatic nonunion of the calcaneal osteotomy 14 months after the initial surgery. (*B*) Revision surgery was performed using a hybrid screw-staples fixation.

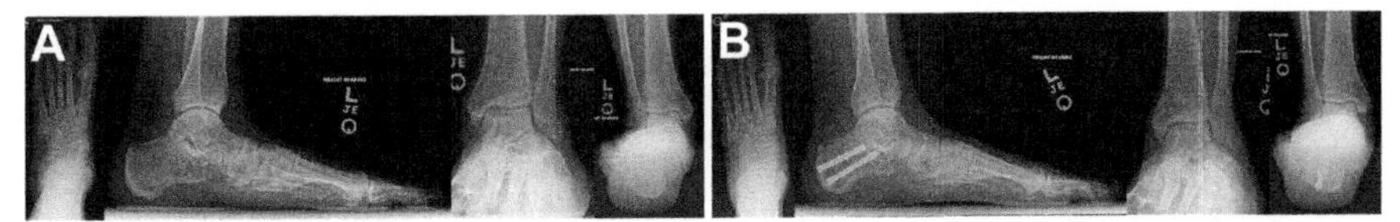

Fig. 21. (*A*) A 66-year-old male patient with substantial progressive collapsing foot deformity. (*B*) At 6-month follow-up, the patient reported substantial pain relief and symptoms improvement; however, especially hindfoot alignment view demonstrated substantial undercorrection of the underlying deformity.

first study analyzing three-dimensional hindfoot and midfoot parameters. All measurements demonstrated very high intraobserver and interobserver reliability. The mean calcaneal shift was 8.3 $\pm$ 4.2 mm. A linear relationship was observed between the amount of osteotomy shift and the three-dimensional hindfoot angle.[58] The same researcher group used WBCT for a detailed three-dimensional measurement of the MDCO in 16 consecutive patients.[84] The medial and inferior displacements were 7.4 $\pm$ 2.1 mm (range, 3.3–11.5 mm) and 3.2 $\pm$ 1.3 mm (range, 1.2–5.4 mm), respectively, resulting in a total displacement of 8.2 $\pm$ 1.9 mm (range, 5.9–11.7 mm). The orientation of the osteotomy has been analyzed in all three major planes with sagittal, axial, and coronal angles of 54.6° $\pm$ 5.6° (range, 45.7° to 64.3°), 80.5° $\pm$ 10.7° (range, 59.8° to 96.3°), and −13.7° $\pm$ 15.7° (range, −37.6° to 6.9°), respectively. The three-dimensional hindfoot angle improved postoperatively from 13.1° $\pm$ 4.6° (range, 6.4° to 20.7°) to 5.7° $\pm$ 4.3° (range, −4.0° to 11.6°). A statistically significant positive correlation was found between the preoperative hindfoot valgus angle, the axial osteotomy inclination, and the inferior displacement.[84]

Usuelli and colleagues[85] analyzed return to sports activities in 42 patients who underwent the MDCO and FDL tendon transfer. Preoperatively, 27 out of 42 patients participated in sport or recreational activities with mostly (57.2%) low-to mid-impact activities. At the minimum follow-up of 24 months (range, 18–31 months), 36 out of 42 patients returned to the sport or recreational activities. The average time to return

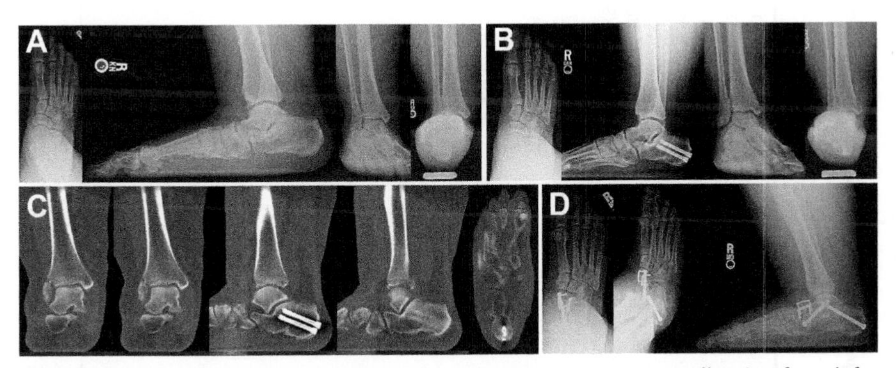

Fig. 22. (*A*) A 50-year-old female patient with substantial progressive collapsing foot deformity. (*B*) At 18-month follow-up, substantial improvement of the underlying deformity was observed; however, the patient was complaining about persisting hindfoot pain. (*C*) Weightbearing computed tomography demonstrated substantial subluxation of the medial facet of the subtalar joint with complete union of the calcaneal osteotomy. (*D*) Revision surgery including triple arthrodesis was performed.

Table 1
Clinical/radiographic outcomes and complications in patients who underwent medial displacement calcaneal osteotomy

Study	Patients (Feet)	Additional Surgeries	Follow-up	Complications	Clinical Outcomes	Radiographic Outcomes
Burssens et al, 2019[58]	18 (18)	• TMT-I AD (2) • Cotton OT (4) • Evans OT (1) • Gastrocnemius recession (11) • FDL tendon transfer (9) • Spring ligament repair (3) • Deltoid ligament repair (1)	3 mo	n.r.	n.r.	• 3D hindfoot angle: 18.2 ± 6.6 → 9.3 ± 6.1° • 3D anatomic tibia axis: 6.8 ± 3.3 → 5.3 ± 2.7° • 3D talocalcaneal axis: 11.4 ± 6.4 → 5.3 ± 6.5° • 3D rotation of tibia: 27.7 ± 4.7 → 28.8 ± 5.8° • 3D navicular height: 33.1 ± 7.6 → 37.1 ± 7.5 mm • 3D navicular rotation: 16.3 ± 5.1 → 22.7 ± 6.5° • 3D Meary angle: 20.2 ± 7.8 → 15.0 ± 9.3°

Cao et al, 2014[86]	16 (21)	• Reconstruction of PTT (21)	28.5 mo (18–48)	None	• AOFAS: 53.3 ± 6.5 → 90.8 ± 1.4	• WB radiographs • Arch height: 21.9 ± 1.4 → 30.8 ± 1.9 mm • CI angle: 12.5 ± 1.3 → 21.9 ± 2.3° • Lat TC angle: 47.3 ± 3.2 → 36.9 ± 2.9° • AP TC angle: 37.2 ± 2.2 → 23.4 ± 2.8° • Lat TFMT angle: 11.7 ± 1.5 → 3.3 ± 1.0° • AP TFMT angle: 11.5 ± 1.8 → 3.6 ± 0.7°
Cantanyariti et al, 2000[87]	24 (24)	• ATT transfer (4) • ATL (21) • FDL tendon transfer (19) • NC AD (4)	27 mo (13–51)	• Sural neuritis (6) • Achilles tendon rupture (2)	n.r.	• Lat TMT angle: 22.1 ± 3.6 → 8.5 ± 2.9° • AP TMT angle: 23.3 ± 3.6 → 11.0 ± 3.4°
Chadwick et al, 2015[88]	31 (31)	• FDL tendon transfer (31)	15.2 y (11.4–16.5)	• PE (1), DVT (1) • Superficial wound infection (3)	• AOFAS: 48.8 → 90.3 • VAS pain: 7.3 → 1.3	n.r.

(continued on next page)

Table 1
(continued)

Study	Patients (Feet)	Additional Surgeries	Follow-up	Complications	Clinical Outcomes	Radiographic Outcomes
				• Symptomatic hardware requiring ROH (5) • Progression of deformity requiring AD (4)		
Guyton et al, 2001[89]	16 (16)	• FDL tendon transfer (16)	31.8 mo (12–70)	• Failure of FDL tendon transfer requiring revision surgery (2)	• AOFAS pain[a]: 35.2 ± 7.1 • AOFAS function[b]: 26.8 ± 2.8	• Lat TFMT angle: 20.4 ± 10.6 → 12.7 ± 8.9° • AP TFMT angle: 21.1 ± 8.1 → 7.2 ± 9.9° • AP TN coverage angle: 22.1 ± 10.3 → 10.3 ± 11.0°
Ivanic et al, 2006[90]	29 (30)	• FDL tendon transfer (30)	58.5 mo (35–97)	• Persisting pain requiring AD (1) • Symptomatic hardware requiring ROH (5)	• AOFAS: 88.8 ± 10.7 • AOFAS pain[a]: 34.0 ± 6.0	n.r.

Kou et al, 2012[40]	24 (24)	• Gastrocnemius recession (24) • FDL tendon transfer (24) • Lat lengthening OT of calcaneus (24) • Medial column stabilization (12)	24 mo		• Symptomatic hardware requiring ROH (7) • DVT (1) • Wound healing problems (2)	• VAS pain: 5.2 ± 2.0 → 1.1 ± 1.4 • VAS mobility: 6.5 ± 2.0 → 8.7 ± 1.5 • VAS strength: 4.8 ± 2.3 → 8.1 ± 1.9 • VAS function: 5.6 ± 2.1 → 8.7 ± 1.6 • VAS overall health: 6.4 ± 2.4 → 8.7 ± 1.7 • VAS satisfaction with results of surgery: 8.9 ± 1.8 • FAOS pain: 60.3 ± 17.9 → 87.3 ± 12.3 • FAOS symptoms: 66.8 ± 22.0 → 85.6 ± 12.2 • FAOS activities of daily living: 65.5 ± 20.2 → 89.7 ± 10.6 • ROFPAQ sensory:	• Hindfoot valgus: 15.6 → 4.1° • Lat TFMT angle: 25.0 → 9.1° • AP TN coverage angle: 27.7 → 8.7°

(continued on next page)

Table 1
(continued)

Study	Patients (Feet)	Additional Surgeries	Follow-up	Complications	Clinical Outcomes	Radiographic Outcomes
					2.5 ± 0.5 → 1.7 ± 0.4 • ROFPAQ affective: 3.3 ± 0.7 → 2.0 ± 0.8 • ROFPAQ cognitive: 3.1 ± 0.5 → 1.7 ± 0.7 • SF-12 physical component summary: 35.9 ± 10.8 → 47.2 ± 10.1	
Marks et al, 2009[32]	14 (14)	n.r.	23.1 ± 21.5 mo	n.r.	• Stride length: 1.0 → 1.1 m • Cadence: 95.9 → 102.3 steps/min • Walking speed: 0.8 → 1.0 m/s • Stance duration: 65.2 → 64.9%	• Lat TFMT angle: −12 ± 9 → −11 ± 12° • Calcaneal pitch: 15 ± 5 → 19 ± 6° • mCun-MT5 distance: −2±4 → 6 ± 7 mm • AP TFMT angle: 15 ± 8 → 12 ± 10°

Myerson et al, 1995[91]	18 (18)	• FDL tendon transfer (18)	20 mo (12–26)	n.r.	n.r.	• AP TFMT angle: 21 → 8.5° • AP TN coverage angle: 34 → 21° • Lat TFMT angle: −22 → −9° • mCun to floor distance: 9 → 16 mm
Myerson et al, 2004[92]	129 (129)	• FDL tendon transfer (129)	5.2 y (0.5–7.0)	• Progressive deformity requiring triple AD (1) • Overcorrection of deformity with secondary ankle instability requiring OT (2) • Sural neuritis (3) • Medial plantar nerve numbness (5) • Wound healing problems (5)	• AOFAS: 79 • SF-12 physical component summary: 32 ± 9.4	• AP TFMT angle: 25 → 6° • AP TN coverage angle: 37 → 16° • Lat TFMT angle: −27 → −12° • mCun to floor distance: 7 → 19 mm

(*continued on next page*)

Table 1
(continued)

Study	Patients (Feet)	Additional Surgeries	Follow-up	Complications	Clinical Outcomes	Radiographic Outcomes
Niki et al. 2012[93]	25 (25)	• FDL tendon transfer (25) • Spring ligament repair (10)	5.6 y (2.6–10.2)	• Wound healing problems (2) • Reduced sensation lateral to the scar (4)	• JSSF: 37.5 → 46.9 • VAS pain: 75 → 9 • SF-36 physical functioning: 44.9 ± 13.5 • SF-36 physical role: 42.8 ± 11.9 • SF-36 bodily pain: 42.3 ± 10.7 • SF-36 general health: 48.2 ± 13.7 • SF-36 vitality: 48.7 ± 12.8 • SF-36 social functioning: 44.5 ± 10.7 • SF-36 emotional role: 47.8 ± 10.2 • SF-36 mental health: 49.0 ± 12.1	• AP TFMT angle: 15.8 ± 6.9 → 13.4 ± 4.9° • AP talocalcaneal angle: 17.0 ± 6.2 → 18.0 ± 6.2° • AP TN coverage: 30.8 ± 5.1 → 27.1 ± 5.6° • Lat TFMT angle: 23.7 ± 8.8 → 14.0 ± 6.7° • Lat TC angle: 50.3 ± 5.0 → 50.9 ± 6.4° • mCun-MT5 distance: 8.8 ± 4.8 → 11.8 ± 3.9 mm • Lat tibiocalcaneal angle: 15.9 ± 4.3 → 4.2 ± 3.5°

Oh et al, 2011[94]	10 (16)	• FDL tendon transfer (8) • Lat lengthening OT of calcaneus (16) • Excision of accessory navicular (6) • Gastrocnemius recession (7) • Cotton OT (4) • Lapidus AD (4)	5.2 y (2–10)	• Symptomatic adhesions around FDL/ PTT transfers requiring surgical lysis (1)	• AOFAS: 49.1 → 93.4 • SF-36 physical component summary: 55.1 • SF-36 mental component summary: 55.7 • FAOS pain: 92.6 • FAOS symptoms: 87.4 • FAOS sports activities: 92.7	• AP TFMT angle: 16.6 → 3.6° • AP TN coverage: 21.8 → 0.6° • Lat TFMT angle: 15.5 → 3.1° • Calcaneal pitch: 12.3 → 15.8°
Pomeroy & Manoli, 1997[95]	17 (20)	• FDL tendon transfer (20) • Lat lengthening OT of calcaneus (20)	17.5 mo (6–36)	• Symptomatic hardware requiring ROH (4) • Sural nerve numbness (2)	• AOFAS: 51.4 → 82.8	n.r.
Ruffilli et al, 2018[96]	63 (102)	• Reconstruction of PTT (53) • FDL tendon transfer (41)	125.1 ± 14.9 mo	• Wound healing problems (5) • Progressive deformity requiring revision surgery (4)	• AOFAS: 89 ± 10	• AP TN coverage: 22.4 ± 7.1 → 15.5 ± 5.6° • Lat TFMT angle: 17.1 ± 9 → 5.7 ± 6.2°
Sammarco & Hockenbury, 2001[97]	17 (17)	• FDL tendon transfer (17) • Tarsal tunnel release (1)	18 mo (12–25)	• Hardware failure with consecutive	• AOFAS: 62.4 → 83.6	• Lat TFMT angle: −17.9 → −14.7°

(continued on next page)

Table 1
(continued)

Study	Patients (Feet)	Additional Surgeries	Follow-up	Complications	Clinical Outcomes	Radiographic Outcomes
		• Excision of accessory navicular (1)		loss of correction (2) • Wound healing problems (2) • Symptomatic hardware requiring ROH (4)		• mCun to floor distance: 19.4 → 19.8 mm • AP TN coverage: 20 → 26.8° • Calcaneal pitch: 16.3 → 12.5°
Tellisi et al, 2008[98]	30 (34)	• FDL tendon transfer (34) • Lat lengthening OT of calcaneus (14) • Spring ligament repair (22) • Deltoid ligament repair (2) • Reconstruction of PTT (16) • ATL (5)	44.5 mo (24–65)	• Complex regional pain syndrome (1) • DVT (1) • Wound healing problems (2) • Overcorrection of deformity requiring revision surgery (1)	• AOFAS: 53.1 ± 14.5 → 83.2 ± 12.3	• AP TN coverage: 29.4 → 16.9° • Lat TFMT angle: −20.0 → 14.2° • mCun to floor distance: 15.3 → 21.2 mm
Wacker et al, 2002[99]	44 (44)	• FDL tendon transfer (44)	51 mo (38–62)	• Progressive deformity requiring revision surgery (2)	• AOFAS: 48.8 → 88.5 • VAS pain: 7.3 → 1.7	n.r.

- DVT (2)
- PE (1)
- Symptomatic hardware requiring ROH (5)
- Wound healing problems (3)
- Sural neuritis (1)
- Reduced sensation around the scar (6)

Abbreviations: 3D, three-dimensional; AD, arthrodesis; AOFAS, American orthopedic foot and ankle society; AP, anteroposterior; ATL, Achilles tendon lengthening; ATT, anterior tibial tendon; CI, calcaneal inclination; DVT, deep vein thrombosis; FAOS, foot and ankle outcome survey; FDL, flexor digitorum longus; JSSF, Japanese society for surgery of the foot; Lat, lateral; mCun, medial cuneiform; mo, months; MT, metatarsal; NC, naviculocuneiform; n.r., not reported; OT, osteotomy; PE, pulmonary embolism; PTT, posterior tibial tendon; ROFPAQ, rowan foot pain assessment questionnaire; ROH, removal of hardware; SF-12/SF-36, short form health survey; TC, talocalcaneal; TFMT, talar first metatarsal; TMT, tarsometatarsal; TN, talonavicular; VAS, visual analog scale; WB, weightbearing; y, years.

[a] AOFAS pain subscale with maximum of 40 possible points.

[b] AOFAS function subscale with maximum of 28 possible points.

to low-to mid-impact and to high-impact activities was 3.6 ± 0.7 months (range, 3–5 months) and 4.3 ± 0.9 months (range, 3–6 months), respectively.[85]

SUMMARY

The MDCO is a reliable surgical technique for the correction of valgus alignment of the heel in patients with PCFD. The osteotomy should be carefully planned preoperatively using weightbearing imaging (radiographs and WBCT). Different surgical techniques with different fixation methods have been described in the current literature. Mostly, the MDCO results in good clinical and radiographic results. However, complications are common.

CLINICS CARE POINTS

- Progressive collapsing foot deformity is often very complex with deviations in several planes.
- Radiographic assessment and preoperative planning includes weightbearing radiographs and weightbearing computed tomography (if available).
- Anatomy knowledge is crucial to avoid intraoperative injuries of neurovascular structures.
- The intraoperative shifting of tuber calcanei should be performed exactly according to the preoperative planning to avoid under- or overcorrection of the underlying deformity.
- The available literature demonstrates reliable clinical and radiographic outcomes in patients who underwent medial displacement calcaneal osteotomy.

SUPPLEMENTARY DATA

Supplementary data related to this article can be found online at https://doi.org/10.1016/j.fcl.2021.05.003.

REFERENCES

1. De Cesar Netto C, Deland JT, Ellis SJ. Guest editorial: Expert consensus on adult-acquired flatfoot deformity. Foot Ankle Int 2020;41(10):1269–71.
2. Whitman R. Observations on seventy-five cases of flat foot, with particular reference to treatment. Trans Am Orthop Assoc 1889;s1-1(1):122–37.
3. Myerson MS, Thordarson DB, Johnson JE, et al. Classification and nomenclature: Progressive collapsing foot deformity. Foot Ankle Int 2020;41(10):1271–6.
4. Greenfield S, Cohen B. Calcaneal osteotomies: Pearls and pitfalls. Foot Ankle Clin 2017;22(3):563–71.
5. Schon LC, De Cesar Netto C, Day J, et al. Consensus for the indication of a medializing displacement calcaneal osteotomy in the treatment of progressive collapsing foot deformity. Foot Ankle Int 2020;41(10):1282–5.
6. Tennant JN, Carmont M, Phisitkul P. Calcaneus osteotomy. Curr Rev Musculoskelet Med 2014;7(4):271–6.
7. Gleich A. Beitrag zur operativen Plattfußbehandlung. Arch Klin Chir 1893;46(1):358–62.
8. Obalinski. Eine Modifikation des Gleichschen Operationsverfahrens beim Plattfuß. Wien Med Press 1895;41(1):1538–40.
9. Ellis SJ, Johnson JE, Day J, et al. Titrating the amount of bony correction in progressive collapsing foot deformity. Foot Ankle Int 2020;41(10):1292–5.

10. Stufkens SA, Knupp M, Hintermann B. Medial displacement calcaneal osteotomy. Tech Foot Ankle 2009;8(2):85–90.
11. Weinfeld SB. Medial slide calcaneal osteotomy. Technique, patient selection, and results. Foot Ankle Clin 2001;6(1):89–94.
12. Den Hartog BD. Flexor digitorum longus transfer with medial displacement calcaneal osteotomy. Biomechanical rationale. Foot Ankle Clin 2001;6(1):67–76.
13. Dipaola M, Raikin SM. Tendon transfers and realignment osteotomies for treatment of stage II posterior tibial tendon dysfunction. Foot Ankle Clin 2007;12(2):273–85.
14. Giza E, Cush G, Schon LC. The flexible flatfoot in the adult. Foot Ankle Clin 2007;12(2):251–71.
15. Guha AR, Perera AM. Calcaneal osteotomy in the treatment of adult acquired flatfoot deformity. Foot Ankle Clin 2012;17(2):247–58.
16. Hockenbury RT, Sammarco GJ. Medial sliding calcaneal osteotomy with flexor hallucis longus transfer for the treatment of posterior tibial tendon insufficiency. Foot Ankle Clin 2001;6(3):569–81.
17. Hunt KJ, Farmer RP. The undercorrected flatfoot reconstruction. Foot Ankle Clin 2017;22(3):613–24.
18. Rodriguez RP. Medial displacement calcaneal tuberosity osteotomy in the treatment of posterior tibial insufficiency. Foot Ankle Clin 2001;6(3):545–67.
19. Michelson JD, Mizel M, Jay P, et al. Effect of medial displacement calcaneal osteotomy on ankle kinematics in a cadaver model. Foot Ankle Int 1998;19(3):132–6.
20. Thordarson DB, Hedman T, Lundquist D, et al. Effect of calcaneal osteotomy and plantar fasciotomy on arch configuration in a flatfoot model. Foot Ankle Int 1998;19(6):374–8.
21. Horton GA, Myerson MS, Parks BG, et al. Effect of calcaneal osteotomy and lateral column lengthening on the plantar fascia: a biomechanical investigation. Foot Ankle Int 1998;19(6):370–3.
22. Hadfield MH, Snyder JW, Liacouras PC, et al. Effects of medializing calcaneal osteotomy on Achilles tendon lengthening and plantar foot pressures. Foot Ankle Int 2003;24(7):523–9.
23. Hadfield M, Snyder J, Liacouras P, et al. The effects of a medializing calcaneal osteotomy with and without superior translation on Achilles tendon elongation and plantar foot pressures. Foot Ankle Int 2005;26(5):365–70.
24. Otis JC, Deland JT, Kenneally S, et al. Medial arch strain after medial displacement calcaneal osteotomy: an in vitro study. Foot Ankle Int 1999;20(4):222–6.
25. Arangio GA, Salathé EP. Medial displacement calcaneal osteotomy reduces the excess forces in the medial longitudinal arch of the flat foot. Clin Biomech (Bristol, Avon) 2001;16(6):535–9.
26. Iaquinto JM, Wayne JS. Effects of surgical correction for the treatment of adult acquired flatfoot deformity: a computational investigation. J Orthop Res 2011;29(7):1047–54.
27. Spratley EM, Matheis EA, Hayes CW, et al. Effects of degree of surgical correction for flatfoot deformity in patient-specific computational models. Ann Biomed Eng 2015;43(8):1947–56.
28. Davitt JS, Beals TC, Bachus KN. The effects of medial and lateral displacement calcaneal osteotomies on ankle and subtalar joint pressure distribution. Foot Ankle Int 2001;22(11):885–9.

29. Patrick N, Lewis GS, Roush EP, et al. Effects of medial displacement calcaneal osteotomy and calcaneal Z osteotomy on subtalar joint pressures: a cadaveric flatfoot model. J Foot Ankle Surg 2016;55(6):1175–9.
30. Steffensmeier SJ, Saltzman CL, Berbaum KS, et al. Effects of medial and lateral displacement calcaneal osteotomies on tibiotalar joint contact stresses. J Orthop Res 1996;14(6):980–5.
31. Nyska M, Parks BG, Chu IT, et al. The contribution of the medial calcaneal osteotomy to the correction of flatfoot deformities. Foot Ankle Int 2001;22(4):278–82.
32. Marks RM, Long JT, Ness ME, et al. Surgical reconstruction of posterior tibial tendon dysfunction: prospective comparison of flexor digitorum longus substitution combined with lateral column lengthening or medial displacement calcaneal osteotomy. Gait Posture 2009;29(1):17–22.
33. Arbab D, Lüring C, Mutschler M, et al. [Adult acquired flatfoot deformity-operative management for the early stages of flexible deformities]. Orthopade 2020;49(11):954–61.
34. Dohle J. [Joint-preserving surgical correction of advanced flexible planovalgus deformity of the adult foot]. Orthopade 2020;49(11):976–84.
35. Hintermann B, Valderrabano V, Kundert HP. Lengthening of the lateral column and reconstruction of the medial soft tissue for treatment of acquired flatfoot deformity associated with insufficiency of the posterior tibial tendon. Foot Ankle Int 1999;20(10):622–9.
36. Thordarson DB, Schon LC, De Cesar Netto C, et al. Consensus for the indication of lateral column lengthening in the treatment of progressive collapsing foot deformity. Foot Ankle Int 2020;41(10):1286–8.
37. Boffeli TJ, Abben KW. Double calcaneal osteotomy with percutaneous Steinmann pin fixation as part of treatment for flexible flatfoot deformity: a review of consecutive cases highlighting our experience with pin fixation. J Foot Ankle Surg 2015;54(3):478–82.
38. Chan JY, Williams BR, Nair P, et al. The contribution of medializing calcaneal osteotomy on hindfoot alignment in the reconstruction of the stage II adult acquired flatfoot deformity. Foot Ankle Int 2013;34(2):159–66.
39. Didomenico LA, Haro AA 3rd, Cross DJ. Double calcaneal osteotomy using single, dual-function screw fixation technique. J Foot Ankle Surg 2011;50(6):773–5.
40. Kou JX, Balasubramaniam M, Kippe M, et al. Functional results of posterior tibial tendon reconstruction, calcaneal osteotomy, and gastrocnemius recession. Foot Ankle Int 2012;33(7):602–11.
41. Moseir-Laclair S, Pomeroy G, Manoli A 2nd. Intermediate follow-up on the double osteotomy and tendon transfer procedure for stage II posterior tibial tendon insufficiency. Foot Ankle Int 2001;22(4):283–91.
42. Mosier-Laclair S, Pomeroy G, Manoli A 2nd. Operative treatment of the difficult stage 2 adult acquired flatfoot deformity. Foot Ankle Clin 2001;6(1):95–119.
43. Aebi J, Horisberger M, Frigg A. Radiographic study of pes planovarus. Foot Ankle Int 2017;38(5):526–31.
44. Barg A, Brunner S, Zwicky L, et al. Subtalar and naviculocuneiform fusion for extended breakdown of the medial arch. Foot Ankle Clin 2011;16(1):69–81.
45. Hintermann B, Deland JT, De Cesar Netto C, et al. Consensus on indications for isolated subtalar joint fusion and naviculocuneiform fusions for progressive collapsing foot deformity. Foot Ankle Int 2020;41(10):1295–8.
46. Knupp M, Stufkens SA, Hintermann B. Triple arthrodesis. Foot Ankle Clin 2011;16(1):61–7.

47. Röhm J, Zwicky L, Horn Lang T, et al. Mid- to long-term outcome of 96 corrective hindfoot fusions in 84 patients with rigid flatfoot deformity. Bone Joint J 2015; 97-b(5):668–74.
48. De Cesar Netto C, Godoy-Santos AL, Saito GH, et al. Subluxation of the middle facet of the subtalar joint as a marker of peritalar subluxation in adult acquired flatfoot deformity: A case-control study. J Bone Joint Surg Am 2019;101(20): 1838–44.
49. De Cesar Netto C, Silva T, Li S, et al. Assessment of posterior and middle facet subluxation of the subtalar joint in progressive flatfoot deformity. Foot Ankle Int 2020;41(10):1190–7.
50. Sripanich Y, Barg A. Imaging of peritalar instability. Foot Ankle Clin 2021;26(2): 269–89.
51. Saltzman CL, El-Khoury GY. The hindfoot alignment view. Foot Ankle Int 1995; 16(9):572–6.
52. Arena CB, Sripanich Y, Leake R, et al. Assessment of hindfoot alignment comparing weightbearing radiography to weightbearing computed tomography. Foot Ankle Int 2021. epub ahead of print.
53. Braus H, Elze C. Anatomie des Menschen. Erster Band: Bewegungsapparat. Berlin Göttingen Heidelberg: Springer; 1954.
54. Geng X, Xu J, Ma X, et al. Anatomy of the sural nerve with an emphasis on the incision for medial displacement calcaneal osteotomy. J Foot Ankle Surg 2014; 54(3):341–4.
55. Talusan PG, Cata E, Tan EW, et al. Safe zone for neural structures in medial displacement calcaneal osteotomy: a cadaveric and radiographic investigation. Foot Ankle Int 2015;36(12):1493–8.
56. Greene DL, Thompson MC, Gesink DS, et al. Anatomic study of the medial neurovascular structures in relation to calcaneal osteotomy. Foot Ankle Int 2001;22(7): 569–71.
57. Bruce BG, Bariteau JT, Evangelista PE, et al. The effect of medial and lateral calcaneal osteotomies on the tarsal tunnel. Foot Ankle Int 2014;35(4):383–8.
58. Burssens A, Barg A, Van Ovost E, et al. The hind- and midfoot alignment computed after a medializing calcaneal osteotomy using a 3D weightbearing CT. Int J Comput Assist Radiol Surg 2019;14(8):1439–47.
59. Deland JT, Page AE, Kenneally SM. Posterior calcaneal osteotomy with wedge: cadaver testing of a new procedure for insufficiency of the posterior tibial tendon. Foot Ankle Int 1999;20(5):290–5.
60. Sahranavard B, Hudson PW, De Cesar Netto C, et al. A comparison of union rates and complications between single screw and double screw fixation of sliding calcaneal osteotomy. Foot Ankle Surg 2019;25(1):84–9.
61. Lucas DE, Simpson GA, Berlet GC, et al. Screw size and insertion technique compared with removal rates for calcaneal displacement osteotomies. Foot Ankle Int 2015;36(4):395–9.
62. Konan S, Meswania J, Blunn GW, et al. Mechanical stability of a locked step-plate versus single compression screw fixation for medial displacement calcaneal osteotomy. Foot Ankle Int 2012;33(8):669–74.
63. Saxena A, Patel R. Medial displacement calcaneal osteotomy: a comparison of screw versus locking plate fixation. J Foot Ankle Surg 2016;55(6):1164–8.
64. Haggerty EK, Chen S, Thordarson DB. Review of calcaneal osteotomies fixed with a calcaneal slide plate. Foot Ankle Int 2020;41(2):183–6.
65. Abbasian A, Zaidi R, Guha A, et al. Comparison of three different fixation methods of calcaneal osteotomies. Foot Ankle Int 2013;34(3):420–5.

66. Kunzler D, Shazadeh Safavi P, Jupiter D, et al. A comparison of removal rates of headless screws versus headed screws in calcaneal osteotomy. Foot Ankle Spec 2018;11(5):420–4.
67. Hintermann B. [Lateral column lengthening osteotomy of calcaneus]. Oper Orthop Traumatol 2015;27(4):298–307.
68. Desai S. Bicortical structural autograft harvest during medializing calcaneal osteotomy: technique tip. Foot Ankle Int 2011;32(6):644–7.
69. Demetracopoulos CA, Deorio JK, Easley ME, et al. Equivalent pain relief with and without resection of the posterior tibial tendon in adult flatfoot reconstruction. J Surg Orthop Adv 2014;23(4):184–8.
70. Rosenfeld PF, Dick J, Saxby TS. The response of the flexor digitorum longus and posterior tibial muscles to tendon transfer and calcaneal osteotomy for stage II posterior tibial tendon dysfunction. Foot Ankle Int 2005;26(9):671–4.
71. Schuh R, Gruber F, Wanivenhaus A, et al. Flexor digitorum longus transfer and medial displacement calcaneal osteotomy for the treatment of stage II posterior tibial tendon dysfunction: kinematic and functional results of fifty one feet. Int Orthop 2013;37(9):1815–20.
72. Guyton GP. Minimally invasive osteotomies of the calcaneus. Foot Ankle Clin 2016;21(3):551–66.
73. Sherman TI, Guyton GP. Minimal incision/minimally invasive medializing displacement calcaneal osteotomy. Foot Ankle Int 2018;39(1):119–28.
74. Walther M, Hörterer H, Harrasser N, et al. [Minimally invasive components of the treatment of tibialis posterior insufficiency in adults : Tendoscopy of the Achilles tendon, minimally invasive calcaneus displacement osteotomy and the sinus tarsi spacer]. Orthopade 2020;49(11):962–7.
75. Walther M, Kriegelstein S, Altenberger S, et al. [Percutaneous calcaneal sliding osteotomy]. Oper Orthop Traumatol 2016;28(4):309–20.
76. Didomenico LA, Anain J, Wargo-Dorsey M. Assessment of medial and lateral neurovascular structures after percutaneous posterior calcaneal displacement osteotomy: a cadaver study. J Foot Ankle Surg 2011;50(6):668–71.
77. Durston A, Bahoo R, Kadambande S, et al. Minimally invasive calcaneal osteotomy: does the Shannon burr endanger the neurovascular structures? A Cadaveric Study. J Foot Ankle Surg 2015;54(6):1062–6.
78. Gutteck N, Haase K, Kielstein H, et al. Biomechanical results of percutaneous calcaneal osteotomy using two different osteotomy designs. Foot Ankle Surg 2020;26(5):551–5.
79. Jowett CR, Rodda D, Amin A, et al. Minimally invasive calcaneal osteotomy: A cadaveric and clinical evaluation. Foot Ankle Surg 2016;22(4):244–7.
80. Kheir E, Borse V, Sharpe J, et al. Medial displacement calcaneal osteotomy using minimally invasive technique. Foot Ankle Int 2015;36(3):248–52.
81. Mourkus H, Prem H. Double calcaneal osteotomy with minimally invasive surgery for the treatment of severe flexible flatfeet. Int Orthop 2018;42(9):2123–9.
82. Coleman MM, Abousayed MM, Thompson JM, et al. Risk factors for complications associated with minimally invasive medial displacement calcaneal osteotomy. Foot Ankle Int 2021;42(2):121–31.
83. Catani O, Cautiero G, Sergio F, et al. Medial displacement calcaneal osteotomy for unilateral adult acquired flatfoot: Effects of minimally invasive surgery on pain, alignment, functioning, and quality of life. J Foot Ankle Surg 2021;60(2):358–61.

84. Peiffer M, Belvedere C, Clockaerts S, et al. Three-dimensional displacement after a medializing calcaneal osteotomy in relation to the osteotomy angle and hindfoot alignment. Foot Ankle Surg 2020;26(1):78–84.
85. Usuelli FG, Di Silvestri CA, D'ambrosi R, et al. Return to sport activities after medial displacement calcaneal osteotomy and flexor digitorum longus transfer. Knee Surg Sports Traumatol Arthrosc 2018;26(3):892–6.
86. Cao HH, Tang KL, Lu WZ, et al. Medial displacement calcaneal osteotomy with posterior tibial tendon reconstruction for the flexible flatfoot with symptomatic accessory navicular. J Foot Ankle Surg 2014;53(5):539–43.
87. Catanzariti AR, Lee MS, Mendicino RW. Posterior calcaneal displacement osteotomy for adult acquired flatfoot. J Foot Ankle Surg 2000;39(1):2–14.
88. Chadwick C, Whitehouse SL, Saxby TS. Long-term follow-up of flexor digitorum longus transfer and calcaneal osteotomy for stage II posterior tibial tendon dysfunction. Bone Joint J 2015;97-b(3):346–52.
89. Guyton GP, Jeng C, Krieger LE, et al. Flexor digitorum longus transfer and medial displacement calcaneal osteotomy for posterior tibial tendon dysfunction: a middle-term clinical follow-up. Foot Ankle Int 2001;22(8):627–32.
90. Ivanic GM, Hofstaetter SG, Trnka HJ. [The acquired flatfoot: mid-term results of the medial displacement calcaneal-osteotomy with flexor digitorum longus transfer]. Z Orthop Ihre Grenzgeb 2006;144(6):619–25.
91. Myerson MS, Corrigan J, Thompson F, et al. Tendon transfer combined with calcaneal osteotomy for treatment of posterior tibial tendon insufficiency: a radiological investigation. Foot Ankle Int 1995;16(11):712–8.
92. Myerson MS, Badekas A, Schon LC. Treatment of stage II posterior tibial tendon deficiency with flexor digitorum longus tendon transfer and calcaneal osteotomy. Foot Ankle Int 2004;25(7):445–50.
93. Niki H, Hirano T, Okada H, et al. Outcome of medial displacement calcaneal osteotomy for correction of adult-acquired flatfoot. Foot Ankle Int 2012;33(11):940–6.
94. Oh I, Williams BR, Ellis SJ, et al. Reconstruction of the symptomatic idiopathic flatfoot in adolescents and young adults. Foot Ankle Int 2011;32(3):225–32.
95. Pomeroy GC, Manoli A 2nd. A new operative approach for flatfoot secondary to posterior tibial tendon insufficiency: a preliminary report. Foot Ankle Int 1997;18(4):206–12.
96. Ruffilli A, Traina F, Giannini S, et al. Surgical treatment of stage II posterior tibialis tendon dysfunction: ten-year clinical and radiographic results. Eur J Orthop Surg Traumatol 2018;28(1):139–45.
97. Sammarco GJ, Hockenbury RT. Treatment of stage II posterior tibial tendon dysfunction with flexor hallucis longus transfer and medial displacement calcaneal osteotomy. Foot Ankle Int 2001;22(4):305–12.
98. Tellisi N, Lobo M, O'malley M, et al. Functional outcome after surgical reconstruction of posterior tibial tendon insufficiency in patients under 50 years. Foot Ankle Int 2008;29(12):1179–83.
99. Wacker JT, Hennessy MS, Saxby TS. Calcaneal osteotomy and transfer of the tendon of flexor digitorum longus for stage-II dysfunction of tibialis posterior. Three- to five-year results. J Bone Joint Surg Br 2002;84(1):54–8.

The Importance of the Medial Column in Progressive Collapsing Foot Deformity: Osteotomies and Stabilization

Christopher E. Gross, MD[a,*], J. Benjamin Jackson III, MD, MBA[b]

KEYWORDS

- Medial column • Naviculocuneiform fusion • Lapidus • Cotton osteotomy

INTRODUCTION

Understanding progressive collapsing foot deformity (PCFD) is a complex undertaking with its varied presentations and spectrum of the disease. The pathologic condition of PCFD is multifactorial, and its surgical solutions are varied and elusive.[1] Technical considerations must take into account the variable degree of hindfoot valgus, forefoot abduction, and forefoot supination (varus).

The complexity of the pathologic process of PCFD is only partially understood. The medial longitudinal arch of the foot is dynamically supported by the posterior tibial tendon (PTT), whereas static restraints include the spring, talocalcaneal cervical and interosseus, and the superficial and deep deltoid ligaments.[2,3] The PTT acts at the navicular tuberosity and other tarsal/metatarsal structures to plantarflex and invert the foot.[4] On a granular level, this foot inversion causes the locking of the transverse tarsal joints to allow for foot stability during push-off.[4,5] The deltoid and spring ligament act as a functional unit and may even be a large confluent ligament according to recent anatomic studies.[6,7] Relative to the deltoid-spring ligament complex, the PTT acts as a secondary stabilizer of the medial arch.[8,9] Researchers do not yet know the exact step-by-step sequence of the kinematic progression of the progressive collapse of the foot. The new PCFD classification system accounts for this in which the only "sequence" would be the staging on flexible (I) and rigid (II), but the classes of deformity can happen concomitantly (A, B, C, D, and E).[10]

We are still elucidating the interaction of the PTT and the deltoid-spring ligament complex. When this dynamic support fails, the transverse tarsal joints become unstable, allowing the peroneus brevis unopposed action, contributing to forefoot abduction. The medial column can collapse at any or all of the following joints:

[a] Medical University of South Carolina, 96 Jonathon Lucas Drive, Charleston, SC 209403, USA; [b] University of South Carolina, Prisma Orthopaedics, 2 medical park, Suite 404, Columbia, SC 29203, USA
* Corresponding author.
E-mail address: cgross144@gmail.com

Foot Ankle Clin N Am 26 (2021) 507–521
https://doi.org/10.1016/j.fcl.2021.06.001
foot.theclinics.com

talonavicular (TN), naviculocuneiform (NC), and first tarsometatarsal joints (first TMT). As the forefoot abducts and the tarsal joints destabilize, the Achilles' tendon's force is displaced, further contributing to hindfoot valgus and eversion of the subtalar joint. This sequence may not happen in every patient. Persistent hindfoot valgus causes compensatory forefoot varus/supination (first ray elevation), which at first is supple, but becomes fixed as the pathologic condition progresses.[10,11]

As the midfoot strains, the static stabilizers attenuate. When the spring ligament fails, there is a loss of peritalar stability causing the talus to assume a more medial and plantarflexed position relative to the navicular.[4,10–12] Interestingly, this may not be sequential at all, as multiple patients show up with extremely flexible deformities, with a relatively preserved PTT and a significant valgus talar tilt. As the pathologic condition progresses, the deltoid ligament attenuates, leading to an increase in tibiotalar valgus angulation and disturbances in talar axial rotation.

Preoperative Planning

Clinical examination

It is important for the clinician to understand that the clinical presentation and physical examination evolve as the pathologic condition progresses. In simple terms, in the early stages of the disease, the deformities are flexible; however, in the latter stages of the disease, the deformities become fixed.[10,13,14] However, this duality may not be representative of all disease presentations. A thorough physical examination diagnoses PCFD while at the same time helps to grade and stage it.[15] For the purposes of this article, the authors focus on assessing the medial column as it relates to the new classification scheme set forth by the PCFD consensus group (de Cesar Netto C and colleagues).[15] First, the patient must have the rigidity of the hindfoot, midfoot, and forefoot recorded (stage I, flexible or stage II, rigid). One must evaluate the patient with PCFD during weight-bearing.[15] Hindfoot alignment is measured with the examiner standing behind the patient.[16] At the same time, excessive abduction of the forefoot can be noted by the "too many toes" sign. In this test, the clinician can see more than the fifth and part of the fourth toe when checking for hindfoot alignment. Single- and double-limb heel rise tests must be performed to assess the strength and competence of the PTT.[17] If the PTT is competent and the subtalar joint is mobile, this deformity of the foot is partially or totally corrected during the maneuver.[18,19] Ankle and subtalar motions are recorded with an emphasis on evaluating a gastrocnemius contracture with a Silfverskiöld test and also on how motion is affected by correction of the hindfoot valgus.

Forefoot supination or first-ray elevation (only in the sagittal plane) can be assessed with the patient seated. The clinician reduces the hindfoot valgus and forefoot abduction as described above with 1 hand. With the other hand, the ankle is brought to neutral by placing the fingers under the fourth and fifth metatarsal heads. If there is persistent forefoot varus (class C), the great toe will remain elevated relative to the base of the fifth ray as the examiner views the foot head-on. Furthermore, the patient will be unable to perform a single-limb heel rise, indicating that the PTT has either elongated past its effective excursion length or degenerated. When either the hindfoot valgus or the forefoot abduction deformity becomes rigid, the patient now has stage II disease.[10] The patient will be unable to perform a single-limb heel rise. The hindfoot cannot be reduced through the subtalar joints, whereas forefoot abduction cannot be reduced through the transverse tarsal joints. Instability of the first TMT joint should be assessed. A patient may have pain while assessing its stability and may also have symptomatic dorsal bossing at the first TMT. Traditionally, one tests first-ray hypermobility by holding and stabilizing the intermediate and lateral columns of the foot with 1 hand while the other produces a translates the medial column in a dorsal-plantar direction.[20,21] There is no 1 universally accepted standard. More than 8 mm in dislocation dorsally is considered a positive result in certain studies.[22]

Radiographic examination

Standing anteroposterior (AP) and lateral radiographs of the foot and ankle (including a hindfoot alignment view) are perfunctory. They help to refine the staging and surgical correction of patients with PCFD. Most importantly, it helps one determine the apex of deformity.[23] One must examine the medial column stability critically. On lateral radiographs, any collapse seen on radiographs indicates insufficiency of the pertaining ligaments of that joint (**Fig. 1**). Collapse can occur through the TN, NC, cuneometatarsal, or a combination of these joints. On the lateral radiographs, the medial column position and alignment are assessed by the talo-first metatarsal or Meary angle.[24] The angle is subtended by the longitudinal axis of the talus and first metatarsal. A measurement of 15° to 30° is considered moderate PCFD.[24] The pes planus deformity is considered severe if the Meary angle is greater than 30°.[24,25] On lateral radiographs, one must note if there is plantar gapping or arthritis at the first TMT (see **Fig. 1**), indicating medial column instability. TN and NC arthritis or sagging should also be noted, which may impact the surgical correction and stabilization of the medial column. Any collapse through these joints represents an insufficiency of the ligaments associated with stabilizing the joint. Overlap of the talus and calcaneus should also be noted. The medial arch sag can also be quantified by the medial arch sag angle.[26] It is measured by the angle created by a line drawn along the articular surface of the navicular and by a line drawn parallel to the first TMT joint.[26]

On AP films, the TN coverage angle should be measured because it indicates the severity of the forefoot abduction and dorsolateral peritalar subluxation (see **Fig. 1**).[24,27] The talar incongruency angle is another reliable and validated radiographic measurement used to assess severity of forefoot abduction.[27] As medial column support fails, the TN joint abducts and the subtalar joint everts and pronates. On normal films, the calcaneocuboid (CC) and TN joints are parallel and even. If the lateral column is short, the TN joint will appear to be 3 to 5 mm distal to the CC joints.[1,23,28,29]

Operative Treatment of Medial Column Instability

There are a myriad of soft tissue, osteotomy, and arthrodesis procedures to address the complex deformity seen in PCFD, but there is no clear optimal treatment algorithm that

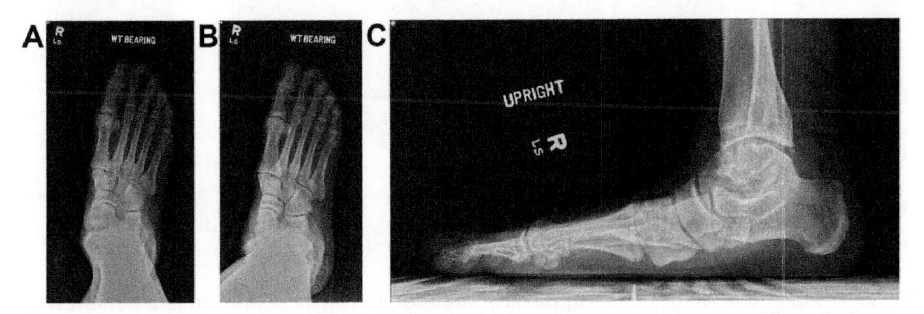

Fig. 1. Three weight-bearing views of the foot of a patient with medial column deficiency and gapping of the first TMT joint. In addition, there is some underlying arthritis with early osteophyte formation at the TN joint. On the AP view, TN uncoverage and lateral peritalar subluxation can be noted.

addresses its totality.[30] If the deformities are supple, then soft tissue procedures (medial soft tissue reconstruction) and osteotomies (to correct passively correctible deformities and protect the medial soft tissue procedures) are often the mainstay in treatment.[31] Once the deformity is not passively correctible or it is rigid, then arthrodeses of the subtalar and TN and/or the CC and/or the naviculocuneiform joints are needed.

Medial column procedures are often supplemented by a medializing calcaneal osteotomy and/or a lateral column lengthening owing to the complex nature of PCFD and its resultant peritalar instability.[2,30–33] The weight-bearing tripod of the foot must be reestablished.[34] If forefoot varus is not corrected after a medializing calcaneus osteotomy and lateral column lengthening, then additional procedures may be performed, including a dorsal opening wedge osteotomy through the medial cuneiform (Cotton osteotomy) or varied medial column arthrodeses[23,34] (**Fig. 2**). Undercorrection of the varus forefoot can lead to an excessive valgus moment to the hindfoot, which can lead to recurrence of deformity.[35,36] NC and first TMT arthrodeses do not restrict motion of the hindfoot, but an isolated TN fusion reduces hindfoot motion by roughly 80%.[37] In later discussion, the authors describe the merits of a NC fusion, Cotton osteotomy, and plantarflexion Lapidus, which are the most commonly

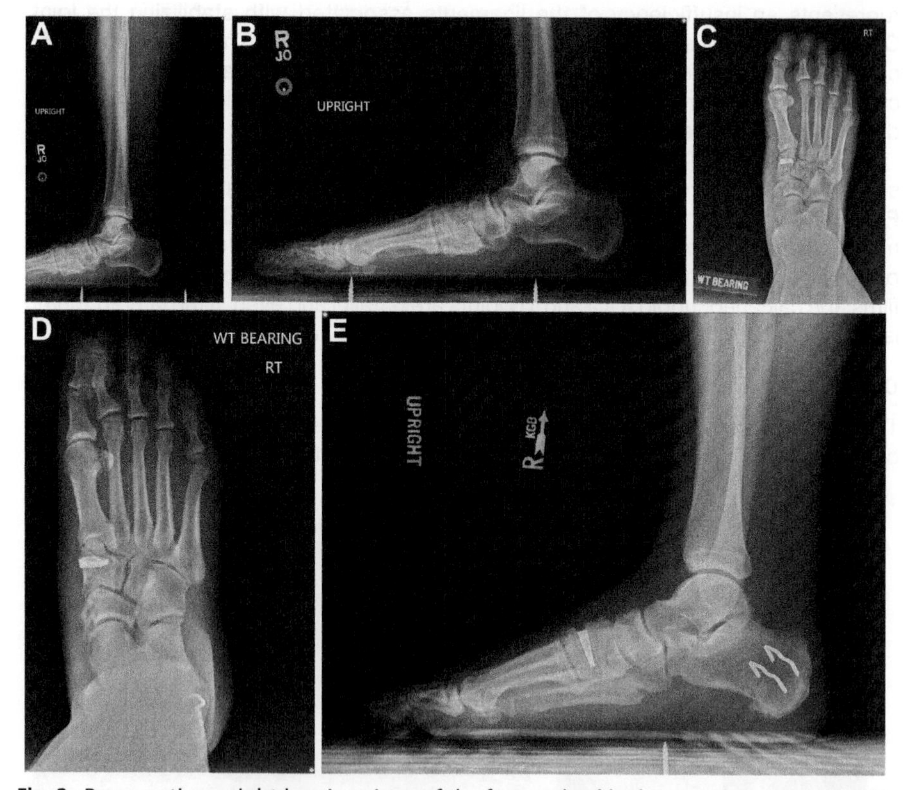

Fig. 2. Preoperative weight-bearing views of the foot and ankle demonstrate a patient with planovalgus alignment with plantar gapping at the first TMT joint and lateral peritalar subluxation. This patient underwent a medial displacement calcaneal osteotomy and a Cotton osteotomy of the medial cuneiform. Note the improvement of the AP and lateral talo-first metatarsal line on the postoperative weight-bearing radiographs of the foot.

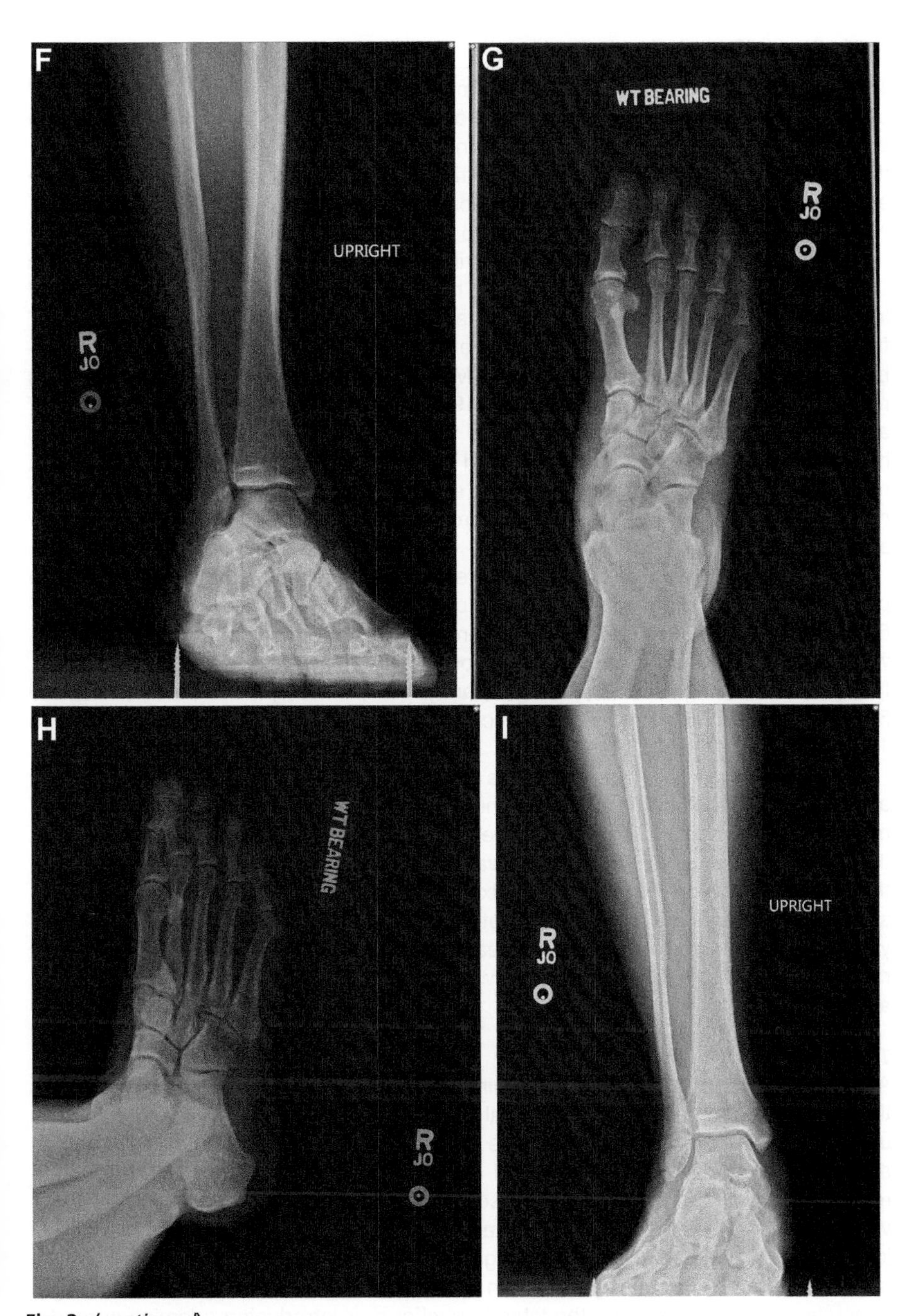

Fig. 2. (*continued*).

performed procedures to address medial column stability and return the height and alignment to the arch of the foot. The appropriate choice of a medial column procedure is based on recognizing arthritic joints and the location of deformity. These surgeries help to improve arch height while maintaining hindfoot motion.

Naviculocuneiform Arthrodesis

The NC arthrodesis has gone through many iterations beginning in 1927. Miller[38] described a surgical solution in pediatric or adolescent patients in which attenuation of the medial support structures resulted in a pes planus deformity. In order to correct the alignment of the medial column, he arthrodesed the NC and first TMT joints while advancing the insertion of the PTT via an osteoperiosteal flap. At 30-month follow-up, he noted symptomatic improvement in 16 patients.

The first article in the literature to describe treating a PCFD with an NC fusion was Greisberg and colleagues.[33] Each patient had a gastrocnemius recession or Achilles' lengthening and flexor digitorum augmentation to the PTT and an NC and/or first TMT fusion. The medial and middle NC joints were prepared, followed by reduction and stabilization with 3.5-mm screws. If first TMT arthritis or sagging was noted, it was reduced and fused as well. Thirteen of 19 patients had both the NC and first TMT arthrodesed. Of the 13 patients who had fusion of the NC and first TMT joints, two had nonunions of the NC joint and one had a nonunion of the TMT joint (15% nonunion rate). Radiographically, the patients had excellent correction of the lateral talo-first metatarsal angle (3°) and significant improvement of the AP TN coverage angle by an average of 14°.

In 2014, Ajis and Geary[12] evaluated 33 feet that had isolated NC fusions (20 had the procedure for PCFD). The mean time to union was 21.7 $\pm$ 2.0 weeks (range, 10.4–60.3 weeks) with a union rate of 97%. There was 1 symptomatic nonunion that underwent revision and healed at 60.3 weeks. For the PCFD patients, the mean lateral talus–first metatarsal angle improved significantly preoperatively from 12.3° $\pm$ 1.3° to 5.2° $\pm$ 1.2° ($P<.05$). The mean TN coverage angle improved significantly from 14.1° $\pm$ 1.8° to 7.4° $\pm$ 1.3° ($P<.05$).

A systematic review of all NC fusions was performed in 2019.[13] Of the 7 reviewed articles, radiographically confirmed nonunion rate was 6.5% (n = 9 of 139 feet) at a mean follow-up of 73.2 months. The revision rate of nonunion was 4.2%, whereas the overall incidence of reoperation was 4%. The most common form of fixation that led to nonunion was all staple fixation at 33.3%.[14] A combined staple-and-screw fixation yielded a nonunion rate of 0%, and combined screw-and-plate fixation yielded a nonunion rate of 2.3%, whereas Kirschner wire fixation yielded a nonunion rate of 5.4%. This systematic review was hindered by the low quality of the data assessed.

Technique

A popliteal and saphenous block is administered. The patient is placed supine and has the leg bumped to neutral in case lateral work needs to be done. A thigh tourniquet is used. Fluoroscopy is used to center the incision and localize the NC joint. The tibialis anterior is encountered and mobilized dorsally but may need to be divided to be repaired later. Subperiosteal sharp dissection exposes the NC joint medially. The investigators then use a Hintermann retractor to distract the NC joint and expose the joint surfaces. The dorsal and plantar ligaments are released. The medial and middle facets are prepared routinely. One can assess the lateral facet by either making a separate dorsal incision over the lateral cuneiform or introducing a lamina spreader into NC joint medially. The intercuneiform spaces are prepared if one can access them. The joint is prepared in the standard fashion, and the joint is reduced by plantarflexion and derotation of the joint (using the K-wires used for the pin distractors as joysticks). Typically, 1 hand rotates clockwise, and the other hand rotates counterclockwise to achieve good correction. One cannot simply fuse the joints in situ without proper reduction. Autograft or allograft with a biologic is used to enhance healing. An assistant holds the great toe in dorsiflexion, activating the windlass mechanism, further compressing the joint. Rigid internal fixation is placed with either screws, staples, compression plate, or a combination thereof.

The patient remains non–weight-bearing for 8 weeks.[33] Sutures are removed, and wounds are inspected after 2 weeks, and a full below-knee cast is applied. At 6 weeks, the cast is removed, and the patient is placed into a CAM walker boot. They start weight-bearing 2 weeks later. At 12 weeks, the patient no longer wears any protective devices.

Cotton Osteotomy

A medial opening wedge osteotomy of the medial cuneiform has been termed a Cotton osteotomy after being first described in a 1936 article by Dr Cotton.[39] In this article, he describes the "triangle of support" for the foot. However, his worked started with an earlier 1898 publication in the *Journal of the Boston Medical Society*.[40] In this work, they describe the importance of rotation around the talus and measuring the ability of the foot to "roll over its inner border" because of excessive pronation in the pathologic state of flatfoot. The understanding of the importance of the medial column of the foot lead to his proposed osteotomy of the medial cuneiform. The opening wedge osteotomy plantarflexes the first ray, increases longitudinal arch height, and corrects of the pronation of the forefoot seen with PCFD. Because of the high rates of union, the ability to improve medial arch height, and stabilize the medial column, this osteotomy has become the "work horse" for medial column restoration in the surgical treatment of PCFD.[35,41,42] It preserves the motion of the medial column most importantly.

Reconstruction of the PCFD begins proximally and moves distally.[23] Oftentimes, a compensatory forefoot varus is last seen intraoperatively relative to the other deformities. At the same time, forefoot varus that is seen preoperatively can be corrected by fixing the more proximal deformities.[23] If there is instability of the first ray or a fixed forefoot varus deformity, a first TMT fusion or NC fusion must be considered, respectively.[43] However, if the deformity is flexible, a Cotton osteotomy is a powerful tool.[43]

In a cadaveric model of an open wedge osteotomy of the medial cuneiform following lateral column lengthening, the investigators measured specimens radiographically and pedobarographically.[44] In patients who had an added Cotton osteotomy, the Meary angle improved significantly while at the same time the TN coverage angle improved. Furthermore, the medial cuneiform height improved. A lateral column lengthening alone increased the lateral column pressure in a flatfoot model. Most importantly, lateral column pressure was normalized after a Cotton and lateral column lengthening relative to intact specimens.

There is no consensus as to the correct type of fixation for a Cotton osteotomy.[23] Multiple strategies have been described, including screws,[43,45] Kirschner wires,[36] dorsal wedge plates, or no fixation.[45] An autograft wedge is not routinely used in this procedure given the robustness of other viable options, including trabecular titanium wedges[46] or allograft bone wedges[46] (fixated with or without a plate or staple). The use of allograft in this situation decreases donor site morbidity and can be easier to perform in the ambulatory surgical setting. In a biomechanical analysis of the use of a femoral head allograft versus a thin dorsal plate with a metal wedge,[47] both techniques offered similar radiographic and pedobarographic results.

Technique

The patient is placed supine and has the leg bumped to neutral in case lateral work needs to be done. A thigh tourniquet is used. A dorsal approach centered on the central aspect of the medical cuneiform allows for efficient access. Commonly, the dorsal medical nerve to the hallux branches off the intermediate branch of the superficial peroneal nerve under the incision. Care must be taken to avoid this nerve. Often it can be freed and retracted medially and inferiorly. The deep dissection is just medial to the extensor hallucis longus, which is then retracted laterally. Fluoroscopy is then used to confirm the central position on the medial cuneiform. An oscillating saw is taken two-thirds to three-quarters of the way down to the plantar surface of the bone. Care should be taken to angle the blade of the saw medially, as the medial cuneiform is shaped such that, to the less experienced, a direct dorsal to plantar cut will result in the saw errantly cutting the intermediate cuneiform or the second metatarsal. A short cut may also affect not reaching the desired plantarflexion. A combination of pin distractor and wide straight osteotome is then used to complete the osteotomy. The pin distractor is then used to progressively increase the size of the opening wedge until, with simulated weight-bearing, there is appropriate balance of the forefoot. Trail wedges are helpful to determine the most appropriate size graft by ensuring that the first ray is neutral relative to the fifth ray, and an allograft or metal wedge can be used. The authors' preferred technique is to use a porous titanium wedge. The variety of available sizes and widths allow for appropriate fit and correction for the vast majority of PCFD reconstructions.

The patient remains non–weight-bearing for 4 weeks. Sutures are removed, and wounds are inspected after 2 weeks; a CAM walker boot is applied so the patient may perform ankle range-of-motion exercises. At 4 weeks, the patient then initiates progressive weight-bearing. At 12 weeks, the patient no longer wears any protective devices.

Plantarflexion Lapidus

Although a first TMT arthrodesis was popularized by Dr Lapidus in 1934, it had previously been described by Albrecht, Truslow, and Kleinberg.[48–51] The initial description of the procedure was described as a fusion of the first TMT joint and the second metatarsal base combined with a distal soft tissue procedure. Others, including Lapidus, continued to modify the technique to only include the first TMT joint in the arthrodesis.[25]

Since the popularization of the procedure in the 1950s, there has been technical refinement in the surgical technique and fixation methods in order to improve the outcome and reduce complications.[52] Further modifications of the technique were created to address the shortening of the first ray that occurs with joint preparation. Surgeons then began to plantarflex their first TMT fusions to address this issue with their hallux valgus correction. Then, additional plantarflexion was added to address patients with forefoot supination/varus during PCFD surgical correction.[53,54] Understanding of first ray instability or hypermobility in the setting of supple or fixed PCFD is evolving.[52]

The Lapidus procedure appears to stabilize the medial column in several biomechanical studies.[55–57] In a cadaver study of the effect of the peroneus longus on the medial column, eversion of the medial cuneiform and dorsiflexion of the talus improved after a Lapidus. Therefore, the authors suggest that the peroneus longus had a stabilizing effect on the medial column after first TMT instability was removed. In a radiographic study[58] of structural radiographic changes of the medial longitudinal arch after a modified Lapidus, the medial cuneiform height and Meary angle both improved. In a pedobarographic comparison of the Lapidus versus the Chevron osteotomy for hallux valgus,[56] the first TMT fusion group had increased fifth metatarsal head plantar pressure in total as well a percentage of the total forefoot pressure. In

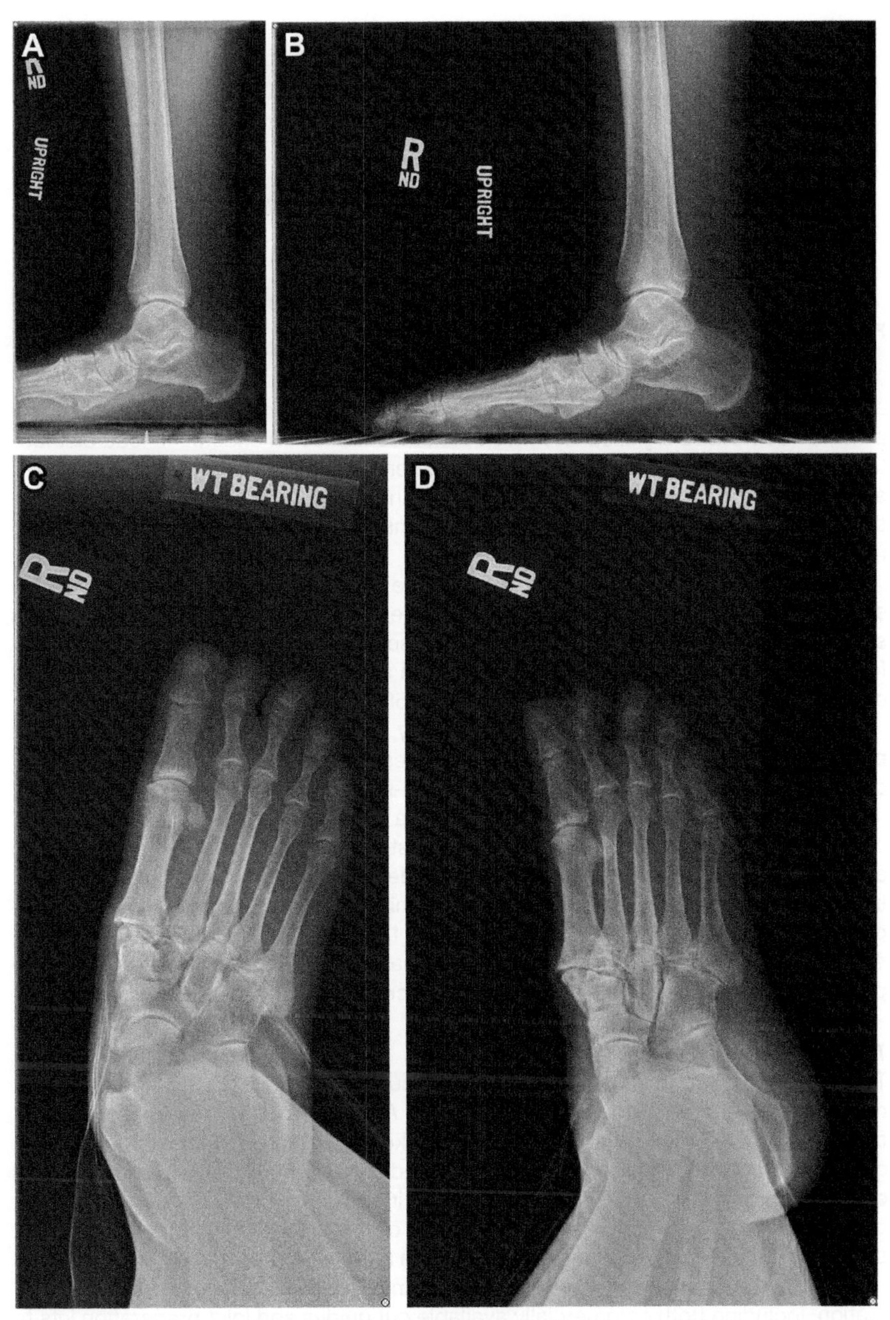

Fig. 3. Preoperative weight-bearing views of the foot and ankle demonstrate a patient with planovalgus alignment with significant lateral peritalar subluxation and first TMT arthritis. This patient was treated with a plantarflexion Lapidus using a tantalum wedge and staple construct in addition to a medial displacement calcaneal osteotomy. One of the staples failed at the plantarflexion Lapidus site, but the patient still progressed to healing. However, not the undercorrection of the AP talo-first metatarsal angle. An Evans osteotomy of the lateral column may have provided this patient with a better correct of all of their deformity.

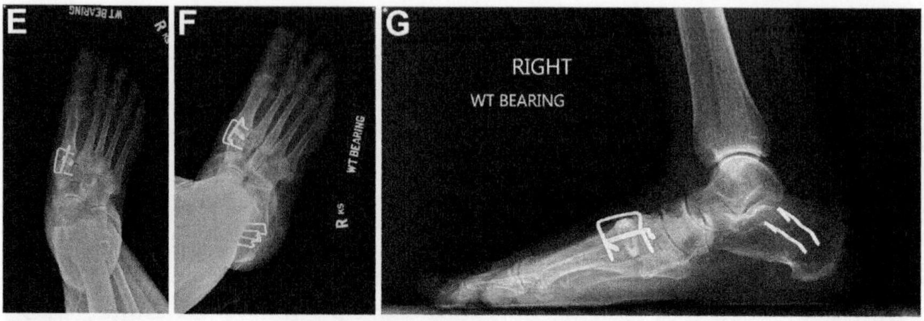

Fig. 3. (*continued*).

addition, pressure under the second metatarsal as a percentage of the total forefoot pressure decreased significantly, which indicates the fusion effects the load distribution of the foot. In a 3-dimensional finite element foot model of a first TMT fusion,[57] stress through the first ray during push-off and midstance significantly improved, thereby transferring weight from other portions of the foot to the more stabilized medial column.

Ideal methods of fixation are highly debatable. Historically, a crossed compression screw technique has been used, but some experts argue that a second compression screw decreases the compression of the first screw placed.[52] Some surgeons argue for 1 compression screw and 1 static screw. In a clinical study of a plantar plate and compression screw,[59] fusion was achieved in 58 of 59 feet.

Plate fixation can be used and placed dorsally, dorsomedially, or medially. In a comparison of plate alone versus dorsal compression screw followed by a plate,[60] compression force over time in the plate-and-screw construct was 7 times longer than the plate alone. Staple constructs have a theoretic advantage over traditional plate-and-screw techniques given that nitinol staples can increase the surface force and contact across the fusion site and provide continuous compression[61] (**Fig. 3**). In a radiographic study of varied hindfoot and midfoot fusions treated with Nitinol staples, 94% of patients achieved fusion across the first TMT with a 4-legged staple. Another option for fixation is an intramedullary nail that reduces hardware irritation, improves compression, and reduces external forces across the joint in 3 planes.[52,62]

Technique

The patient is placed supine and has the leg bumped to neutral in case lateral work needs to be done. A thigh tourniquet is used. A dorsal approach is made centered over the first TMT joint. Sharp dissection is taken down through the skin, and blunt dissection is used to ensure that the dorsal medial nerve to the hallux is not coursing obliquely through the proximal aspect of the incision. Once this is ensured, sharp dissection is used to perform a capsulotomy of the first TMT joint. Attention must be given on the medial side to ensure the tibialis anterior tendon or insertion is not disrupted with the dissection.[52] There are several methods and techniques for joint preparation, including both commercially available cut guides and joint preparation kits to assist the surgeon. Alternatively, the joint can be prepared manually with a sharp osteotome, curette, and then drill bit or bits to pierce the subchondral bone. Simple curette preparation minimizes first ray shortening and allows for correction of the first intermetatarsal angle, hallux valgus angle, and tibial sesamoid position.[63] After the joint is fully denuded of cartilage, fixation methods vary. Step plates exist that have a built-in plantarflexion to them in progressive increments. Another option is to

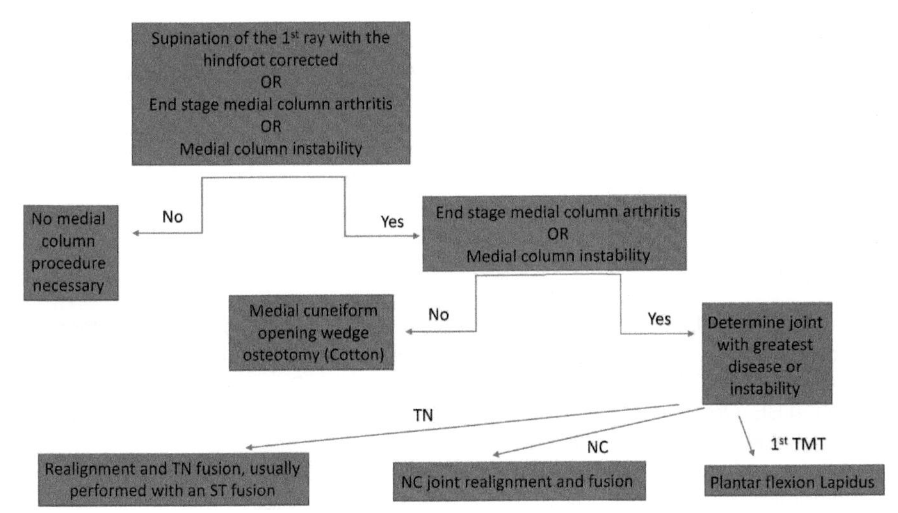

Fig. 4. A conceptual treatment algorithm for evaluating and treating patients with medical column insufficiency, with or without arthritis of the medial column joints. ST, subtalar.

interpose a dorsally wide and plantarly narrow allograft, autograft, or metal wedge to plantarflex the medial column.[64] This "Lapicotton technique"[64] offers the benefit of offsetting the shortening that was created by joint preparation (see **Fig. 3**). Fixation of the wedge can vary from plates, screws, staples, or a combination thereof. Notably, the authors have had a poor experience with an interposed porous titanium wedge combined with staple fixation because of an unexpectedly high rate of nonunion.

Postoperatively, the patient remains non–weight-bearing for 6 weeks, although some investigators argue for earlier partial weight-bearing as early as 2 weeks postoperatively.[65] Sutures are removed; wounds are inspected after 2 weeks, and a below-knee cast is applied. At 6 weeks, the cast is removed, and the patient is placed into a CAM walker boot. They then initiate progressive weight-bearing. At 12 weeks, the patient no longer wears any protective devices.[65]

In conclusion, stabilization procedures of the medial column correct forefoot varus and abduction while increasing the load-bearing capabilities of the medial arm of the foot tripod. Surgeons must be conscientious of the medial column after correcting proximal PCFD deformities, as success of the construct hinges on correcting forefoot varus and abduction (**Fig. 4**).

CLINICS CARE POINTS

- It is important for the clinician to understand that the clinical presentation and physical examination evolve as the pathologic condition progresses. In simple terms, in the early stages of the disease, the deformities are flexible; however, in the latter stages of the disease, the deformities become fixed.
- There is no clear optimal treatment algorithm that addresses the deformities in progressive collapsing foot deformity.
- If the deformities are supple, then soft tissue procedures (medial soft tissue reconstruction) and osteotomies (to correct passively correctible deformities and protect the medial soft tissue procedures) are often the mainstay in treatment.

- Once the deformity is not passively correctible or it is rigid, then arthrodeses of the subtalar and talonavicular and/or the calcaneocuboid and/or the naviculocuneiform joints are needed.

DISCLOSURE STATEMENT

The authors have nothing to disclose.

REFERENCES

1. Sangeorzan BJ, Hintermann B, de Cesar Netto C, et al. Progressive collapsing foot deformity: consensus on goals for operative correction. Foot Ankle Int 2020;41:1299–302.
2. Cohen BE, Ogden F. Medial column procedures in the acquired flatfoot deformity. Foot Ankle Clin 2007;12. 287-299, vi.
3. Willegger M, Seyidova N, Schuh R, et al. The tibialis posterior tendon footprint: an anatomical dissection study. J Foot Ankle Res 2020;13:25.
4. Hintermann B, Ruiz R. Biomechanics of medial ankle and peritalar instability. Foot Ankle Clin 2021;26:249–67.
5. Wiseman ALA, Stringer CB, Ashton N, et al. The morphological affinity of the early Pleistocene footprints from Happisburgh, England, with other footprints of Pliocene, Pleistocene, and Holocene age. J Hum Evol 2020;144:102776.
6. Campbell KJ, Michalski MP, Wilson KJ, et al. The ligament anatomy of the deltoid complex of the ankle: a qualitative and quantitative anatomical study. J Bone Joint Surg Am 2014;96:e62.
7. Cromeens BP, Kirchhoff CA, Patterson RM, et al. An attachment-based description of the medial collateral and spring ligament complexes. Foot Ankle Int 2015; 36:710–21.
8. Bastias GF, Dalmau-Pastor M, Astudillo C, et al. Spring ligament instability. Foot Ankle Clin 2018;23:659–78.
9. Brodell JD Jr, MacDonald A, Perkins JA, et al. Deltoid-spring ligament reconstruction in adult acquired flatfoot deformity with medial peritalar instability. Foot Ankle Int 2019;40:753–61.
10. de Cesar Netto C, Deland JT, Ellis SJ. Guest editorial: expert consensus on adult-acquired flatfoot deformity. Foot Ankle Int 2020;41:1269–71.
11. Cifuentes-De la Portilla C, Larrainzar-Garijo R, Bayod J. Biomechanical stress analysis of the main soft tissues associated with the development of adult acquired flatfoot deformity. Clin Biomech (Bristol, Avon) 2019;61:163–71.
12. Hintermann B, Deland JT, de Cesar Netto C, et al. Consensus on indications for isolated subtalar joint fusion and naviculocuneiform fusions for progressive collapsing foot deformity. Foot Ankle Int 2020. 1071100720950738.
13. Parsons S, Naim S, Richards PJ, et al. Correction and prevention of deformity in type II tibialis posterior dysfunction. Clin Orthop Relat Res 2010;468:1025–32.
14. Bluman EM, Title CI, Myerson MS. Posterior tibial tendon rupture: a refined classification system. Foot Ankle Clin 2007;12. 233-249, v.
15. de Cesar Netto C, Myerson MS, Day J, et al. Consensus for the use of weight-bearing CT in the assessment of progressive collapsing foot deformity. Foot Ankle Int 2020;41:1277–82.
16. de Cesar Netto C, Kunas GC, Soukup D, et al. Correlation of clinical evaluation and radiographic hindfoot alignment in stage II adult-acquired flatfoot deformity. Foot Ankle Int 2018;39:771–9.

17. Johnson KA, Strom DE. Tibialis posterior tendon dysfunction. Clin Orthop Relat Res 1989;196–206.
18. Hintermann B. Medial ankle instability. Foot Ankle Clin 2003;8:723–38.
19. Ruiz R, Hintermann B. Clinical appearance of medial ankle instability. Foot Ankle Clin 2021;26:291–304.
20. Voellmicke KV, Deland JT. Manual examination technique to assess dorsal instability of the first ray. Foot Ankle Int 2002;23:1040–1.
21. Glasoe WM, Allen MK, Saltzman CL, et al. Comparison of two methods used to assess first-ray mobility. Foot Ankle Int 2002;23:248–52.
22. Glasoe WM, Grebing BR, Beck S, et al. A comparison of device measures of dorsal first ray mobility. Foot Ankle Int 2005;26:957–61.
23. Johnson JE, Sangeorzan BJ, de Cesar Netto C, et al. Consensus on indications for medial cuneiform opening wedge (Cotton) osteotomy in the treatment of progressive collapsing foot deformity. Foot Ankle Int 2020;41:1289–91.
24. Flores DV, Mejia Gomez C, Fernandez Hernando M, et al. Adult acquired flatfoot deformity: anatomy, biomechanics, staging, and imaging findings. Radiographics 2019;39:1437–60.
25. Sangeorzan BJ, Mosca V, Hansen ST Jr. Effect of calcaneal lengthening on relationships among the hindfoot, midfoot, and forefoot. Foot Ankle 1993;14:136–41.
26. Aiyer A, Dall GF, Shub J, et al. Radiographic correction following reconstruction of adult acquired flat foot deformity using the Cotton medial cuneiform osteotomy. Foot Ankle Int 2016;37:508–13.
27. Ellis SJ, Yu JC, Williams BR, et al. New radiographic parameters assessing forefoot abduction in the adult acquired flatfoot deformity. Foot Ankle Int 2009;30: 1168–76.
28. Myerson MS, Thordarson DB, Johnson JE, et al. Classification and nomenclature: progressive collapsing foot deformity. Foot Ankle Int 2020;41:1271–6.
29. Hintermann B, Deland JT, de Cesar Netto C, et al. Consensus on indications for isolated subtalar joint fusion and naviculocuneiform fusions for progressive collapsing foot deformity. Foot Ankle Int 2020;41:1295–8.
30. McCormick JJ, Johnson JE. Medial column procedures in the correction of adult acquired flatfoot deformity. Foot Ankle Clin 2012;17:283–98.
31. Wagner E, Wagner P. Current concepts in treatment of ligament incompetence in the acquired flatfoot. Foot Ankle Clin 2021;26:373–89.
32. Ajis A, Geary N. Surgical technique, fusion rates, and planovalgus foot deformity correction with naviculocuneiform fusion. Foot Ankle Int 2014;35:232–7.
33. Greisberg J, Assal M, Hansen ST Jr, et al. Isolated medial column stabilization improves alignment in adult-acquired flatfoot. Clin Orthop Relat Res 2005;197–202.
34. Hirose CB, Johnson JE. Plantarflexion opening wedge medial cuneiform osteotomy for correction of fixed forefoot varus associated with flatfoot deformity. Foot Ankle Int 2004;25:568–74.
35. Conti MS, Garfinkel JH, Kunas GC, et al. Postoperative medial cuneiform position correlation with patient-reported outcomes following Cotton osteotomy for reconstruction of the stage II adult-acquired flatfoot deformity. Foot Ankle Int 2019;40: 491–8.
36. Lutz M, Myerson M. Radiographic analysis of an opening wedge osteotomy of the medial cuneiform. Foot Ankle Int 2011;32:278–87.
37. O'Malley MJ, Deland JT, Lee KT. Selective hindfoot arthrodesis for the treatment of adult acquired flatfoot deformity: an in vitro study. Foot Ankle Int 1995;16: 411–7.

38. Miller OL. A plastic flat foot operation. JBJS 1927;9:84–91.
39. Cotton FJ. Foot statistics and surgery. N Engl J Med 1936;214:352–62.
40. Lovett RW, Cotton FJ. Pronation of the foot, considered from an anatomical standpoint. J Boston Soc Med Sci 1898;2:155–61.
41. Boffeli TJ, Schnell KR. Cotton osteotomy in flatfoot reconstruction: a review of consecutive cases. J Foot Ankle Surg 2017;56:990–5.
42. Kunas GC, Do HT, Aiyer A, et al. Contribution of medial cuneiform osteotomy to correction of longitudinal arch collapse in stage IIb adult-acquired flatfoot deformity. Foot Ankle Int 2018;39:885–93.
43. Tankson CJ. The Cotton osteotomy: indications and techniques. Foot Ankle Clin 2007;12:309–15, vii.
44. Benthien RA, Parks BG, Guyton GP, et al. Lateral column calcaneal lengthening, flexor digitorum longus transfer, and opening wedge medial cuneiform osteotomy for flexible flatfoot: a biomechanical study. Foot Ankle Int 2007;28:70–7.
45. Wang CS, Tzeng YH, Lin CC, et al. Comparison of screw fixation versus non-fixation in dorsal opening wedge medial cuneiform osteotomy of adult acquired flatfoot. Foot Ankle Surg 2020;26:193–7.
46. Romeo G, Bianchi A, Cerbone V, et al. Medial cuneiform opening wedge osteotomy for correction of flexible flatfoot deformity: trabecular titanium vs. bone allograft wedges. Biomed Res Int 2019;2019:1472471.
47. League AC, Parks BG, Schon LC. Radiographic and pedobarographic comparison of femoral head allograft versus block plate with dorsal opening wedge medial cuneiform osteotomy: a biomechanical study. Foot Ankle Int 2008;29:922–6.
48. Albrecht A. The pathology and treatment of hallux valgus. Tussk Vracht 1911;10:14–9.
49. Kleinberg S. The operative cure of hallux valgus and bunions. Am J Surg 1932;15:75–81.
50. Truslow W. Metatarsus primus varus or hallux valgus? JBJS 1925;7:98–108.
51. Lapidus PW. Operative correction of metatarsus primus varus in hallux valgus. Surg Gynecol Obstet 1934;58:183–91.
52. Li S, Myerson MS. Evolution of thinking of the Lapidus procedure and fixation. Foot Ankle Clin 2020;25:109–26.
53. Alshalawi S, Teoh KH, Alrashidi Y, et al. Lapidus arthrodesis by an anatomic dorsomedial plate. Tech Foot Ankle Surg 2020;19:89–95.
54. Habbu R, Holthusen SM, Anderson JG, et al. Operative correction of arch collapse with forefoot deformity: a retrospective analysis of outcomes. Foot Ankle Int 2011;32:764–73.
55. Bierman RA, Christensen JC, Johnson CH. Biomechanics of the first ray. Part III. Consequences of Lapidus arthrodesis on peroneus longus function: a three-dimensional kinematic analysis in a cadaver model. J Foot Ankle Surg 2001;40:125–31.
56. King CM, Hamilton GA, Ford LA. Effects of the Lapidus arthrodesis and chevron bunionectomy on plantar forefoot pressures. J Foot Ankle Surg 2014;53:415–9.
57. Wai-Chi Wong D, Wang Y, Zhang M, et al. Functional restoration and risk of non-union of the first metatarsocuneiform arthrodesis for hallux valgus: a finite element approach. J Biomech 2015;48:3142–8.
58. Avino A, Patel S, Hamilton GA, et al. The effect of the Lapidus arthrodesis on the medial longitudinal arch: a radiographic review. J Foot Ankle Surg 2008;47:510–4.

59. Klos K, Wilde CH, Lange A, et al. Modified Lapidus arthrodesis with plantar plate and compression screw for treatment of hallux valgus with hypermobility of the first ray: a preliminary report. Foot Ankle Surg 2013;19:239–44.
60. Garas PK, DiSegna ST, Patel AR. Plate alone versus plate and lag screw for lapidus arthrodesis: a biomechanical comparison of compression. Foot Ankle Spec 2018;11:534–8.
61. Aiyer A, Russell NA, Pelletier MH, et al. The impact of nitinol staples on the compressive forces, contact area, and mechanical properties in comparison to a claw plate and crossed screws for the first tarsometatarsal arthrodesis. Foot Ankle Spec 2016;9:232–40.
62. Shofoluwe A, Fowler B, Marques L, et al. The relationship of the Phantom(R) Lapidus Intramedullary Nail System to neurologic and tendinous structures in the foot: an anatomic study. Foot Ankle Surg 2021;27:231–4.
63. McAlister JE, Peterson KS, Hyer CF. Corrective realignment arthrodesis of the first tarsometatarsal joint without wedge resection. Foot Ankle Spec 2015;8:284–8.
64. de Cesar Netto C, Ahrenholz S, Iehl C, et al. Lapicotton technique in the treatment of progressive collapsing foot deformity. J Foot Ankle 2020;14:301–8.
65. Schipper ON, Ford SE, Moody PW, et al. Radiographic results of nitinol compression staples for hindfoot and midfoot arthrodeses. Foot Ankle Int 2018;39:172–9.

I am Afraid of Lateral Column Lengthening. Should I Be?

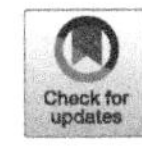

Alexander W. Crawford, MD[a], Amgad M. Haleem, MD, PhD[a,b,*]

KEYWORDS

- Progressive collapsing foot deformity • Lateral column lengthening
- Evans osteotomy

KEY POINTS

- Midforefoot abduction with talar head uncoverage at the Chopart joint is the key feature of class B progressive collapsing foot deformity (PCFD).
- Lateral column lengthening remains a viable option for correction for midfoot abduction in progressive collapsing foot deformity (PCFD).
- Different types of lateral column lengthening procedures have been described including Evans, Z-cut, Hintermann osteotomies, and calcaneocuboid arthrodesis.
- In this article we describe the techniques, graft types, outcomes, controversies, and complications of each lateral column lengthening procedure.

INTRODUCTION

Progressive collapsing foot deformity (PCFD), formerly known as adult-acquired flatfoot deformity, is a common cause of pain and medial longitudinal arch flattening in an estimated 5 million people within the United States.[1] Historically, posterior tibial tendon dysfunction was identified as a key pathologic process in PCFD.[2–4] The posterior tibial tendon is a crucial part of effective gait, providing hindfoot inversion on contraction. It has been hypothesized that this tendon has a hypovascular watershed region inferior to the medial malleolus, thus causing an area susceptible to tendinosis or rupture.[3–5] However, recent consensus has been reached that posterior tibial tendon dysfunction is no longer the key pathology in the classification of this three-dimensional deformity.[6] Johnson and Strom[2] first described a classification system for pes planovalgus deformity secondary to posterior tibial tendon dysfunction in

[a] Department of Orthopedic Surgery, Oklahoma University Health Sciences Center, University of Oklahoma College of Medicine, 800 Stanton L Young Boulevard, Suite 3400, Oklahoma City, OK 73104, USA; [b] Department of Orthopedic Surgery, Kasr Al-Ainy Hospitals, College of Medicine, Cairo University, Cairo, Egypt

* Corresponding author. Department of Orthopedic Surgery, Oklahoma University Health Sciences Center, University of Oklahoma College of Medicine, 800 Stanton L Young Boulevard, Suite 3400, Oklahoma City, OK 73104.

E-mail addresses: haleem@kasralainy.edu.eg; amgad-haleem@ouhsc.edu

Foot Ankle Clin N Am 26 (2021) 523–538
https://doi.org/10.1016/j.fcl.2021.06.003
1083-7515/21/Published by Elsevier Inc.

1989. These stages correlate to disease severity and each requires a unique treatment plan. Stage IIb adult-acquired flatfoot deformity, as initially described, involved moderate pain with or without lateral pain, flexible deformity, an inability to perform a heel-rise test, elongated tendon with longitudinal tears, and more than 30% talar head uncoverage with significant midforefoot abduction.[1] Recently, a new classification system has replaced the Johnson-Strom system as the understanding of this deformity has evolved.[6] This system refines the Johnson-Strom system by classifying the deformity as flexible (stage 1) versus rigid (stage II), with modifiers A, B, C, and D added based on the anatomic deformities that are present on clinical examination: hindfoot, midfoot, forefoot, and sinus tarsi impingement, respectively.[6] This system allows for actionable classification and more effective communication surrounding each patient's deformity. Class B PCFD under the new system therefore defines the midfoot/forefoot abduction component that was present in the previous stage IIb classification. Abduction most frequently occurs at the level of the talonavicular joint as the navicular rotates in eversion around the curved talar head (hindfoot), or at the level of the naviculocuneiform joint (midfoot) and tarsometatarsal joint (forefoot). This eventually leads to abduction of one segment of the foot (mid/forefoot) over the hindfoot, with subsequent peritalar subluxation.[6–8]

The operative approach to treating class B PCFD requires an anatomic and biomechanical approach to ensure the best functional outcomes for patients. Over the past four decades, such operative management has transformed drastically, with current treatment involving a medializing displacement calcaneal osteotomy (MDCO), lateral column lengthening (LCL), and/or first ray plantarflexion procedures.[9] Each of these procedures is used to correct a biomechanical aspect of the collapsed medial longitudinal arch, hindfoot valgus angulation, or midforefoot abduction. LCL, used in conjunction with these procedures, allows for the correction of midforefoot abduction component of the deformity.[10]

LCL was first described by Evans in 1975.[10] The importance of the lateral column was discovered by chance when Evans first noticed that patients with shortened lateral columns produced lateral rotation of the navicular leading to midforefoot abduction. The lateral column, made up of the anterior facet of the calcaneus, the cuboid, and the fourth and fifth metatarsal, held the key for Evans to correct the midforefoot abduction component of PCFD. By performing an osteotomy with a graft insertion in between the anterior and middle facet of the calcaneus, Evans was able to correct this deformity and re-establish the medial longitudinal arch.[10] This finding supports the biomechanical understanding of today with midforefoot abduction in class B PCFD.

An adult flatfoot deformity may manifest in one or many forms, either individually or combined: a medial collapsing arch, hindfoot valgus, and/or midforefoot abduction. Besides the bony pathology, soft tissue factors include a tight soleus-gastrocnemius complex leading a valgus vector force on the calcaneus, and the historically proposed previously mentioned loss of medial dynamic stabilizer of the hindfoot: the posterior tibial tendon. As one or more of these develop, a hindfoot calcaneovalgus deformity develops with talocalcaneal joint subluxation during weightbearing. This ultimately leads to peritalar subluxation with the midforefoot assuming an abducted position around the talar head.[8]

Over the years, variations of Evan's initial procedure have been developed to allow for correction of midforefoot abduction, and improved talar-head uncoverage.[11–14] Currently used variations of Evans osteotomy to lengthen the lateral column are the step-cut osteotomy (also known as Z-osteotomy or Z-cut osteotomy), Hintermann osteotomy, and calcaneocuboid (CC) arthrodesis.

Generally, patients who receive LCL in the operative treatment of PCFD class B have favorable radiographic and functional outcomes. Although LCL when used in combination with other soft tissue procedures often yields excellent outcomes for patients with class B PCFD, it is not without complications. Complications range from CC joint arthritis, overcorrection leading to lateral foot overload, sural nerve injury, peroneus longus tendon damage, and fifth metatarsal stress fractures.[15–18] Each of the techniques discussed later has implications that must be addressed when approaching a patient with class B PCFD. In this review article we describe the techniques, graft types, outcomes, controversies, and complications of each LCL approach to help answer the question: Should I be afraid of LCL?

SURGICAL TECHNIQUES

In the treatment of class B PCFD, there are several different techniques used for LCL to correct midforefoot abduction. In this review, we discuss the Evans osteotomy, step-cut osteotomy, Hintermann osteotomy, and CC distraction arthrodesis. In each of these procedures, autografts, allografts, and titanium wedges are all implant options.

INDICATIONS

Clinically, the visible abduction foot deformity on physical examination guides in the decision making of performing an LCL procedure. Preoperative imaging confirms this through quantification of midforefoot abduction. The most commonly used radiographic parameters are talar head (talonavicular) uncoverage of 40% on weightbearing anteroposterior (AP) radiographs of the foot, AP talar–first metatarsal angle, talar–second metatarsal angle, and lateral incongruency angle (LIA).[19–22] A derived linear equation relating the change in LIA is used to titrate the amount of required LCL. Every 1 mm of LCL corresponds to a 6.8° change in LIA.[23]

Although titrating the correction is possible and is factored in preoperative planning, indications for each LCL technique are not clearly defined in the literature and rely heavily on clinical judgment, abduction deformity severity, and surgeon preference. As with all reconstructive options in PCFD, the deformity must be flexible (that is, class B1) to perform an LCL procedure. Although not always the case, a more severe deformity may become stiff (class B2) directing the surgeon to a fusion. For patients with significant hindfoot valgus accompanying midforefoot abduction, an LCL procedure combined with an MDCO could be appropriate for the treatment plan. A step-cut osteotomy as described here is also a good option in such a situation because it serves as an MDCO and an LCL procedure, with more powerful correction. In patients with minimal hindfoot valgus, an Evans osteotomy, Hintermann osteotomy, or CC distraction arthrodesis is the preferred surgical treatment, because these three surgical techniques have a negligible effect on hindfoot valgus and primarily correct midforefoot abduction through LCL.

EVANS OSTEOTOMY

In 1975, Evans first described the operative management of the "calcaneovalgus deformity" in pediatric patients.[10] In this paper, Evans not only describes his surgical technique but also determines that the length of the lateral column plays a significant role in determining the physiologic shape of the foot. Currently, the Evans osteotomy is used by surgeons as an LCL technique for class B PCFD to correct the midforefoot abduction component of this disease. The surgical technique includes making an incision over the lateral surface of the hindfoot that is parallel and just superior to the peroneal tendons.[10] During the surgery, the sural nerve and peroneal tendons are relevant anatomic structures and should be avoided because an injury to them can lead to complications.[17] The cut into the calcaneus should be made 11 to 15 mm proximal to the CC joint and in the lateromedial direction, hinging on the medial cortex without violation.[10] The osteotomy site is then opened and a wedge graft laterally based is inserted. If the medial hinge is kept intact, no fixation is required. However, wedge grafts have been traditionally fixed with a single fully threaded screw, placed in non-compression mode, or a two-hole plate or a staple. The use of compression screws has the theoretic risk of splitting/breakage of bone-based corticocancellous grafts (**Fig. 1**). A theoretical disadvantage of the plate or staple constructs is proximity to the peroneal tendons with potential irritation if a non-low-profile surface implant is used. Another option is relying on an intact medial cortical hinge with nonfixation of the osteotomy. An adjustment to the Evans osteotomy was proposed years later to orient the lateromedial cut in between the anterior and middle facet of the calcaneus, which allows better preservation of those joints.[24–26]

HINTERMANN OSTEOTOMY

In 1999, Hintermann and coworkers[14] proposed a novel LCL osteotomy as a treatment of class B PCFD. In this surgical technique, an oblique incision is made over the lateral surface of the hindfoot. The cut into the calcaneus is made 12 to 20 mm proximal to the CC joint and in the lateromedial direction oriented between the middle and posterior joint facet of the calcaneus,[14,27] therefore focusing on the talonavicular joint axis, which is considered the main center of rotation of the hindfoot complex. Hintermann proposed that an Evan osteotomy, close to the CC joint, has the theoretic disadvantage of destabilizing the anterior calcaneus, provoking CC incongruency and an increase of pressure across the CC joint. This has ramifications in the operative setting because frequent CC dorsal subluxation is encountered not infrequently intraoperatively during the performance of an Evans osteotomy requiring K-wire stabilization of the joint, either prophylactically or therapeutically if subluxation occurs. The Hintermann osteotomy avoids such a problem and moreover, focuses on the center of rotation of the subtalar joint as previously mentioned by shifting the plane of the osteotomy posteriorly. The sural nerve and peroneal tendons are anatomic structures

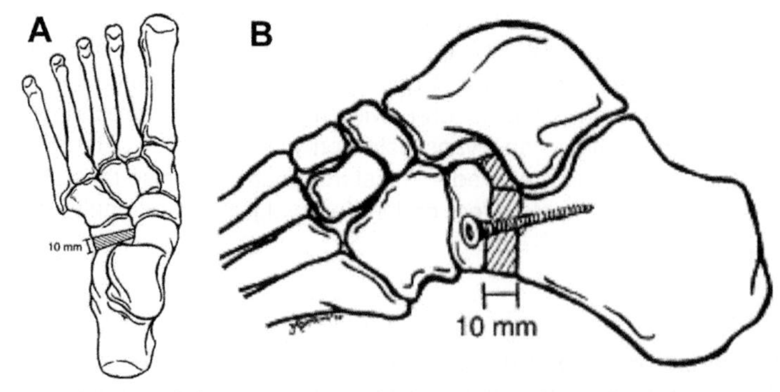

Fig. 1. Evans osteotomy. (*A*) An osteotomy of the calcaneus is performed 10 mm proximal to the calcaneocuboid joint. Using a lamina spreader, grafts are inserted into the osteotomy site. (*B*) A 3.5-mm cortical screw is fixed through the graft of choice and is placed at a right angle to the osteotomy. Splitting and graft breakage can occur with the use of compression screws. (*From* Mosier-Laclair et al., with permission.[54])

at risk of injury during this surgery. After the cut is made, a spreader or multiple chisels are used to provide space for the specific graft material (**Fig. 2**).[14,27] Grafting and subsequent fixation is similar as in the aforementioned Evans technique.

STEP-CUT OSTEOTOMY (Z-OSTEOTOMY)

Griend[11] first proposed the step-cut osteotomy as a surgical technique for management of class B PCFD in 2008. The purpose of this technique is to provide an alternative LCL technique; afford a more robust correction of the deformity, including the hindfoot valgus component; and minimize the known complications with LCL.[11] Theoretically, the step-cut osteotomy lowers symptoms of lateral column pain by using the axial rotation of the distal fragment rather than translational forces, which are present in other LCL procedures. In this technique, the lateral incision is centered over the neck of the calcaneus in preparation for three separate cuts to be made into the calcaneus.[11] A distal vertical cut is made 8 to 12 mm proximal to the CC joint and in the dorsal half of the calcaneus.[11,28] Next, the proximal vertical cut is made at approximately the same level as the peroneal tubercle and in the plantar portion of the calcaneus.[11,28] Finally, a longitudinal cut connects the two vertical cuts, which completes the "Z" (**Fig. 3**).[11] Two wedge grafts are required for this technique, proximally and distally (**Fig. 4**). Although fixation might not be required because of the press-fit nature of

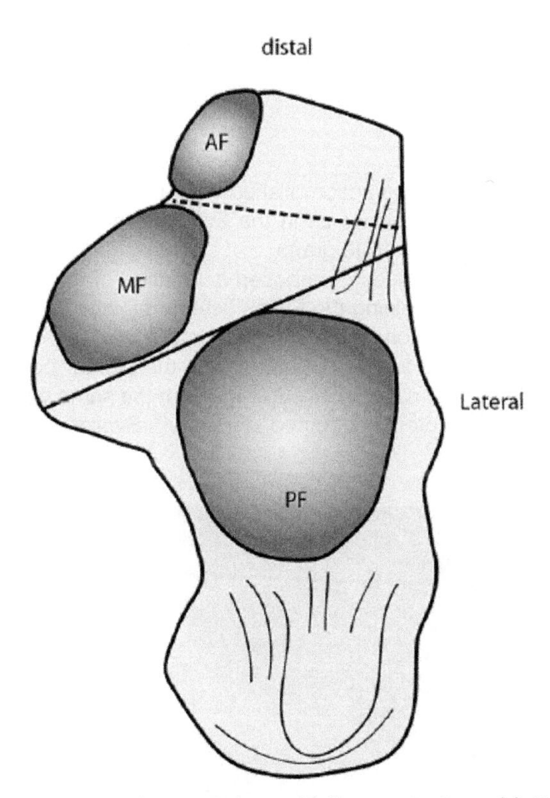

Fig. 2. Hintermann osteotomy. In comparison with Evans osteotomy (*dotted line*) across the anterior and medial facets of the subtalar joint, the Hintermann osteotomy is performed across the anterior border of the posterior facet (*solid line*). AF, anterior facet; MF, medial facet; PF, posterior facet. (*From* Ettinger et al., with permission.[27])

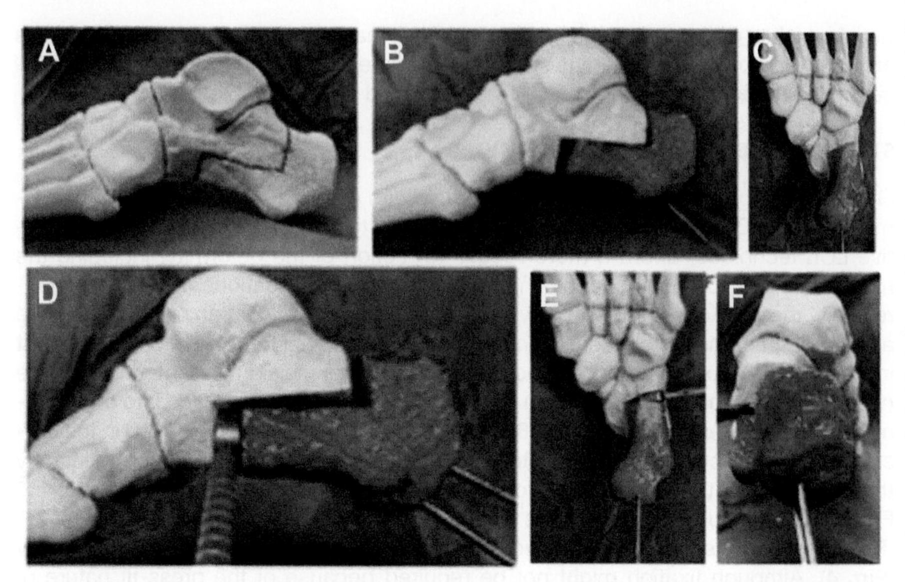

Fig. 3. Step-cut osteotomy technique. (*A*) Outline of the step-cut drawn sagittally. (*B, C*) With this technique, one continuous osteotomy is performed allowing for axial rotation of the horizontal arm. (*D–F*) Trial wedges are used to gauge the correction of the lateral column. The taper of the wedge graft allows for axial rotational forces to be used rather than translational forces, which can lead to lateral column pain. (*From* Ebaugh et al., with permission.[29])

the wedge graft, it could also be accomplished with a single noncompression screw from the anterior calcaneal tubercle as in the Evans technique directed posteriorly and plantarly to engage both wedge grafts.

In 2019, Ebaugh and colleagues[29] proposed a variation of the step-cut osteotomy with hopes of effectively combining the Evans osteotomy with the medializing calcaneal osteotomy. In this variation of the step-cut osteotomy, the distal vertical cut is made 10 to 15 mm proximal to the CC joint and in the plantar portion of the calcaneus.[29] In addition, the proximal vertical cut is made at the same point as a traditional medializing calcaneal osteotomy, directed dorsally.[29] Similar to Griend's step-cut

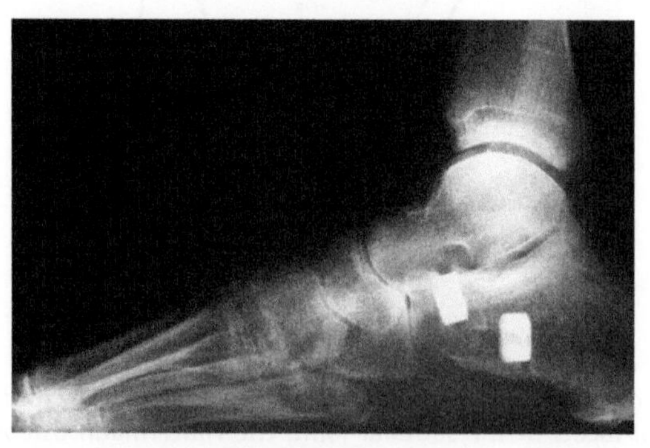

Fig. 4. Step-cut osteotomy. Lateral radiograph showing two unified wedge grafts at separate osteotomy sites. (*From* Scott et al., with permission.[55])

osteotomy, Ebaugh's longitudinal cut centrally connects the two vertical cuts (see **Fig. 3**).[11,29] A newer variation of the step-cut osteotomy has been described by Wapner and colleagues[30] in which a full-thickness transverse is cut along the long axis of the calcaneus to allow for correction of the hindfoot valgus deviation in addition to the midforefoot abduction in a single incision. With this modification, although two wedge grafts are still preferable, a single wedge graft can be used distally and transfixed with a larger diameter single screw and the posterior cut can be left without grafting. This is because of its location in robust cancellous bone with good healing potential.

CALCANEOCUBOID DISTRACTION ARTHRODESIS

Since the end of the last century, distraction arthrodesis of the CC joint has also been an operative technique used for LCL and treating stage class B PCFD.[12,16] However, this technique is not preferred and is solely indicated in patients with anticipated increased lateral column overload because of the anticipated use of a large-sized wedge graft to correct a significantly larger abduction deformity, stiffer deformities (PCFD class B2), or in patients with early CC arthritic changes. In this surgical technique, a lateral incision is made over the CC joint.[12,16] After all articular cartilage has been debrided from the joint, a lamina spreader is used to lengthen the lateral column in preparation for graft placement (**Fig. 5**).[12,16] A wide variety of fixation techniques have previously been described for this procedure, including crossing compression screws, hindfoot staples, and lateral plates, although the latter have a high risk of peroneal tendon irritation and are not preferred.[12,16,31,32]

GRAFT CHOICE

Using standard technique, tricortical autografts are frequently harvested from the iliac crest for LCL procedures. Although these remain the most cost-effective, donor site morbidity is a factor that cannot be overlooked. This is specifically true in the outpatient setting where postoperative pain control from the iliac crest donor site might be more cumbersome for the patient than the operated foot, which is usually managed with postoperative anesthetic lower extremity nerve blockade.

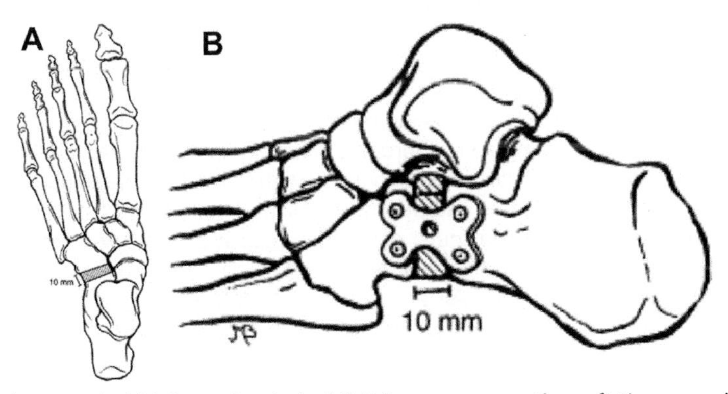

Fig. 5. Calcaneocuboid joint arthrodesis. (*A*) Using a rongeur, the soft tissue overlying the calcaneocuboid joint is removed. The joint cartilage is then removed with a curette. To facilitate osteogenesis, the subchondral bone is curetted until bleeding. Using the lamina spreader, the joint is distracted 10 mm to allow for graft placement. (*B*) Although various fixation methods are available, such as crossing 3.5-mm screws or lateral plates, complications, such as peroneal tendon rubbing, are more common with lateral plates. (*From* Mosier-Laclair et al., with permission.[54])

This popularized the use of allografts in LCL procedures. Allografts are used alone or in combination with biologics, such as platelet-rich plasma or autologous bone marrow aspirate concentrate to autopopulate the noncellularized allograft with autologous growth factors and mesenchymal stem cells to promote graft/host incorporation. Although there are no studies showing superior results when incorporating any of these biologics with allografts compared with allografts alone, Grier and Walling[33] found allografts with platelet-rich plasma to be at least equivalent to autologous grafts. Different metal trials are available for intraoperative trialing to determine appropriate allograft wedge size needed to correct the deformity, clinically and radiographically, by simulated weightbearing intraoperative fluoroscopic imaging. However, several studies have recommended not exceeding 8 mm in wedge size to avoid lateral column overload, even in face of an undercorrected deformity.[23,34]

Finally, with the advent of porous trabecular metal technology in total joint arthroplasty, porous titanium wedges (PTW) became available for foot and ankle procedures, including tantalum metal wedges for LCL. Similarly, these can be trialed to determine the size needed to provide adequate correction of the deformity.[35–37] Once the osteotomy has been widened using chisels or lamina spreaders, adjustments have been made to the biologic graft, and the appropriate graft size is selected, the implant is hammered into an appropriate depth and overall position.[35] If the medial cortical hinge is intact and a press-fit is achieved, no fixation is required. However, various fixation options are available.

CLINICAL OUTCOMES

Evans osteotomy, as originally described, corrects the relative shortening of the lateral column to correct the midforefoot abduction around the talonavicular joint. This procedure and its outcomes have been a focal point for clinical and cadaveric research surrounding the biomechanics and functional outcomes for patients.[27,38] Chan and colleagues[23] demonstrated that every millimeter of LCL corresponded with a 6.8° change in the LIA. These researchers also noted that the correction of midforefoot abduction is primarily determined by LCL and is modeled linearly.[23] Ten-year clinical outcome data published by Ruffilli and colleagues[18] demonstrated an 86% patient satisfaction rate in patients who received LCL in conjunction with soft tissue procedures and medializing calcaneal osteotomies. Tellisi and colleagues[39] described a statistically significant improvement in the American Orthopaedic Foot and Ankle Society Hindfoot-Score from 53.1 $\pm$ 14.5 points preoperatively to 83.2 $\pm$ 12.2 points postoperatively for patients receiving an LCL procedure. In addition to improved clinical outcomes, many radiographic outcomes associated with PCFD have been shown to have significant increases after Evans osteotomy. Ruffilli and colleagues[18] demonstrated a significant increase in the talonavicular coverage angle in patients with class B PCFD after receiving LCL. In a recent retrospective cohort study Tsai and colleagues[36] found a significant improvement in the AP and talo–first metatarsal angle, calcaneal pitch, talocalcaneal angle, and the talonavicular uncoverage angle. These radiographic findings support the clinical improvements that have been seen after LCL surgeries. In general, Evans osteotomy has a good safety profile and has low nonunion rates.[17] In regards to graft size, studies have found that incrementally increasing graft sizes greater than 8 mm is associated with an increased risk of lateral column overload and recommended caution when exceeding such graft size.[40,41]

Complications of Evans osteotomy include nonunion, excessive foot stiffness, CC joint arthritis, lateral column overload, sural nerve injury, peroneus longus tendon damage, and fifth metatarsal stress fractures.[17] These complications range in prevalence with lateral column overload being a major source of postoperative pain. In a study recently comparing the combination of LCL, flexor digitorum longus transfer, and medializing calcaneal osteotomy versus medializing calcaneal osteotomy paired with tendon transfer, 45% of the patients undergoing the LCL procedure reported lateral-sided foot pain in comparison with the 17% of the patients without the lateral column procedure.[23]

Using Evans osteotomy, Grier and Walling[33] determined allografts are a viable alternative to autografts and demonstrated allografts have a lower complication rate and higher union rate when compared with autografts. Vosseller and colleagues[34] found no significant differences in failure[36] (defined as nonunion or loss of 50% or greater correction) rates of patients undergoing either an Evans osteotomy with an autograft or allograft implant. In regards to healing time, Vosseller's study showed that the median time to radiographic healing for autograft was 17.3 weeks, and the median time to radiographic healing for allograft was 21 weeks.[34] Although the difference in median time to radiographic healing was statistically significant, the difference in median time was not statistically significant for clinical healing.[34] Vosseller's work demonstrated a statistically significant difference in median graft size between the allografts and autografts of cases that failed the surgery, but there is a question as to whether it is clinically significant because the size difference was less than 1 mm. Dolan and colleagues[42] found in a randomized prospective study that tricortical iliac crest allografts maintain equal efficacy when compared with iliac crest autografts in LCL. Dolan and colleagues[42] identified prolonged graft donor site pain as a significant postoperative complication in patients who received an autologous graft for their LCL procedure.

PTW has also been assessed for efficacy and safety when used in Evans osteotomies. In several studies, PTWs were found to have high union rates, maintain comparable safety profiles to allografts and autografts, and provide adequate correction of the deformity.[35–37,43] Gross and Tsai individually and retrospectively reviewed 71 patients and only three patients experienced nonunion and one patient experienced a PTW fracture.[35,36] Similarly to autografts and allografts, pain and arthritis within the CC joint was observed as a significant complication of using PTWs with Evans osteotomies.[35,36]

The Hintermann and Evans osteotomy were found to provide significant improvement in clinical outcome scores and radiographic correction of PCFD.[27] Ettinger and coworkers[27] noted that fewer degenerative features of the CC joint were observed with the Hintermann osteotomy, but there was uncertainty if differences in the fixation method had a significant role in this observation. The average graft size for the Evans and Hintermann osteotomies were 11 mm and 9.4 mm, respectively.[27] In a cadaveric study conducted by Ettinger and coworkers,[24] they found there is potential for anatomic structures to be damaged in the Evans and Hintermann osteotomy. For the Hintermann osteotomy, 100% of anterior calcaneal and 85.7% of medial calcaneal articular facets remained intact, whereas 42.9% of anterior calcaneal and 71.4% of medial calcaneal articular facets remain intact for cadavers undergoing the Evans osteotomy.[24] The posterior calcaneal articular facet remained intact for all cadavers in the study. Although this technique has seen recent renewed interest, there remains a paucity of literature comparing the Hintermann and Evans osteotomies in regards to clinical and radiographic outcomes.

The step-cut osteotomy has been described as a single-incision, single-osteotomy alternative to Evans osteotomy. Demetracopoulos and colleagues[28] support this approach in a recent retrospective review evaluating the step-cut osteotomy in 37 patients for radiographic and clinical improvement based on functionality scores. Demetracopoulos and Ebaugh both found the step-cut osteotomy achieved and usually maintained radiographic correction of PCFD with a high union rate.[28,29] Specifically, only one nonunion was identified between both of these studies, totaling 54 successful unions.[28,29] Ebaugh implemented a variation of the step-cut osteotomy, which is set posteriorly when compared with the more traditional step-cute technique outlined by Griend. The purpose of this variation is to functionally combine the Evans osteotomy with a medializing calcaneal osteotomy, and Ebaugh's results mirrored findings from studies that evaluated a traditional step-cut osteotomy in combination with a medializing calcaneal osteotomy. In Demetracopoulos' study, the traditional step-cut osteotomy was completed and then a medializing calcaneal osteotomy was provisionally performed to correct residual hindfoot valgus.

The step-cut osteotomy and Evans osteotomy achieved a union rate of 98.7% and 92.3%, respectively, in Saunders' and coworkers[44] retrospective study comparing the two. In addition, there was no increase in the incidence of lateral-sided foot pain, and the step-cut osteotomy did have a shorter healing time. The Evans' group showed greater improvement of the talonavicular percent uncoverage and talonavicular coverage angle, but the authors concluded this may have been caused by larger graft size and overcorrection.

CC arthrodesis serves as an alternative method for lengthening the lateral column through the distraction of the CC joint. This procedure was hypothesized because of the potential CC arthrosis seen with LCL.[45] However, this procedure has been considered a less favorable option for LCL because of increased complications after sufficient follow-up occurred.[31] This procedure has been associated with decreased subtalar joint range of motion, less ankle range of motion, less favorable long-term outcomes, and graft collapse.[23,31]

DISCUSSION

In selecting the appropriate technique of LCL, modeling the approach based on variations in clinical presentation is vital. Because of the lack of level 1 evidence comparing the efficacy of each treatment modality, one must rely on case series and studies to help guide preoperative planning for class B PCFD. This inherently creates controversy in the proper management of this disease. Pairing the patient's degree of clinical severity and anatomy, one procedure may be favored over another. Although Evans osteotomy has been thoroughly studied, newer techniques, such as the step-cut osteotomy, have become popularized recently. Recent variations in the step-cut osteotomy have been hypothesized and older techniques, such as the Hintermann osteotomy, are making new waves.[11,27] When evaluating the outcomes of LCL in literature, true attribution of improvement is hard to establish because of the concomitant procedures that occur with LCL. Although clinical outcomes may be multifactorial, research on lateral column procedures has proven radiographically the changes caused by lengthening the lateral column.

Evans osteotomy is satisfactorily performed with allograft, autograft, or PTW.[33,34,42,43,46,47] With all providing comparable union rates and functioning as viable implant options for LCL, there are several factors to consider when selecting the best choice for a specific patient. When comparing associated risks of allografts with autografts, allografts maintain a 12% risk of bacterial infection, and autografts have a significant risk of graft harvest site morbidity.[33,48] The graft harvest site morbidity not only has the potential to cause significant pain months after the LCL procedure, but it also could lead to increased medical expenses and increased use of health services postoperatively. Grier and Walling[33] determined that allografts and platelet-rich plasma cost +$2500 more than an autograft for LCL. Still, other researchers speculate that allografts are the more cost-effective option when compared with autografts.[42]

In regards to other graft material options, it has been speculated within the literature that allografts and PTWs provide a more uniform operative experience, which can theoretically shorten operative time and expenses.[35,49] Both allow a surgeon to trial a wedge before implantation, which is used to determine the specific wedge size needed to achieve the appropriate degree of radiographic correction.[36] However, this is overcome with autologous grafts by measuring the distraction gap, achieving clinical and radiographic correction intraoperatively with laminar spreaders in the osteotomy site, and downsizing the iliac crest tricortical wedge to fit this measured gap. In addition, autografts only have the capability of downsizing, whereas allografts and PTWs have the capability of downsizing and upsizing within surgery because of the variable selection sizes available.[36] Because PTWs are not biologic, one negative to consider is the risk of implant removal caused by postoperative infections.[35,43] Finally, when deciding which graft to use in LCL, it is important to keep in mind the apparent relative costs of graft material. Unfortunately, limited objective data are available for comparison of these procedures because of the integrated nature of treating class B PCFD. Future studies should focus on the cost analysis of using autograft, allograft, and PTW.

Although the Evans osteotomy has a good safety profile and low nonunion rates, the osteotomy can increase the pressure placed on the CC joint, which can result in pain and arthritis. An independent factor that remains congruent across graft types is the size of graft used. The ideal graft size has been studied thoroughly in clinical and cadaveric studies. The most frequently used graft sizes range from 8 to 12 mm.[10,12] Choosing the graft size correctly enables for correction of the midforefoot abduction component with minimizing complications.[40] Oversizing a graft can lead to a common side effect of lateral foot overload. A prospective study by Kou and colleagues[50] demonstrated the incidence of lateral-sided pain after surgery at 6 months to be 76%, with a subsequent drop to 28% at 1 year and 12% at 2 years. These authors hypothesize that this pain is caused by subfibular impingement. Conti and colleagues[51] noted that correction of midforefoot position to an LIA of fewer than 5° was associated with a poorer clinical outcome, which was hypothesized to be secondary to symptoms of lateral overload. Ellis and colleagues[52] also described increased pressures on the lateral side of the foot of patients who have undergone LCL. This correlation highlights the importance of careful graft size selection to minimize overload and thus minimize future lateral-sided pain. In the case of undersizing a graft, the midforefoot abduction component may not be fully corrected. This can lead to unsatisfactory results for patients and retained impairment of function. Finally, the consensus group on PCFD recommends ideal graft size to be 5 to 10 mm. The osteotomy site should be gradually distracted (possibly with a pin distractor or laminar spreader) until correction of the abduction deformity is obtained, measured by talar head coverage via simulated AP weightbearing intraoperative fluoroscopy. Once this correction is achieved, it is imperative that passive hindfoot motion, especially eversion, be evaluated. If significant hindfoot stiffness is encountered, then the amount of distraction at the osteotomy is reduced until passive eversion is unrestricted.[53]

Ettinger and coworkers[27] found the Hintermann osteotomy to be a viable surgical technique for LCL, and it seemed to have fewer degenerative changes in the CC joint. This is a promising finding because lateral-sided pain and arthritis of the CC joint is a significant complication of LCL. Further studies are needed to evaluate the efficacy of the Hintermann osteotomy in class B PCFD treatment and to further validate its rates of degenerative changes postoperatively seen in the CC joint.

The theoretic benefits of step-cut osteotomy over Evans osteotomy include the improvement of lateral column symptoms, fewer nonunions, and faster healing times.[11,28,29,44] This procedure replaces the dual calcaneal osteotomy (posterior calcaneal displacement osteotomy and Evans osteotomy) with an isolated calcaneal osteotomy, allowing for translation and rotation with less lengthening.[11] Studies have shown it to have high union rates, comparable complication rates, and long-term maintenance of radiographic correction.[28,29,44] For patients with hindfoot valgus, the posteriorly set step-cut osteotomy could be considered as an operative approach to correct midforefoot abduction and hindfoot valgus with one single osteotomy.[29] Saunders and colleagues[44] described the theoretic benefit of faster healing because of the horizontal limb involvement in the step-cut osteotomy versus in an Evans osteotomy but failed to find a statistically significant impact on overall healing outcomes. This finding indicates the lack of sufficient support to perform one procedure over another. Given these data, nonunion rates seem to be impressively low in patients receiving the step-cut osteotomy. However, more prospective studies should be performed to determine efficacy and superiority.

Nevertheless, because of the step-cut location on the calcaneus, extra caution must be taken to avoid iatrogenic damage to the peroneal tendons from plate placement and screw head proximity to the tendons inferiorly. In a recent retrospective review, Saunders and colleagues[44] described this complication in 3 of the 111 patients (143 feet) receiving a step-cut osteotomy. Although Demetracopolous and colleagues[28] demonstrated statistically significant improvement in patients' outcomes undergoing step-cut osteotomy, they also noted iatrogenic peroneal tendon injury and lateral-sided foot pain as complications in their cohort. This theoretic risk of step-cut osteotomies is improved by proper retraction of the peroneal tendons during the operation, avoidance of the dorsal to plantar screws, and the use of two longitudinal screws.[44] Another disadvantage to using the step-cut osteotomy is the necessity for correction of hindfoot valgus in patients with severe class A and B PCFD. Demetracopolous and colleagues demonstrated that an additional MDCO may be necessary after a step-cut osteotomy to correct residual hindfoot valgus deformity. This finding may indicate that an isolated step-cut osteotomy may not be the correct procedure for all patients depending on the degree of midforefoot abduction and hindfoot valgus around Chopart joint.

The learning curve required for these procedures is an important and often undervalued metric. The classic Evans osteotomy has been taught for more than 30 years and is the most common form of LCL used. The invention and adaptation of new approaches, such as the step-cut osteotomy, requires a learning curve and a sound surgical comprehension of previous LCL techniques to achieve the outcomes seen by the large cohort retrospective studies performed by skilled senior authors.

SUMMARY

LCL has long been used in conjunction with other soft tissue and bony procedures to correct the midforefoot abduction seen in class B PCFD. Although the procedure has changed since its inception, the effectiveness of this osteotomy to restore the physiologic shape of the foot has been used in the reconstructive algorithm of the abduction component of the deformity. The innovation of novel techniques to address complications, such as lateral column overload, has led to newer procedures with fewer nonunions, improved functional outcomes, and decreased complications. Although LCL certainly is not complication free, it is an effective and safe way to restore the collapsed arch seen in PCFD and improve the talonavicular head uncoverage seen in advanced PCFD. The overall low complication rates, low nonunion rates, and improved radiographic and functional outcomes provided by LCL make this a valuable option for the treatment of class B progressive collapsing foot deformity. The Evans osteotomy is a procedure that no foot and ankle surgeon should be afraid to perform to correct the midforefoot abduction seen in this deformity.

CLINICS CARE POINTS

- Lateral column lengthening is a reliable and safe method of correcting the midforefoot abduction in class B progressive collapsing foot deformity.
- Evans osteotomy is a well-studied method of lateral column lengthening that provides satisfactory results with autograft, allograft, or porous titanium wedges.
- Evans osteotomy complications include notable rates of lateral column pain, calcaneocuboid arthritis, and foot stiffness.
- Step-cut osteotomy is a viable alternative to Evans osteotomy and provides a robust deformity correction with decreased complications of lateral column overload.
- Calcaneocuboid distraction arthrodesis is generally not preferred and is reserved for select indications.
- Autograft, allograft, and titanium wedges have all been proven to be viable graft choices and consideration should be given for graft size to decrease lateral column overload.

ACKNOWLEDGMENTS

The authors thank Brandon Moritz, Dr Cameron Shirazi, and Dr Wade Schwerdtfeger for their contributions to the article and editing they performed.

DISCLOSURE

The authors have no disclosures relevant to the topic of this article.

REFERENCES

1. Hadfield MH, Snyder JW, Liacouras PC, et al. Effects of medializing calcaneal osteotomy on Achilles tendon lengthening and plantar foot pressures. Foot Ankle Int 2003;24(7):523–9.
2. Johnson KA, Strom DE. Tibialis posterior tendon dysfunction. Clin Orthop Relat Res 1989;239:196–206.
3. Supple KM, Hanft JR, Murphy BJ, et al. Posterior tibial tendon dysfunction. Semin Arthritis Rheum 1992;22(2):106–13.
4. Frey C, Shereff M, Greenidge N. Vascularity of the posterior tibial tendon. J Bone Joint Surg Am 1990;72(6):884–8.
5. Petersen W, Hohmann G, Stein V, et al. The blood supply of the posterior tibial tendon. J Bone Joint Surg Br 2002;84(1):141–4.
6. Myerson MS, Thordarson DB, Johnson JE, et al. Classification and nomenclature: progressive collapsing foot deformity. Foot Ankle Int 2020;41(10):1271–6.
7. Probasco W, Haleem AM, Yu J, et al. Assessment of coronal plane subtalar joint alignment in peritalar subluxation via weight-bearing multiplanar imaging. Foot Ankle Int 2015;36(3):302–9.
8. Ananthakrisnan D, Ching R, Tencer A, et al. Subluxation of the talocalcaneal joint in adults who have symptomatic flatfoot. J Bone Joint Surg Am 1999;81(8): 1147–54.

9. Abousayed MM, Alley MC, Shakked R, et al. Adult-acquired flatfoot deformity: etiology, diagnosis, and management. JBJS Rev 2017;5(8):e7.
10. Evans D. Calcaneo-valgus deformity. J Bone Joint Surg Br 1975;57-B(3):270–8.
11. Griend RV. Lateral column lengthening using a "Z" osteotomy of the calcaneus. Tech Foot Ankle Surg 2008;7(4):257–63.
12. Thomas RL, Wells BC, Garrison RL, et al. Preliminary results comparing two methods of lateral column lengthening. Foot Ankle Int 2001;22(2):107–19.
13. Kitaoka HB, Kura H, Luo ZP, et al. Calcaneocuboid distraction arthrodesis for posterior tibial tendon dysfunction and flatfoot: a cadaveric study. Clin Orthop Relat Res 2000;(381):241–7.
14. Hintermann B, Valderrabano V, Kundert HP. Lengthening of the lateral column and reconstruction of the medial soft tissue for treatment of acquired flatfoot deformity associated with insufficiency of the posterior tibial tendon. Foot Ankle Int 1999;20(10):622–9.
15. Bolt PM, Coy S, Toolan BC. A comparison of lateral column lengthening and medial translational osteotomy of the calcaneus for the reconstruction of adult acquired flatfoot. Foot Ankle Int 2007;28(11):1115–23.
16. Haeseker GA, Mureau MA, Faber FW. Lateral column lengthening for acquired adult flatfoot deformity caused by posterior tibial tendon dysfunction stage II: a retrospective comparison of calcaneus osteotomy with calcaneocuboid distraction arthrodesis. J Foot Ankle Surg 2010;49(4):380–4.
17. Jara ME. Evans osteotomy complications. Foot Ankle Clin 2017;22(3):573–85.
18. Ruffilli A, Traina F, Giannini S, et al. Surgical treatment of stage II posterior tibialis tendon dysfunction: ten-year clinical and radiographic results. Eur J Orthop Surg Traumatol 2018;28(1):139–45.
19. Deland JT. Adult-acquired flatfoot deformity. J Am Acad Orthop Surg 2008;16(7): 399–406.
20. Sangeorzan BJ, Mosca V, Hansen ST Jr. Effect of calcaneal lengthening on relationships among the hindfoot, midfoot, and forefoot. Foot Ankle 1993;14(3): 136–41.
21. Haddad SL, Myerson MS, Younger A, et al. Adult acquired flatfoot deformity. Foot Ankle Int 2011;32(1):95–101.
22. Vulcano E, Deland JT, Ellis SJ. Approach and treatment of the adult acquired flatfoot deformity. Curr Rev Musculoskelet Med 2013;6(4):294–303.
23. Chan JY, Greenfield ST, Soukup DS, et al. Contribution of lateral column lengthening to correction of forefoot abduction in stage IIB adult acquired flatfoot deformity reconstruction. Foot Ankle Int 2015;36(12):1400–11.
24. Ettinger S, Sibai K, Stukenborg-Colsman C, et al. Comparison of anatomic structures at risk with 2 lateral lengthening calcaneal osteotomies. Foot Ankle Int 2018; 39(12):1481–6.
25. Mosca VS. Calcaneal lengthening for valgus deformity of the hindfoot. Results in children who had severe, symptomatic flatfoot and skewfoot. J Bone Joint Surg Am 1995;77(4):500–12.
26. Hyer CF, Lee T, Block AJ, et al. Evaluation of the anterior and middle talocalcaneal articular facets and the Evans osteotomy. J Foot Ankle Surg 2002;41(6):389–93.
27. Ettinger S, Mattinger T, Stukenborg-Colsman C, et al. Outcomes of Evans versus Hintermann calcaneal lengthening osteotomy for flexible flatfoot. Foot Ankle Int 2019;40(6):661–71.
28. Demetracopoulos CA, Nair P, Malzberg A, et al. Outcomes of a stepcut lengthening calcaneal osteotomy for adult-acquired flatfoot deformity. Foot Ankle Int 2015;36(7):749–55.

29. Ebaugh MP, Larson DR, Reb CW, et al. Outcomes of the extended Z-cut osteotomy for correction of adult acquired flatfoot deformity. Foot Ankle Int 2019;40(8): 914–22.
30. Wapner K, Freeland E, Kirwan G, et al. A retrospective radiographic evaluation of a modified method of lateral column lengthening. Foot Ankle Spec 2020. 1938640020919187.
31. Beimers L, Louwerens JW, Tuijthof GJ, et al. CT measurement of range of motion of ankle and subtalar joints following two lateral column lengthening procedures. Foot Ankle Int 2012;33(5):386–93.
32. Kobayashi H, Kageyama Y, Shido Y. Calcaneocuboid distraction arthrodesis with synthetic bone grafts: preliminary results of an innovative bone grafting procedure in 13 patients. J Foot Ankle Surg 2017;56(6):1223–31.
33. Grier KM, Walling AK. The use of tricortical autograft versus allograft in lateral column lengthening for adult acquired flatfoot deformity: an analysis of union rates and complications. Foot Ankle Int 2010;31(9):760–9.
34. Vosseller JT, Ellis SJ, O'Malley MJ, et al. Autograft and allograft unite similarly in lateral column lengthening for adult acquired flatfoot deformity. HSS J 2013; 9(1):6–11.
35. Gross CE, Huh J, Gray J, et al. Radiographic outcomes following lateral column lengthening with a porous titanium wedge. Foot Ankle Int 2015;36(8):953–60.
36. Tsai J, McDonald E, Sutton R, et al. Severe flexible pes planovalgus deformity correction using trabecular metallic wedges. Foot Ankle Int 2019;40(4):402–7.
37. Matthews M, Cook EA, Cook J, et al. Long-term outcomes of corrective osteotomies using porous titanium wedges for flexible flatfoot deformity correction. J Foot Ankle Surg 2018;57(5):924–30.
38. Zhou H, Ren H, Li C, et al. Biomechanical analysis of cuboid osteotomy lateral column lengthening for stage II B adult-acquired flatfoot deformity: a cadaveric study. Biomed Res Int 2017;2017:4383981.
39. Tellisi N, Lobo M, O'Malley M, et al. Functional outcome after surgical reconstruction of posterior tibial tendon insufficiency in patients under 50 years. Foot Ankle Int 2008;29(12):1179–83.
40. Oh I, Imhauser C, Choi D, et al. Sensitivity of plantar pressure and talonavicular alignment to lateral column lengthening in flatfoot reconstruction. J Bone Joint Surg Am 2013;95(12):1094–100.
41. Momberger N, Morgan JM, Bachus KN, et al. Calcaneocuboid joint pressure after lateral column lengthening in a cadaveric planovalgus deformity model. Foot Ankle Int 2000;21(9):730–5.
42. Dolan CM, Henning JA, Anderson JG, et al. Randomized prospective study comparing tri-cortical iliac crest autograft to allograft in the lateral column lengthening component for operative correction of adult acquired flatfoot deformity. Foot Ankle Int 2007;28(1):8–12.
43. Moore SH, Carstensen SE, Burrus MT, et al. Porous titanium wedges in lateral column lengthening for adult-acquired flatfoot deformity. Foot Ankle Spec 2018; 11(4):347–56.
44. Saunders SM, Ellis SJ, Demetracopoulos CA, et al. Comparative outcomes between step-cut lengthening calcaneal osteotomy vs traditional evans osteotomy for stage IIB adult-acquired flatfoot deformity. Foot Ankle Int 2018;39(1):18–27.
45. Hill K, Saar WE, Lee TH, et al. Stage II flatfoot: what fails and why. Foot Ankle Clin 2003;8(1):91–104.

46. Foster JR, McAlister JE, Peterson KS, et al. Union rates and complications of lateral column lengthening using the interposition plating technique: a radiographic and medical record review. J Foot Ankle Surg 2017;56(2):247–51.
47. Muller SA, Barg A, Vavken P, et al. Autograft versus sterilized allograft for lateral calcaneal lengthening osteotomies: comparison of 50 patients. Medicine (Baltimore) 2016;95(30):e4343.
48. Lord CF, Gebhardt MC, Tomford WW, et al. Infection in bone allografts. Incidence, nature, and treatment. J Bone Joint Surg Am 1988;70(3):369–76.
49. Sagherian BH, Claridge RJ. Porous tantalum as a structural graft in foot and ankle surgery. Foot Ankle Int 2012;33(3):179–89.
50. Kou JX, Balasubramaniam M, Kippe M, et al. Functional results of posterior tibial tendon reconstruction, calcaneal osteotomy, and gastrocnemius recession. Foot Ankle Int 2012;33(7):602–11.
51. Conti MS, Garfinkel JH, Ellis SJ. Outcomes of reconstruction of the flexible adult-acquired flatfoot deformity. Orthop Clin North Am 2020;51(1):109–20.
52. Ellis SJ, Yu JC, Johnson AH, et al. Plantar pressures in patients with and without lateral foot pain after lateral column lengthening. J Bone Joint Surg Am 2010;92(1):81–91.
53. Thordarson DB, Schon LC, de Cesar Netto C, et al. Consensus for the indication of lateral column lengthening in the treatment of progressive collapsing foot deformity. Foot Ankle Int 2020;41(10):1286–8.
54. Mosier-Laclair S, Pomeroy G, Manoli A. Operative treatment of the difficult stage 2 adult acquired flatfoot deformity. Foot Ankle Clin 2001;6(1):95–119.
55. Scott RT, Berlet GC. Calcaneal Z osteotomy for extra-articular correction of hindfoot valgus. J Foot Ankle Surg 2013;52(3):406–8.

Flexible Progressive Collapsing Foot Deformity

Is There Any Role for Arthroereisis in the Adult Patient?

Kaan Suleyman Irgit, MD[a,*], Atanas Zhivkov Katsarov, MD, PhD[b]

KEYWORDS

• Arthroereisis • Adult • Flatfoot • Flexible • Talus • Subtalar joint
• Progressive collapsing foot deformity

KEY POINTS

- Arthroereisis is a minimally invasive procedure originally designed for the treatment of pediatric patients that may be used as adjunct or stand-alone procedure in the treatment of adult flexible pes planus.
- It is a volume-obtaining procedure that blocks excessive pronation of the heel in a less invasive manner, preserves foot function, and spares the subtalar joint.
- One of the main areas of concern of subtalar arthroereisis is the postoperative rate of discomfort in sinus tarsi.

INTRODUCTION

Progressive collapsing foot deformity (PCFD) is one of the most common problems challenging the foot and ankle surgeon today. Its importance and management have been the subject of debate for many years.[1] PCFD is a complex deformity and various treatment modalities have been used to treat it when it is symptomatic. Arthroereisis has been developed and used successfully in treating pediatric flatfeet cases for decades.[2] Influenced by this success, surgeons started using arthroereisis as an isolated or adjunct procedure in adult patients with PCFD. Over the last two decades, there is a substantial increase in clinical research of the use of arthroereisis in PCFD. At the same time, there has been an improvement in the imaging and surgical techniques, and new types of implants and technology have emerged. Despite these advances, it is still a debate how to classify the disease, when to operate, how much correction to achieve, which implant to use, necessity and timing of

[a] Orthopedics and Traumatology, Marmara School of Medicine, Fevzi Cakmak Mah, Muhsin Yazicioglu Cad No 10, PK 34899, Pendik, İstanbul, Turkey; [b] Ortomedica Clinic, "G. Washington" Street 22, Sofia 1000, Bulgaria
* Corresponding author.
E-mail address: kaanirgit@yahoo.com

Foot Ankle Clin N Am 26 (2021) 539–558
https://doi.org/10.1016/j.fcl.2021.06.004 foot.theclinics.com

removal, and whether to use the technique as an isolated or adjunct procedure.[3] The focus of this article is directed to the role of arthroereisis in the treatment of PCFD.

DEFINITION

Arthroereisis (*arthron* [joint], *ereisis* [lifting], from Latin) is defined as an operative procedure with the goal of limiting the overpronation in the subtalar joint (STJ).[2] Subtalar arthroereisis refers to the use of an implant positioned in the sinus tarsi, used as an endo-orthosis, to limit the pathologic motion at the STJ. This procedure is extra-articular because the implant is situated in tarsal sinus and/or tarsal canal where there is no presence of cartilage.

HISTORY OF ARTHROEREISIS

Chambers[4] (1946) was the first to develop the concept and perform arthroereisis with a bone block graft to fill the sinus tarsi. He believed that by elevating the floor of the sinus tarsi one could limit the plantarflexion and anterior excursion of the talus and thereby prevent excessive pronation.[4,5] This original procedure was implemented with a posterior facet osteotomy.[4] In 1970, LeLievre[6] first described a method of blocking the sinus tarsi, restricting subtalar motion without bone fusions. LeLievre used a free-floating bone graft obtained from the base of the proximal phalanx and inserted a temporary staple across the STJ. He introduced the term lateral arthroereisis. Later, Subotnick[7] (1974) described the use of a silicon made, free-floating, sinus tarsi implant. Viladot[8] (1992) published a series of 234 surgically treated flatfoot in children. He reported a success rate of 99% and was first to describe a true sinus tarsi implant: the "cuplike" endo-orthosis.

Since the first description of the technique, there are more than 30 types of implants designed for STJ arthroereisis.[4,7,9–11] Some of them have stood the test of time; others have been abandoned. One of the main issues of the technique has been discomfort in sinus tarsi area. To decrease this complaint, design, shape, biomechanics, and the material of the implant have been changed and improved in time. From 1970 to the 1980s many arthroereisis implants were designed mostly to fit into sinus tarsi not the tarsal canal. They were made of silastic, high-molecular-weight polyethylene, Teflon, and stainless steel. In the following years implants made of polyethylene, ultrahigh-molecular-weight polyethylene (UHMWPE), a combination of metal in polyethylene (titanium in UHMWPE), titanium, stainless steel, and bioabsorbable poly-L-lactic acid were introduced.[8,9,12,13]

There have been various implant designs: cylindrical, conical, spherical, pegged, and wineglass shaped.[9,12–15] Recent radiographic studies proved that the tarsal canal morphology is conical.[9] Hence the second-generation implants are more conical than oval and became more threaded for better purchasing and possibility for soft tissue ingrowth. To date, the ideal size of a subtalar arthroereisis implant is still a subject of debate.[16]

BIOMECHANICS OF SUBTALAR ARTHROEREISIS

The talonavicular and talocalcaneal joints form the peritalar joint complex.[17] Talocalcaneal motion is complex and triplanar: inversion, adduction, and plantar flexion occur together (whereas eversion, abduction, and dorsiflexion occur together).[17]

During normal gait, with the initial contact of the heel-strike, peritalar joints move into a more everted or valgus position. The posterior tibialis muscle acts eccentrically as a shock absorber by controlling the arch collapse and eversion of the foot.[5] After heel-strike, during stance, this eversion causes forefoot abduction and the medial arch flattens. The axes between the transverse tarsal joints become parallel and unlocked. As the foot moves from foot-flat to toe-off, the hindfoot inverts and comes to a varus position. When the posterior tibial tendon (PTT) is intact, the Achilles tendon, which contributes largely on cycle, initiates the heel rise. Just before toe-off, transverse tarsal joints become nonparallel and locked, stabilizing the medial longitudinal arch.[18] At this stage of normal gait cycle the forward propulsion force generated by triceps surae should be transmitted through the medial longitudinal arch to the metatarsal heads. If there is a dysfunction on PTT or a disease on supportive structures, the medial longitudinal arch cannot work efficiently to form a rigid lever arm. Triceps surae, via Achilles tendon, provides the most powerful dynamic arch deforming force on the midfoot alignment.[19] The repetitive force on midfoot leads to more collapse, abduction, and eventually arthritis and pain. With a pathologic medial column, an efficient gait may not be possible. Prachgosin and colleagues[20,21] collected data from 28 nonobese adults in a three-dimensional motion analysis laboratory and calculated the medial longitudinal arch biomechanics radiographs. They showed that a flatfoot performed a significantly greater eversion deforming force acting at the medial longitudinal arch structure, greater hindfoot and forefoot motion, and less medial longitudinal arch flexibility, and abnormal ground reaction force during walking.[20]

Subtalar arthroereisis implants aim to stabilize the STJ by limiting its hypermotion. One idea behind the arthroereisis is to prevent talus moving downward and inward on the calcaneus and to correct valgus deformity of the hindfoot in a minimally invasive manner without fusing the STJ. Christensen and coworkers[22] conducted a well-designed biomechanical study on 11 fresh frozen cadaver specimens. After the application of arthroereisis and the tibia was axially loaded to 756 N, they found that the implant significantly inverts and slightly dorsiflexes the navicular, rotates the talus dorsally and externally, inverts the calcaneus and cuboid, and the navicular inverted relative to the cuboid. Arangio and coworkers[23] conducted a biomechanical study and reported that by decreasing the biomechanical stress along the medial column of the foot, arthroereisis shifts the load from the joints of the medial column back toward the lateral column, decreases the moments at the talonavicular joint and the medial cuneiform–navicular joint, and decreases the forces in the medial extensions of the long plantar ligament and plantar aponeurosis.

Schon[9] studied the shape of the sinus tarsi on computed tomography scans and found that the space is more conical than cylindrical (**Fig. 1**). A previous MRI study found that the lateral height of the tarsal canal was small in the adult population (8 ± 1.7 mm).[16]

It is a concern among surgeons whether the use of isolated arthroereisis is an efficient surgery to treat flexible PCFD in adult patients. Wong and colleagues[24] failed to show subtalar arthroereisis alone is strong enough to restore internal load transfer and stress to normal levels. Husain and Fallat[10] found that the tension on the Achilles tendon increases after insertion of an arthroereisis. Furthermore subtalar arthroereisis may not be available to address the transverse plane deformities.[12]

According to their biomechanical properties, Vogler[14] classified implants for the STJ into three types (**Fig. 2**). His classification is the most used until recently. Kirby theorized that all the STJ arthroereisis implants, regardless of design, material, and size, are “axis-altering” devices because they alter the postoperative spatial location of the STJ axis during weightbearing activities.[25] In 2012 Graham and Nikhil[15] proposed a new classification (**Fig. 3**), based on the device geometry, anatomic orientation (fit of the device within the tarsal sinus), primary location at which the device is anchored within the tarsal sinus, and mechanism of talar stabilization and biomechanical

Anterior
Middle facet
Posterior facet

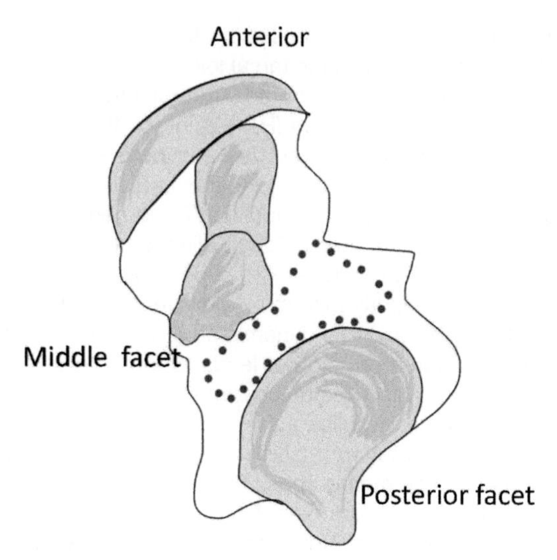

Fig. 1. Sinus tarsi and tarsal canal projection.

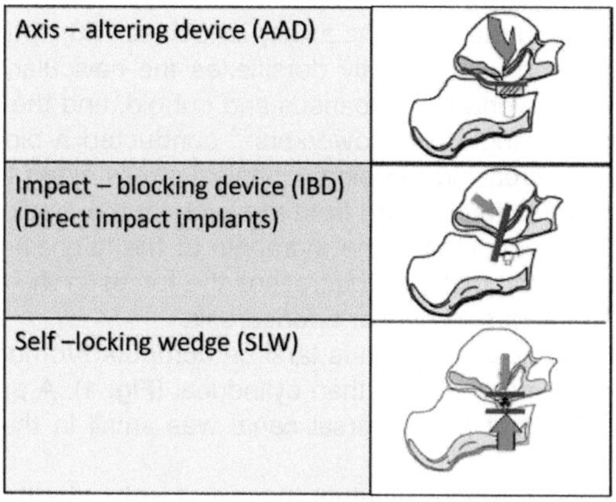

Axis – altering device (AAD)
Impact – blocking device (IBD)
(Direct impact implants)
Self –locking wedge (SLW)

Fig. 2. Vogler biomechanical classification of subtalar implants.[14]

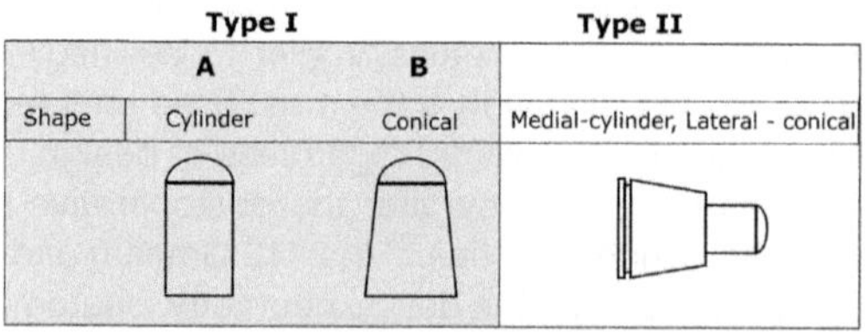

Type I
Type II
A
B
Shape
Cylinder
Conical
Medial-cylinder, Lateral - conical

Fig. 3. Geometry and position classification, Graham and Nikhil classification of subtalar implants.[15]

functioning. The benefits of a conical-shaped STJ implant include a more accurate fit into the sinus tarsi with a narrower trailing end, which can result in less pain and irritation.[9] The blunt thread design offers softer fit into the sinus tarsi with less irritation and less chance of synovitis and inflammation postoperatively. Some of the subtalar implants act in the canal and others in the canal and the sinus. The canal has a lower degree of extrusion than conventional sinus implants.[11]

INDICATIONS

It is debatable and unlikely nowadays that PCFD is caused by PTT dysfunction. Adult acquired flatfoot deformity (AAFD) has been described by Johnson and Strom[26] in four distinct stages. It was lately modified by Myerson and coworkers (**Table 1**).[27,28] At the end of 2019 a group of nine foot and ankle experts, after analysis, discussion, and subsequent voting, suggested a change in terminology. The consensus group advocated for the use of the term PCFD instead of AAFD for various reasons.[3] According to the expert group, PCFD seems a more accurate and comprehensive description of this complex deformity. The world "adult" was taken out, which allows including younger patients. Flattening of the arch and hyperpronation of the rear foot seems to be a process, not a single-stage deterioration. They state that the term "progressive" describes the natural history of the disorder.[3] However, the recent adult arthroereisis literature is based on the previous classification scheme, and the study groups in the literature vary (**Table 2**).

The main indication for STJ arthroereisis for treating PCFD is not yet clear. When conservative treatment is insufficient to control the severe STJ pronation in flexible flatfoot deformity and the pain persists, arthroereisis is used as an adjunct or a stand-alone procedure for stage I, class A, B, or C PCFD. Literature is scarce, with several case series using a variety of implants conducting different methodologies. There are no well-designed prospective randomized studies published and no proper algorithm yet established. The authors propose to use the STJ arthroereisis mostly as an additional procedure; however, it may be used as an isolated procedure for symptomatic patients who have no benefit from conservative management for stage I, class A or B PCFD.

The absolute contraindications are STJ arthritis, peroneal muscle spasm (associated with STJ disease), rigid PCFD, and excessive ligamentous laxity.

SURGICAL TECHNIQUE

The aim of subtalar arthroereisis surgery is to block the hyperpronation of the calcaneus. The anesthesia depends on the additional procedures performed.[29]

Proper entering of the incision and the guidewire are determined either with or without C-arm control. Palpate the soft spot just inferior to the distal tip of the fibula.[29] Make an incision about 15 mm in length, in the skin lines over sinus tarsi. Keep intact the intermediate dorsal cutaneous branch of the superficial peroneal nerve (the communicating branch between the sural nerve and intermediate dorsal cutaneous nerve) and peroneal tendons. Spread gently the subcutaneous tissue after the skin incision. Insert the guide pin in the canal (for cannulated implants), in the direction following the axis of the STJ. Pass along the whole canal until it protrudes the medial skin above the synovial sheath of the PTT. Hold it with a clamp. Sinus tarsi decompression is required when combined cylinder plus conical-shape implants are used. For noncannulated implants a guidewire and sinus tarsi decompression are not necessary. After the soft tissue spreading, a specially designed blunt lever is introduced laterally in sinus tarsi, to correct the collapse of the talus and to put the STJ in

Table 1
AAFD classification described by Johnson and Strom and lately modified by Myerson[26,27]

Stage	A	B	C	D	E	
I	Tenosynovitis with or without osseous deformity	Inflammatory disease	Partial PTT tear with normal hindfoot anatomy	Partial PTT tear with hindfoot valgus	—	—
II	Ruptured PTT and flexible flatfoot	Minimal hindfoot valgus (1,2,3,4)	Severe hindfoot valgus, flexible forefoot supination (5,6 + 2,3,4)	Fixed forefoot supination	Forefoot abduction	Medial ray instability
III	Rigid hindfoot valgus	Hindfoot valgus	Forefoot abduction	Treatment options: 1. Calcaneal osteotomies. 2. Tendon transfers. 3. Arthroereisis procedures. 4. Achilles tendon lengthening. 5. Isolated hindfoot fusions. 6. Medial column procedures.		
IV	Ankle valgus	Flexible ankle valgus	Rigid ankle valgus			

Table 2
Clinical studies including separate results and/or complications for the adult patient population

Author	Study Design	Indication	Patients (n)	Average Age	FU	Implant Type	Implant Material	Additional Procedure	Clinical Result	Radiologic Parameters
Viladot et al,[30] 2003	Retrospective case series	Stage II PTTD	19	56	27.31	Kalix Integra (KalixII, Integra, NJ)	Metal in UHMWPE	C	Postoperative AOFAS 81.6 84% would undergo the same procedure again 17 were satisfied, 2 dissatisfied	Moreau-Costa-Bartani angle and Kite deviation angle Significant improvement in both angles
Needleman,[18,a] 2006	Retrospective case series	Adult flexible flatfoot	28	51	44	MBA (KMI, Carlsbad, CA)	Metal	C	Postoperative AOFAS 87 Haddad telephone questions are 78% satisfied, 4% not sure, 18% not satisfied	Medial longitudinal arch Uncovering of the head of the talus (TN) Difference in standing ankle height Significant improvement in all measurements
Saxena & Nguyen,[16,b] 2007	Retrospective case series	Adult flexible flatfoot and PTTD	8	52.5	24	ACL interference screw (Arthrex, Inc, Naples, FL)	Bio-absorbable	I	NA	MRI
Adelman et al,[34] 2008	Retrospective case series	Stage IIB PTTD	10	57	3.75	MBA (KMI)	Metal	C	VAS significantly improved 78% satisfaction	Calcaneal inclination angle Talar declination angle Meary angle Calcaneal inclination angle Lateral cyma line TN congruity AP talocalcaneal angle Cuboid abduction angle Significant improvement in all measurements

(*continued on next page*)

Table 2
(*continued*)

Author	Study Design	Indication	Patients (n)	Average Age	FU	Implant Type	Implant Material	Additional Procedure	Clinical Result	Radiologic Parameters
Garras et al,[36] 2012	Retrospective case series	Stage II A with an accessory navicular	23	18	54	MBA (KMI)	Metal	C	AOFAS and Visual Analog Pain Scale Both improved significantly after the surgery 19/20 had good or excellent results	Lateral talar–first metatarsal angle (Meary angle) Talus–first metatarsal angle on AP view The degree of talar head uncoverage as a percentage of the entire talar head on the AP view Significant improvement in all measurements
Graham & Nikhil,[15,e] 2012	Retrospective case series	RTTD	83	58	17 d	HyProCure_ EOTTS device	Metal	I	NA	Talar–second metatarsal angle Talar declination angle Calcaneal inclination angle
Zhu & Xu,[35] 2015	Retrospective case series	Stage IIA and IIC AAFD, stage IIB was excluded	24	30	49	Kalix Integra (KalixII)	Metal in UHMWPE	C	Postoperative AOFAS 85.6 67% excellent or good results	Lateral view Talar–first metatarsal angle Lateral standing view of talocalcaneal angle and TNCA Average preoperative talar–first metatarsal angle and TN coverage angle Significant improvement in all measurements

Saxena et al,[38] 2016	Retrospective case series	Adult flexible flatfoot	104	78	53	Prostop (Arthrex, Inc) Arthrex Bio-tenodesis implants (Arthrex, Inc) MBA (Integra LifeSciences, Plainsboro, NJ) Prostop Plus (Arthrex, Inc) Kalix (Integra LifeSciences) Bionix interference implants (now Bioretec, Tampere, Finland) CSI implant (Nexa Orthopedics, San Diego, CA)	Metal, bio-degradable	C	NA	NA
Yasui et al,[50] 2017	Retrospective case series	Stage IIA AAFD	13	13	37.3	NA	NA	C	FAOS, VAS both improved significantly after the surgery	Lateral talus–first metatarsal angle Calcaneal pitch Cuneiform to ground distance
Ozan et al,[31,c] 2015	Retrospective case series	Adult flexible flatfoot	26	24	15	Horizon; BioPro (Port Huron, MI)	Metal	I	AOFAS VAS both improved significantly after the surgery	Calcaneal inclination angle Lateral talocalcaneal angle Meary angle TN angles or Kite angles Significant improvement in all measurements
Voegeli et al,[32] 2018	Retrospective case series	Stage IIA1	37	55	47.5	NA	NA	C	74% excellent or good results	Meary angle Moreau-Costa-Bartani angle Kite angle Coverage of the talar head All parameters significantly improved

(*continued on next page*)

Table 2
(continued)

Author	Study Design	Indication	Patients (*n*)	Average Age	FU	Implant Type	*Implant Material*	*Additional Procedure*	*Clinical Result*	Radiologic Parameters
Aynardi et al,[46] 2017	Case control study	Adult flexible flatfoot Excluded >40% TN joint uncoverage on AP weightbearing radiographs	30 (9 implanted)	55 vs 51	40 vs 28	NEXA implant (Wright Medical, Memphis, TN) ProStop Plus (Arthrex) implant	Metal	C	SF-36 via telephone VAS Both improved significantly after the surgery	TN coverage angle Lateral talar–first metatarsal angle (or Meary angle)
Ceccarini et al,[48] 2018	Retrospective case series	Stage IIA AAFD (20 stage IIA1 and 2 stage IIA2)	31	46	34	RSB calcaneo-stop LIMA Corporate	Bio-absorbable	C	AOFAS 82 VAS-FA 83 Both improved significantly after the surgery 23/29 patients to be excellent-good (79.4%)	Talar–first metatarsal angle in the AP views TN congruence in the AP view Djian Annonier Meary angle
Bernasconi et al,[44,d] 2020	Case control study	Stage IIB AAFD	22	55	11	Futura Conical Subtalar Implant (Tornier/Wright Medical Group)	Metal	C	NA	AP view TNCA Talocalcaneal divergence angle Calcaneo–fifth metatarsal angle the lateral view Talocalcaneal divergence angle Talo–first metatarsal angle Dijan-Annonier angle Calcaneal pitch angle

Junxian et al,[40] 2020	Case control study	Stage IIB AAFD	22	51 vs 53	>12	NA	NA	C	AOFAS SF-36 VAS All significantly improved significantly after the surgery	Medial column length (AP) Lateral column length (AP) Lateral column length (L) Medial column length (L) Lateral column height (L) TN uncoverage angle Calcaneal pitch angle Talus–first metatarsal angle (AP) Talus–first metatarsal angle (L)
Silva et al,[41] 2020	Case control study	Stage IIB AAFD	79	46 vs 47	24	MBA (Integra LifeSciences)	Metal	C	AOFAS, SF-36, VAS were all improved same after 6 mo in both groups All parameters were superior in LCL group vs STJA in 24 m	AP view TN uncoverage angle lateral view Calcaneal pitch angle Talo–first metatarsal angle Medial cuneiform height

Abbreviations: AAFD, adult acquired flatfoot deformity; AOFAS, American Orthopaedic Foot & Ankle Society; AP, anteroposterior; FAOS, Foot and Ankle Outcome Score; FU, follow up; LCL, lateral column lengthening; MBA, Maxwell- Brancheau arthroereisis; NA, Not available; PTTD, posterior tibial tendon dysfunction; RTTD, flexible/reducible talotarsal joint dislocation (partial); SF-36, Short Form-36; STJA, sinus tarsi joint arthroereisis; TN, talonavicular; TNCA, talonavicular coverage angle; VAS, Visual Analog Scale.

[a] Out of 28 patients, 12 were PTTD and one was AAFD.

[b] Out of eight, two fulfilled the postsurgical follow-up criteria.

[c] Congenital, traumatic, and neurologic conditions were excluded.

[d] STJA was performed in 54% and cotton osteotomy in 23%.

[e] Postoperative radiographs were taken at 17 days.

congruent position. It is crucial to make a correction with a proper tool that is placed under the neck of talus, while pronating the forefoot and supinating the hindfoot with the lever.

The next step is to determine the appropriate implant size. Start inserting the cannulated trial sizers or trial devices from the smallest, keeping the guidewire in the canal. Estimate in dorsiflexed foot the passive range of motion of the talonavicular joint after the insertion of every sizer. The position of the sizer/trial device is monitored with C-arm control, anteroposterior and lateral view. The appropriate trial device/sizer is removed and replaced with the implant, with the same size as the last inserted trial device/sizer under C-arm control. The range of motion of the STJ is evaluated again. The surgeon should monitor two key points at all times: the implant position and the STJ movement.

Finally, the guidewire is removed, and the incision is closed. Furthermore, the surgeon could decide the need for an additional procedure to be performed. The residual valgus should not be more than 5° and the dorsiflexion of the ankle should be at least 10°. If the ankle dorsiflexion does not reach this level, an Achilles tendon lengthening should be performed. For isolated procedures postoperative protocol includes 2 weeks of nonweightbearing in a splint, followed by progressive weightbearing in a walker boot and physical therapy. If additional osteotomies are performed 6 weeks of nonweightbearing should be followed by gradual weightbearing depending on the radiologic union seen on the control radiographs.

RESULTS

Clinical studies are focused generally on improvement in radiologic and clinical measurements, implant removal rates, and the causes of implant removal. Most articles show significant improvement in postoperative clinical scores, and visual analog scores (see **Table 2**).[18,31–33] With a belief that arthroereisis alone does not correct every deformity, most authors apply arthroereisis as an adjunct procedure to treat the flexible PCFD.[18,29,30,32,34–37] Additional gastrocnemius recession is generally recommended to improve the clinical results.[35,37,38] Myerson and Kadakia[39] suggested that patients with a large degree of talonavicular uncovering after a calcaneal medial displacement calcaneal osteotomy (MDCO) would benefit from arthroereisis. Adelman and coworkers[34] suggested that arthroereisis is easier to perform and carries no risk of nonunion or malunion, no risk of medial neurovascular damage, and requires less immobilization and not weightbearing. They used arthroereisis in combination with flexor digitorum longus transfer and gastrocnemius recession, and depicting similar results when using STJ arthroereisis instead of an MDCO.[34] Zhu and Xu[35] recommended to add medial calcaneal osteotomy only for more severe deformities. Only in a few studies was STJ arthroereisis used as a stand-alone procedure.[11,31] Christensen and colleagues[22] have shown that the STJ arthroereisis implant not only significantly alters the three-dimensional positions of the talus and calcaneus, but also significantly changes the three-dimensional positions of the cuboid and navicular. Schon[9] postulates that when subtalar arthroereisis is used as an adjunct procedure in conjunction with medial soft tissue stabilizing procedures, the implant typically is no longer needed after soft tissue healing and may be removed without risk to the surgical correction. Saxena and Nguyen[16] recommended that an Evans calcaneal osteotomy should be considered as an adjunctive procedure if instability persists after placement of Maxwell- Brancheau arthroereisis implant.

Some surgeons are reluctant whether PCFD reconstruction involving only MDCO and flexor digitorum longus transfer would undercurrent the deformity, using lateral column lengthening (LCL) to address residual forefoot abduction. However, with LCL there is a risk of nonunion, lateral pain, increased calcaneocuboid pressure, and progression of joint osteoarthritis (up to 40% at 5 years). To compare the efficiency of STJ arthroereisis versus LCL on PCFD, two studies were recently published.[40,41] In both studies, STJ arthroereisis improved clinical and radiologic results, despite the considerable complication rate (**Table 3**). Researchers proposed that STJ arthroereisis be considered as an alternative to restore adequate talonavicular coverage without increasing lateral columns pressure.[42,43]

In a larger case series published by Brancheau and colleagues,[42] significant increase in talocalcaneal, calcaneocuboid, and first and second intermetatarsal angles, and calcaneal inclination and talar declination angles after arthroereisis was performed. In most studies restoring the normal angular relationships between hindfoot and forefoot osseous structures on weightbearing in the transverse and sagittal planes was possible after the use of STJ arthroereisis.[43,44] It was noted, however, that correction of radiographic parameters is not always a reliable predictor of satisfaction with the surgical outcome.

Regarding implant removal, in one case-control study, age, gender, implant characteristics, sizes, surgical error, and surgeon experience did not affect the necessity of implant removal.[12] Saxena and coworkers[38] also found that age was not a risk factor for implant removal.

Table 3
Sinus tarsi pain complication rate and removal rate

Author	Sinus Tarsi Pain Rate (%, n of Patients)	Removal Rate (%)
Viladot et al,[30] 2003	31 (6)	11
Needleman et al,[18] 2006	46 (13)	39
Saxena & Nguyen,[16] 2007	37 (3)	25
Adelman et al,[34] 2008	40 (4)	10
Garras et al,[36] 2012	13 (3)	13
Graham & Nikhil,[15,a] 2014	13 (15)	6
Zhu & Xu,[35] 2015	25 (6)	36
Saxena et al,[38] 2016	NA	22
Yasui et al,[50] 2017	13 (3)	13
Ozan et al,[31] 2015	11.5 (3)	11.5
Voegeli et al,[32] 2018	38 (14)	35
Aynardi et al,[46] 2017	6.7 (1)	6.7
Ceccarini et al,[48] 2018	16.1 (5)	10
Bernasconi et al,[44] 2020	30 (4)	30
Junxian et al,[40] 2020	50 (6)	30
Silva et al,[41] 2020	20.6 (7)	20.6

Abbreviation: NA, Not available.

[a] Authors reported 6% removal of primary implantation; however, total implant-related issues 16/83 = 19%. Nine of 16 were implant related.

A recent survey involving 1818 American Orthopaedic Foot & Ankle Society members and 404 responders showed that surgeons outside of United States have more tendency to use the technique in adult patients.[45] The rates of surgeons who have used the technique and kept on using it are higher in the rest of the world than in the United States (53% vs 24% in the United States).[45]

COMPLICATIONS

Because of its ability to change the osseous geometry of the foot, the arthroereisis procedure also has the potential to produce negative biomechanical effects on the foot and lower extremity.[25] Talar cyst formation, implant migration, overcorrection/undercorrection, infection/wound problems, psychogenic reactions, wearing of nonmetallic implants, unremitting and unresolving pain, avascular necrosis of talus, talar fracture, talar neck fracture, and in situ subtalar fusion are the complications of subtalar arthroereisis.[31,32,35,40,43,46,47,49]

Most of the complications are caused by inadequate surgical technique (large or small implant size), improper patient selection, and poor preoperative clinical assessment (**Fig. 4**). Overall, sinus tarsi pain is the main determinant of clinical well-being and satisfaction. Sinus tarsi pain is the most common complication and the reported discomfort caused by sinus tarsi pain is between 6.7% and 46%.[18,43]

In 6% to 39% of patients, the presence of sinus tarsi pain necessitated implant removal (**Table 4**). Overcorrection via too large of an implant or the use of metal implant is often relieved after removal and it is generally reversible.[47] Advocates of bioabsorbable implants propose some advantages over metallic implants: decreased interference during MRI and no need for implant removal.[16,37,47,48] Aynardi and colleagues[46] stated that proposed bioabsorbable implants have demonstrated few complications and may be a safe adjunct to stage II, AAFD correction in adults. Ideally the absorbable implant should keep the corrected position as the implant degrades over time, requiring less need for removal. Theoretically, biodegradable implants need 9 months to degrade completely.[16] However, such complications as screw breakage, inflammatory responses, foreign body reactions, cyst formation, and local bone lysis have been reported with bioabsorbable screws. With UHMWPE there is a risk of dynamic deformation that is increased with age and body mass index. Saxena and

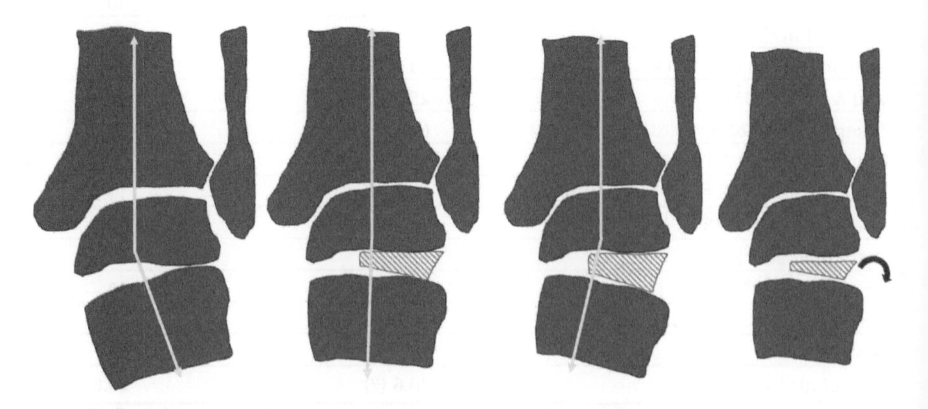

Fig. 4. Proper placement and malposition of the implant with risk of overcorrection and extrusion. STA, Subtalar Arthroereisis.

Table 4
Advantages and disadvantages of subtalar arthroereisis

Advantages	Disadvantages
Extra-articular	Limited evidence for indications
Dynamic	High rate of sinus tarsi pain
Joint-sparing	No objective criteria for proper correction
Removable/reversible	Possibility of loss of correction after removal
Easy to perform	
No risk of nonunion, malunion	
No risk of medial neurovascular damage	

Nguyen[16] reported three patients with discomfort out of eight patients by using Poly (l-lactic acid) implants. Baker and colleagues[37] reported the worst results, with the bioabsorbable implants used as an isolated procedure.

Graham and Nikhil[15] reported a 6% lower removal rate than others. Nonetheless, in this study there were 16 (19%) patients who suffered implant-related issues; seven requiring removal and nine requiring revisions of the implant. The authors reported two cases of removal of implants because of psychogenic reactions.[15] Symptomatic oversizing was stated several times by Graham and Voegeli.[31,48] Too large of an implant may cause too much stress on the lateral side, STJ stiffness, and restriction in ankle dorsiflexion.[48] Too small of an implant may allow migration and undercorrection.[49] Generally, removal is needed when either the implant is too large or malpositioned.[15,47] The reaction and pain occurring after use of a larger implant or use of metal implant is often relieved after removal. Dislocation and extrusion are other indications for removal.[31,37,38] Saxena and coworkers[38] reported 4.7% of the implants were dislocated. Adults do not have the same remodeling capacity of pediatric patients and the loss of correction after extracting the implant might be a concern. However, some studies showed that there is no loss of correction and clinical results are still favorable after removal of implants.[32,35,50] This may be attributed to the effect of the adjunct procedures.[9] In case of sinus tarsi pain, Voegeli and colleagues recommended to remove the implant at least 1 year after surgery for the recovery of soft tissue to prevent loss of reduction. In their series there was no loss of correction in eight cases after implant removal.

Recently Bernasconi and colleagues[44] and Junxain and colleagues[40] reported high removal rates and sinus tarsi pain, 33% and 50%, respectively. Although Bernasconi and colleagues[44] reported resolution of pain after the removal, one patient in this study was clinically worse after the retention of the implant.

Subtalar fusion is another rare complication but hypothetically it may be caused by malposition of the arthroereisis implant, or multiple attempts at guidewire placement.[51] Voegeli and coworkers[32] reported five subtalar fusions as complication. Implant malposition may also contribute to subtalar arthritis, leading to subtalar fusion.

DISCUSSION

PCFD is a complex entity, with patients presenting in different stages or classes. There are several surgical techniques available for treatment, yet there is no consensus regarding the best treatment option.[52] One of the treatment options that has recently attracted attention in adult literature is the subtalar arthroereisis. Subtalar arthroereisis, alone or combined with other soft tissue or osseous procedures, is a reasonable treatment option for flexible PCFD class A, B, or C. However, the exact algorithm is not clear yet. When used alone, subtalar arthroereisis could correct mild to moderate hindfoot valgus. Isolated subtalar arthroereisis may allow quicker return to daily activities with less pain compared with other surgical interventions.

It could be performed along with soft tissue correction/repair and tendon transfers because STJ arthroereisis achieves the necessary three-plane correction. Arthroereisis prevents the talus from displacing onto the calcaneus and eliminates applied tension to the repaired tendon.[30]

It is a less invasive alternative to calcaneal osteotomy or LCL when treating a flexible PCFD. Performing of arthroereisis is easier, quicker, and less invasive compared with arthrodesis, calcaneal osteotomies, or medial column stabilization procedures. Another advantage is that arthroereisis spares the STJ and does not disturb the articulations between the facets of talus and calcaneus.

One major problem of the technique is the high rate of sinus tarsi pain. Yasui and coworkers[50] suggested custom orthoses for supporting footwear would help resolve mild cases and cortisone injection for severe cases. If conservative management fails, removal of the implant generally creates an immediate relief to most patients.[16,29,32,34] Most patients start having symptoms related to the implant between 7 and 18 months after surgery. In the study by Ceccarini and coworkers,[48] removal was done in an average of 14 months after the surgery. However, there is not enough evidence of routine implant removal. After removal generally, no loss of correction is usually observed, which may be attributed to additional surgeries. Improper sizing and implant dislocation are another indication of removal. Zhu and Xu[35] recommended routine implant removal besides the fact that most studies show removal rates of 20% to 30% in short-term and midterm follow-up.

There are no long-term results published in adult patients and literature is lacking retrospective case control studies or prospective randomized studies to prove whether STJ arthroereisis should be used alone or as adjunct treatment of different stages of the deformity. A variety of patient-related scoring systems, additional surgeries, radiologic measurements, and different classification schemes are used in each study, which makes it harder to come up with a proper algorithm.

SUMMARY

Subtalar arthroereisis is a reliable procedure in the treatment of flexible PCFD. In the last two decades there were more studies with adult patients; however, the literature is still scarce. STJ arthroereisis is considered a temporary or definitive internal orthotic implant preventing excessive, nonphysiologic eversion of the hindfoot, without excessively limiting normal motion, while properly orienting the talus over the calcaneus. Patient selection, appropriate planning, concomitant procedures decision, surgical technique, and implant choice are important factors to properly address each case. Conical implants seem to have better results, but data are not sufficient to propose one implant over another.

Results also seem to be better when performed as an adjunctive procedure as opposed to a primary procedure. Implant removal for sinus tarsi pain issues has been reported as a common complication.

In summary, STJ arthroereisis is a minimally invasive, low-risk, and promising technique with good short-term and midterm results. Multicenter, large number, prospective randomized studies are needed for further evaluation of the long-term effects of arthroereisis as an isolated or adjunctive procedure and to determine a proper algorithm.

CLINICS CARE POINTS

Pearls

- STJ arthroereisis has a role in treating symptomatic PCFD patients.
- The implant prevents talus moving downward and inward on the calcaneus and corrects valgus deformity of the hindfoot in a minimally invasive manner.
- Tarsal canal has a more conical morphology.
- It is crucial to make a correction maneuver with a proper tool before inserting the implant.
- The lever should be placed under the neck of the talus; the hindfoot is supinated by the lever while the forefoot is pronated by the surgeon.
- After the surgery it is crucial to limit weightbearing for a short time and physical therapy increases the chance of a successful result.

Pitfalls

- The precise algorithm is not clear in adult PCFD patients.
- The most common complication is pain in sinus tarsi.
- In some patients sinus tarsi pain resolves with conservative management. If conservative management fails, implant can easily be removed.
- There is a slight risk of losing the correction after removal.

FINANCIAL DISCLOSURE

None reported.

CONFLICT OF INTEREST

The authors declare that they have no conflict of interest to report.

REFERENCES

1. Staheli L. Evaluation of planovalgus foot deformities with special reference to the natural history. J Am Podiatr Med Assoc 1987;77(1):2–6.
2. Highlander PD, Sung WH, Weil L Jr. Subtalar arthroereisis. Clin Podiatr Med Surg 2011;28(4):745.
3. de Cesar Netto C, Deland J, Ellis S. Editorial: expert consensus on adult-acquired flatfoot deformity. Foot Ankle Int 2020;41(10):1269–71.
4. Chambers E. An operation for the correction of flexible flat feet of adolescents. West J Surg Obstet Gynecol 1946;54:77–86.
5. Van Boerum D, Sangeorzan B. Biomechanics and pathophysiology of flat foot. Foot Ankle Clin 2003;8(3):419–30.
6. LeLievre J. The valgus foot: current concepts and correction. Clin Orthop Relat Res 1970;70:43–55.
7. Subotnick SI. The subtalar joint lateral extra-articular arthroereisis: a preliminary report. J Am Podiatr Med Assoc 1974;64(9):701–11.
8. Viladot A. Surgical treatment of the child's flatfoot. Clin Orthop Relat Res 1992; 283:34–8.
9. Schon LC. Subtalar arthroereisis: a new exploration of an old concept. Foot Ankle Clin 2007;12(2):329–39.
10. Husain ZS, Fallat LM. Biomechanical analysis of Maxwell-Brancheau arthroereisis implants. J Foot Ankle Surg 2002;41(6):352–8.
11. Graham M, Jawrani N, Chikka A, et al. Surgical treatment of hyperpronation using an extraosseous talotarsal stabilization device: radiographic outcomes in 70 adult patients. J Foot Ankle Surg 2012;51(5):548–55.

12. Cook EA, Cook JJ, Basile P. Identifying risk factors in subtalar arthroereisis explantation: a propensity-matched analysis. J Foot Ankle Surg 2011;50(4): 395–401.
13. Grady JF, Dinnon M. Subtalar arthroereisis in the neurologically normal child. Clin Podiatr Med Surg 2000;17(3):443–57, vi.
14. Vogler HM. Subtalar joint blocking operations for pathological pronation syndromes. In: McGlamry ED, editor. Comprehensive textbook of foot surgery. Baltimore: Williams & Wilkins; 1987. p. 447–65.
15. Graham M, Nikhil T. Extraosseous talotarsal stabilization devices: a new classification system. J Foot Ankle Surg 2012;51:613–9.
16. Saxena A, Nguyen A. Preliminary radiographic findings and sizing implications on patients undergoing bioabsorbable subtalar arthroereisis. J Foot Ankle Surg 2007;46(3):175–80.
17. Sangeorzan A, Sangeorzan B. Subtalar joint biomechanics: from normal to pathologic. Foot Ankle Clin 2018;23(3):341–52.
18. Needleman RL. A surgical approach for flexible flatfeet in adults including a subtalar arthroereisis with the MBA sinus tarsi implant. Foot Ankle Int 2006;27:9–18.
19. Thordarson D, Schmotzer H, Chon J. Reconstruction with tenodesis in an adult flatfoot model: a biomechanical evaluation of four methods. J Bone Joint Surg Am 1995;77-A(10):1557–64.
20. Prachgosin T, Chong DY, Leelasamran W, et al. Medial longitudinal arch biomechanics evaluation during gait in subjects with flexible flatfoot. Acta Bioeng Biomech 2015;17(4):121–30.
21. Langford J, Bozof H, Horowitz B. Subtalar arthroereisis: the Valenti procedure. Clin Podiatr Med Surg 1987;4:153–5.
22. Christensen JC, Campbell N, DiNucci K. Closed kinetic chain tarsal mechanics of subtalar joint arthroereisis. J Am Podiatr Med Assoc 1996 Oct;86(10):467–73.
23. Arangio GA, Reinert KL, Salathe EP. A biomechanical model of the effect of subtalar arthroereisis on the adult flexible flat foot. Clin Biomech 2004;19:847–52.
24. Wong DW, Wang Y, Chen TL, et al. Biomechanical consequences of subtalar joint arthroereisis in treating posterior tibial tendon dysfunction: a theoretical analysis using finite element analysis. Comput Methods Biomech Biomed Engin 2017; 20(14):1525–32.
25. Kirby K. Understanding the biomechanics of subtalar joint arthroereisis. Podiatry Today 2011;24(4):36–45.
26. Johnson KA, Strom DE. Tibialis posterior tendon dysfunction. Clin Orthop Relat Res 1989;259:196–203.
27. Myerson M. Adult acquired flatfoot deformity. J Bone Joint Surg Am 1996;78-A(5): 780–92.
28. Haddad S, Myerson M, Younger A, et al. Adult acquired flatfoot deformity, symposium. Foot Ankle Int 2011;32:95.
29. Zaret DI, Myerson MS. Arthroereisis of the subtalar joint. Foot Ankle Clin N Am 2003;8:605–17.
30. Viladot R, Pons M, Alvarez F, et al. Subtalar arthroereisis for posterior tibial tendon dysfunction: a preliminary report. Foot Ankle Int 2003;24(8):600–6.
31. Ozan F, Doğar F, Gençer K, et al. Symptomatic flexible flatfoot in adults: subtalar arthroereisis. Ther Clin Risk Manag 2015;11:1597–602.
32. Voegeli A, Fontecilla C, Serrá JA, et al. Results of subtalar arthroereisis for posterior tibial tendon dysfunction stage IIA1. Based on 35 patients. Foot Ankle Surg 2018;24(1):28–33.

33. Bresnahan P, Chariton J, Vedpathak A. Extraosseous talotarsal stabilization using HyProCure: preliminary clinical outcomes of a prospective case series. J Foot Ankle Surg 2013;52:195–202.
34. Adelman VR, Szczepanski JA, Adelman RP. Radiographic evaluation of endoscopic gastrocnemius recession, subtalar joint arthroereisis, and flexor tendon transfer for surgical correction of stage II posterior tibial tendon dysfunction: a pilot study. J Foot Ankle Surg 2008;47(5):400–8.
35. Zhu Y, Xu XY. Treatment of stage II adult acquired flatfoot deformity with subtalar arthroereises. Foot Ankle Spec 2015;8(3):194–202.
36. Garras D, Hansen P, Miller A, et al. Outcome of modified Kidner procedure with subtalar arthroereisis for painful accessory navicular associated with planovalgus deformity. Foot Ankle Int 2012;33(11):934–9.
37. Baker J, Klein E, Weil L Jr, et al. Retrospective analysis of the survivability of absorbable versus nonabsorbable subtalar joint arthroereisis implants. Foot Ankle Spec 2013;6(1):36–44.
38. Saxena A, Via AG, Maffulli N, et al. Subtalar arthroereisis implant removal in adults: a prospective study of 100 patients. J Foot Ankle Surg 2016;55(3):500–3.
39. Myerson MS, Kadakia AR. Correction of flatfoot deformity in the adult, Chapter 14. In: Myerson MS, Kadakia AR, editors. Reconstructive foot and ankle surgery: management of complications. 3rd edition. Elsevier; 2019. p. 194–219.
40. Junxian C, Kunnasegaran R, Thevendran G. Surgical management of symptomatic adult pes planovalgus secondary to stage 2B posterior tibial tendon dysfunction: a comparison of two different surgical treatments. Indian J Orthop 2020; 54(1):22–30.
41. Silva M, Koh DTS, Tay KS, et al. Lateral column osteotomy versus subtalar arthroereisis in the correction of Grade IIB adult acquired flatfoot deformity: a clinical and radiological follow-up at 24 months. Foot Ankle Surg 2020. S1268-7731(20)30162-4.
42. Brancheau S, Walker K, Northcutt D. An analysis of outcomes after use of the Maxwell-Brancheau arthroereisis implant. J Foot Ankle Surg 2012;51:3–8.
43. Graham M, Jawrani N, Chikka A. Extraosseous talotarsal stabilization using HyProCure in adults: a 5-year retrospective follow-up. J Foot Ankle Surg 2012; 51:23–9.
44. Bernasconi A, Argyropoulos M, Patel S, et al. Subtalar arthroereisis as an adjunct procedure improves forefoot abduction in stage IIb adult-acquired flatfoot deformity. Foot Ankle Spec 2020. 1938640020951031.
45. Shah NS, Needleman RL, Bokhari O, et al. 2013 subtalar arthroereisis survey the current practice patterns of members of the AOFAS. Foot Ankle Spec 2015;8(3): 180–5.
46. Aynardi M, Walley K, Hallam J, et al. Mid-term outcomes & complications following the use of an arthroereisis implant to aid in stage II flat-foot correction in adults: a case-control study. Foot Ankle Orthop 2017;2(3):122–30.
47. Kempland C, Greene G, Hallam J, et al. Short- to mid-term outcomes following the use of an arthroereisis implant as an adjunct for correction of flexible, acquired flatfoot deformity in adults. Foot Ankle Spec 2018;20(10):1–9.
48. Ceccarini P, Rinonapoli G, Gambaracci G, et al. The arthroereisis procedure in adult flexible flatfoot grade IIA due to insufficiency of posterior tibial tendon. Foot Ankle Surg 2018;24(4):359–64.
49. Corpuz M, Shofler D, Labovitz J, et al. Fracture of the talus as a complication of subtalar arthroereisis. J Foot Ankle Surg 2012;51(1):91–4.

50. Yasui Y, Tonogai I, Rosenbaum AJ, et al. Use of the arthroereisis screw with tendoscopic delivered platelet-rich plasma for early stage adult acquired flatfoot deformity. Int Orthop 2017;41(2):315–21.
51. Lui T. Spontaneous subtalar fusion: an irreversible complication of subtalar arthroereisis. J Foot Ankle Surg 2014;53(5):652–6.
52. Needleman R. Current topic review: subtalar arthroereisis for the correction of flexible flatfoot. Foot Ankle Int 2005;26:336–46.

Surgical Management of Musculotendinous Balance in the Progressive Collapsing Foot Deformity

The Role of Peroneal and Gastrocnemius Contracture

Philip Kaiser, MD*, Daniel Guss, MD, MBA

KEYWORDS

• Progressive collapsing foot deformity • Flexible flatfoot • Tendon balancing
• Gastrocnemius contracture

KEY POINTS

- Progressive collapsing foot deformity (PCFD) is a multiplanar foot deformity comprised of hindfoot valgus, forefoot abduction, forefoot varus, and collapse or hypermobility of the medial column
- Clinical history and physical examination focused on hindfoot alignment, the variable degree of gastrocnemius contracture, medial column hypermobility, and possible pain generators (ie, torn posterior tibialis tendon and subfibular impingement) remain paramount to developing a focused and appropriate treatment plan.
- Weight-bearing radiographs and computed tomography can be helpful diagnostic tools to assess foot and hindfoot alignment, degenerative changes, and areas of bony impingement. In certain cases, magnetic resonance imaging can assess preoperative tendon quality and tearing.
- Surgical correction in cases of PCFD requires a tailored approach for each individual patient. Bony procedures, including osteotomies/realignments (calcaneal osteotomy, lateral column lengthening, and Cotton osteotomy) often are combined with tendon transfers (ie, flexor digitorum longus transfer to the medial navicular) to improve hindfoot alignment, arch height, dynamic inversion strength, and medial column stability. In select cases of PCDF, joint-sacrificing procedures, such as arthrodesis (midfoot/hindfoot), are combined with tendon rebalancing.

Department of Orthopaedic Surgery, Foot and Ankle Service, Harvard Medical School, Massachusetts General Hospital and Newton-Wellesley Hospital, MGH-NWH Foot & Ankle Center, Building 52, Suite 1150, 40 2nd Avenue, Waltham, MA 02451, USA
* Corresponding author.
E-mail address: pkaiser@mgh.harvard.edu

Foot Ankle Clin N Am 26 (2021) 559–575
https://doi.org/10.1016/j.fcl.2021.06.005 foot.theclinics.com

INTRODUCTION

Progressive collapsing foot deformity (PCFD) is a complex foot deformity with varying degrees of hindfoot valgus, forefoot abduction, forefoot varus, and collapse or hypermobility of the medial column.[1] The term PCFD replaces the historical conflation of adult acquired flatfoot deformity (AAFD) and posterior tibial tendon dysfunction (PTTD), whose titular focus on the posterior tibial tendon (PTT) underrepresents that numerous contributors to a collapsing foot, be they bony, soft tissue, or host-related.[1,2] Many cases are multifactorial involving arthritis and deformity to the midfoot or ankle without rupture or dysfunction of the PTT. This updated nomenclature was proposed in a consensus statement by a group of international orthopedic foot and ankle experts in November 2019 and published in *Foot & Ankle International* in August 2020. It aimed to incorporate the evolving understanding of PCFD into a standardized nomenclature to be used for future research and reporting on this topic.[1,2]

The original 3-stage classification systems for PTTD was proposed by Johnson and Strom in 1989[3] (**Table 1**), and later elaborated on by Myerson in 1996, and by Bluman and colleageus, in 2007, to involve a subdivided fourth stage (**Table 2**) of supple tibiotalar valgus (stage IVa) and rigid tibiotalar valgus (stage IVb).[4,5]

PCFD encapsulates the multifactorial nature of the deformity. Flexible or rigid deformity of the ankle, subtalar, transverse tarsal, naviculocuneiform, and tarsometatarsal (TMT) joints as well as gastrocnemius-soleus complex (GSC) contracture; ligamentous insufficiencies involving medial and plantar structures, such as the deltoid, interosseus talocalcaneal, and spring ligaments; and the plantar fascia attenuation now all have been recognized as contributors or sequelae of PCFD.[6,7] The new PCFD classification put forth by the consensus group comprehensively stratifies deformity class by type/location (**Table 3**) and stage by the degree of flexibility at the affected joint (flexible vs rigid) to better describe this complex 3-dimensional deformity.[1] Unlike prior classification systems, the PCFD classification does not imply progression of deformity through the various classes, many of which may coexist in a given patient but nonetheless are anatomically distinct.

As with many foot and ankle disorders, careful history, physical examination, weight-bearing radiographs, and judicious use of advanced imaging remain the cornerstones toward diagnosing PCFD and developing a patient-specific treatment plan. A patient's barefoot gait should be assessed alongside a patient's ability to single toe raise, with an eye toward reconstitution of hindfoot valgus into varus when doing so.[8] Passive range of motion of the ankle and hindfoot should be assessed and compared with the contralateral side, wherein decrease in motion may represent substantial deformity, arthritis, or even coalition, especially in the pediatric or young adult population.[9] Additionally, standing arch height, gastrocnemius contracture with Silfverskiöld testing, and assessment of first ray hypermobility are important components of the physical examination and complement radiographic investigation.[10] Identifying a patient's deformity flexibility (PCFD stage) and patterns (PCFD classes) on both physical examination and imaging is critical toward successful treatment, understanding that there may be multiple contributors, as discussed previously.

This review focuses on the management of muscle and tendon balance in the collapsing foot. Although the most recent literature and research with regard to soft tissue balancing in the collapsing foot still is intertwined with the PTTD classification system, the general principles and concepts of tendon and muscle balance in PCFD are unchanged and remain incredibly important to successful surgical reconstruction. The reader is challenged to interpret the findings of this review in the new lens of PCFD classes and stages. Future studies will examine the interplay between

Table 1
Johnson and Strom classification, 1989[3]

Variable	Stage I—Mild, Medial Pain	Stage II—Moderate, Medial Pain	Stage III—Severe, Medial, and Lateral Pain
Examination	Mild swelling and tenderness	Moderate swelling and	Not much swelling but marked
Swelling and tenderness	Along PTT	Tenderness along PTT	Tenderness along PTT
Heel rise test	Mild weakness	Marked weakness	Marked weakness
Too many toes sign	Absent	Present	Present
Deformity	Absent	Present (flexible)	Present (fixed)
Pathologic features	Normal tendon length paratendinitis	Elongated with longitudinal tears	Disrupted with visible tears
Images	No changes	Gross deformity	Deformity and diffuse arthritic changes
Treatment	Conservative, tenosynovectomy	FDL transfer	Triple arthrodesis

Reproduced with permission from FAI August 2020 article: Classification and Nomenclature: Progressive Collapsing Foot Deformity. Myerson et al.

tendon and muscle balance with joint-sparing procedures, such as ligament reconstructions (deltoid and spring), osteotomies/realignments (calcaneal osteotomy, lateral column lengthening, and Cotton osteotomy), and joint-sacrificing procedures, such as arthrodesis (midfoot/hindfoot/ankle) and even total ankle replacement in PCFD, to create better treatment algorithms for each specific deformity.[11]

GASTROCNEMIUS-SOLEUS COMPLEX

The role of lengthening of the GSC in PCFD has been studied widely and debated. Over time, a hindfoot valgus positioning may lead to contracture of the GSC.[12] On the other hand, the correlate also may be true, wherein a contracted GSC may progressively accentuate a hindfoot valgus in a chicken and egg manner. Accordingly, restoration of hindfoot coronal alignment is one of the key principles in treatment of PCFD.[13] Critically, bipedal motion relies on relative knee extension and ankle dorsiflexion, especially through the second rocker of gait.[14] A GSC contracture limits ankle dorsiflexion, precipitating heel elevation and an increased load transfer to the forefoot and medial column. Therefore, although the GSC anatomically spans the knee, ankle, and subtalar joints, its contribution to arch collapse in the setting of contracture may extend well distal to its attachment sites, including the transverse tarsal and midfoot joints. Any limitation on ankle dorsiflexion places increased pressure on the forefoot and midfoot from the midstance phase to push-off, which can further weaken and stretch the medial column stabilizers, such as the spring and superficial deltoid ligaments, PTT, and capsular ligaments (**Fig. 1**).[12,15–17] Arangio and colleagues[18] studied 22 patients with PCFD with unilateral Achilles contracture by physical examination and found significantly increased radiographic talonavicular uncoverage (**Fig. 2**), increased talo–first metatarsal angle, increased tibiocalcaneal angle (**Fig. 3**), and increased valgus hindfoot alignment (**Fig. 4**) on the laterality of an Achilles contracture.

Table 2
Bluman and colleagues' classification, 2007[4]

Stage	Substage	Most Characteristic Clinical Findings	Most Characteristic Radiographic Findings	Treatment
I	A	Normal anatomy Tenderness along PTT	Normal	Immobilization, NSAIDs, cryotherapy Orthoses Tenosynovectomy ± Systemic disease-specific pharmacotherapy
	B	Normal anatomy Tenderness along PTT	Normal	Immobilization, NSAIDs, cryotherapy Orthoses Tenosynovectomy
	C	Slight HF valgus Tenderness along PTT	Slight HF valgus	Immobilization, NSAIDs, cryotherapy Orthoses Tenosynovectomy
II	AI	Supple HF valgus Flexible forefoot vanjs Possible pain along PTT	HF valgus Meary line disruption Loss of calcaneal pitch	Orthoses Medial displacement calcaneal osteotomy TAL or Strayer and FDL transfer if deformity corrects only with ankle plantarflexion
	A2	Supple HF valgus Fixed forefoot varus Possible pain along PTT	HF valgus Meary line disruption Loss of calcaneal pitch	Orthoses Medial displacement calcaneal osteotomy and FDL transfer Cotton osteoectomy
	B	Supple HF valgus Forefoot abduction	HF valgus Talonavicular uncovering Forefoot abduction	Orthoses Medial displacement calcaneal osteotomy and FDL transfer Lateral column lengthening
	C	Supple HF valgus Fixed forefoot varus Medal column instability First ray	HF valgus First TMT joint plantar gapping	Medial displacement calcaneal osteotomy and FDL transfer Cotton osteotomy

(*continued on next page*)

Table 2
(*continued*)

Stage	Substage	Most Characteristic Clinical Findings	Most Characteristic Radiographic Findings	Treatment
		dorsiflexion with HF correction Sinus tarsi pain		or medial column fusion
III	A	Rigid HF valgus Pain in sinus tarsi	Subtalar joint space loss HF valgus Angle of Gissane sclerosis	Custom bracing if not operative candidate Triple arthrodesis
	B	Rigid HF valgus Forefoot abduction Pain in sinus tarsi	Subtalar joint space loss HF valgus Angle of Gissane sclerosis Forefoot abduction	Custom bracing if not operative candidate Triple arthrodesis ± lateral column lengthening
IV	A	Supple tibiotalar valgus	Tibiotalar valgus HF valgus	Surgery for HF valgus and associated deformity Deltoid reconstruction
	B	Rigid tibiotalar valgus	Tibiotalar valgus HF valgus	TTC fusion or pantalar fusion

Abbreviations: HF, hindfoot; NSAIDs, nonsteroidal anti-inflammatory drugs; TTC, tibiotalocalcaneal.

Reproduced with permission from FAI August 2020 article: Classification and Nomenclature: Progressive Collapsing Foot Deformity. Myerson et al.

The historic distinction between an isolated gastrocnemius contracture versus a contracture of the combined GSC is based on clinical examination with a Silfverskiöld test.[25] A discrepancy of 10° or greater in passive ankle dorsiflexion with the knee bent versus extended suggests a contracture of the gastrocnemius muscle whereas no change can be attributed to a GSC contracture.[15,17] Additionally, at least 10° to 15° of ankle dorsiflexion is typically necessary for normal gait and ascending stairs.[26,27] The GSC can be lengthened at different anatomic locations, depending on the degree of contracture as well as whether it results from a combined gastrocnemius and soleus contracture versus an isolated gastrocnemius contracture.[28] Anatomic zones for doing so include the following: zone 1, which spans the extent to which the medial gastrocnemius muscle belly is anatomically distinct from the soleus; zone 2, which extends from the distal extent of the gastrocnemius muscle to the distal extent of the soleus muscle and where the gastrocnemius aponeurosis can no longer be separated bluntly from the soleus fascia; and zone 3, which extends from the end of the soleus muscle to the Achilles insertion.[28]

In cases of combined gastrocnemius and soleus contracture (ie, Achilles contracture) the Hoke percutaneous hemitransection often is performed in Zone 3.[15,29,30] Alternatively a double hemitransection or an open Z-lengthening may be performed, although the open approach often is not as compatible with concomitant hindfoot

Table 3
Consensus group classification of progressive collapsing foot deformity

	Stage of the Deformity	
Stage I (Flexible)		Stage II (Rigid)
Types of Deformity (Classes—Isolated or Combined)	**Deformity Type/Location**	**Consistent Clinical/Radiographic Findings**
Class A	Hindfoot valgus deformity	Hindfoot valgus alignment Increased hindfoot moment arm, hindfoot alignment angle, foot and ankle offset
Class B	Midfoot/forefoot abduction deformity	Decreased talar head coverage Increased talonavicular coverage angle Presence of sinus tarsi impingement
Class C	Forefoot varus deformity/medial column instability	Increased talo–first metatarsal angle Plantar gapping first TMT joint/NC joints Clinical forefoot varus
Class D	Peritalar subluxation/dislocaoon	Significant subtalar joint subluxation/subfibular impingement
Class E	Ankle instability	Valgus tilting of the ankle joint

Abbreviation: NC, naviculocuneiform.

Reproduced with permission from FAI August 2020 article: Classification and Nomenclature: Progressive Collapsing Foot Deformity. Myerson et al.

or midfoot procedures and generally is reserved for more significant posterior ankle contractures.[31]

If limited ankle dorsiflexion is attributed to isolated gastrocnemius contracture, multiple procedures exist to selectively lengthen the gastrocnemius, but the most commonly described procedure is the Strayer (zone 1), which is the authors' preferred technique.[32] In this procedure, a posteromedial incision is performed and the gastrocnemius fascia selectively transected while leaving the soleus fascia untouched. Care must be taken to protect the sural nerve which courses posteriorly.

Firth and colleagues[28] conducted a study of the surgical anatomy and various surgical techniques for GSC lengthening under controlled loading in cadavers whose preservation was performed with the ankle in equinus generating a fixed contracture. They explored the Bauman, and Strayer (all zone 1); Vulpius and Baker (all zone 2), and White and Hoke (all zone 3) procedures (**Fig. 5**).[29,30,32–39] They found that the more distal the procedure, the more it was able to lengthen the GSC. A Strayer procedure was on average able to achieve approximately 1 cm of lengthening and did so in a relatively linear fashion as the load was increased from 0 kg to 40 kg. The Hoke procedure, in contrast, was able to lengthen to approximately 3.5 cm, but they described a "slide point" when lengthening approached 2 cm, beyond which the Achilles may rupture, leading to an uncontrolled lengthening and ankle dorsiflexion. Care, therefore, must be taken to avoid excessive loads when performing the more distal and powerful Achilles lengthening procedures.

GSC lengthening in PCFD is one of the keys to restoring hindfoot coronal alignment, and often it is combined with medialization of the calcaneus. In a recent study, Chang and colleagues[12] conducted a systematic review evaluating the effect of gastrocnemius recession (GR) and tendo-Achilles lengthening (TAL) in PCFD. Ten level IV

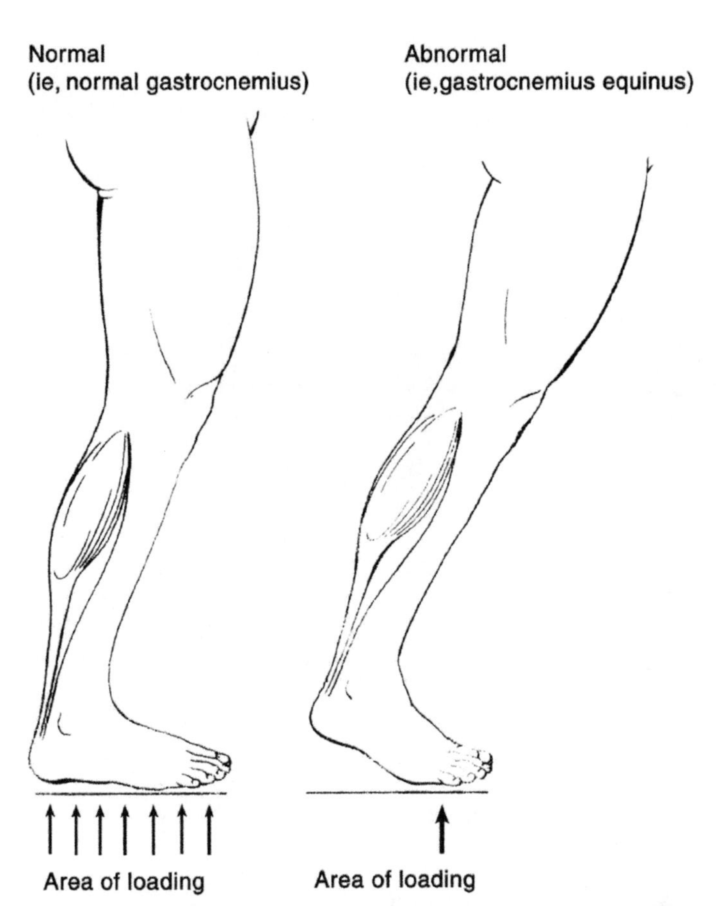

Fig. 1. Graphically depicted load patterns during gait. This illustration demonstrates the anticipated variation in forefoot and midfoot loading during late–stance phase gait between normal subjects (ie, those with normal gastrocnemius length) and patients with an abnormal (ie, contracted) gastrocnemius length. (*From* DiGiovanni CW, Kuo R, Tejwani N, et al. Isolated gastrocnemius tightness. J Bone Joint Surg 2002;84:968; **Reproduced with permission** from the Journal of Bone and Joint Surgery.)

studies were included, comprised of 79 GRs and 111 TALs. They determined that no study in the literature directly compared patients who underwent a GR for PCFD with those who did not nor did any study compare the effects of performing a TAL in place of a GR with regard to ankle range of motion and plantar flexion strength. Studies included in the review demonstrated improvements in ankle range of motion and plantar flexion strength after GR in cases of PCFD correction. Saxena and Widtfeldt demonstrated endoscopic GR helped improved ankle dorsiflexion from −9.3° preoperatively to 3.7° postoperatively, and Kou and colleagues showed improvement in plantarflexion strength from an average of 14.0 Nm preoperatively to 22.4 Nm postoperatively in patients undergoing GR as a component to PCFD correction.[40,41] Seven studies (3 using GR and 4 using TAL) demonstrated radiographic improvement in the postoperative lateral TMT angle, and 3 studies reported improvement in postoperative lateral calcaneal inclination angle (2 using GR and 1 using TAL). All GSC lengthening procedures were performed, however, in combination with various other

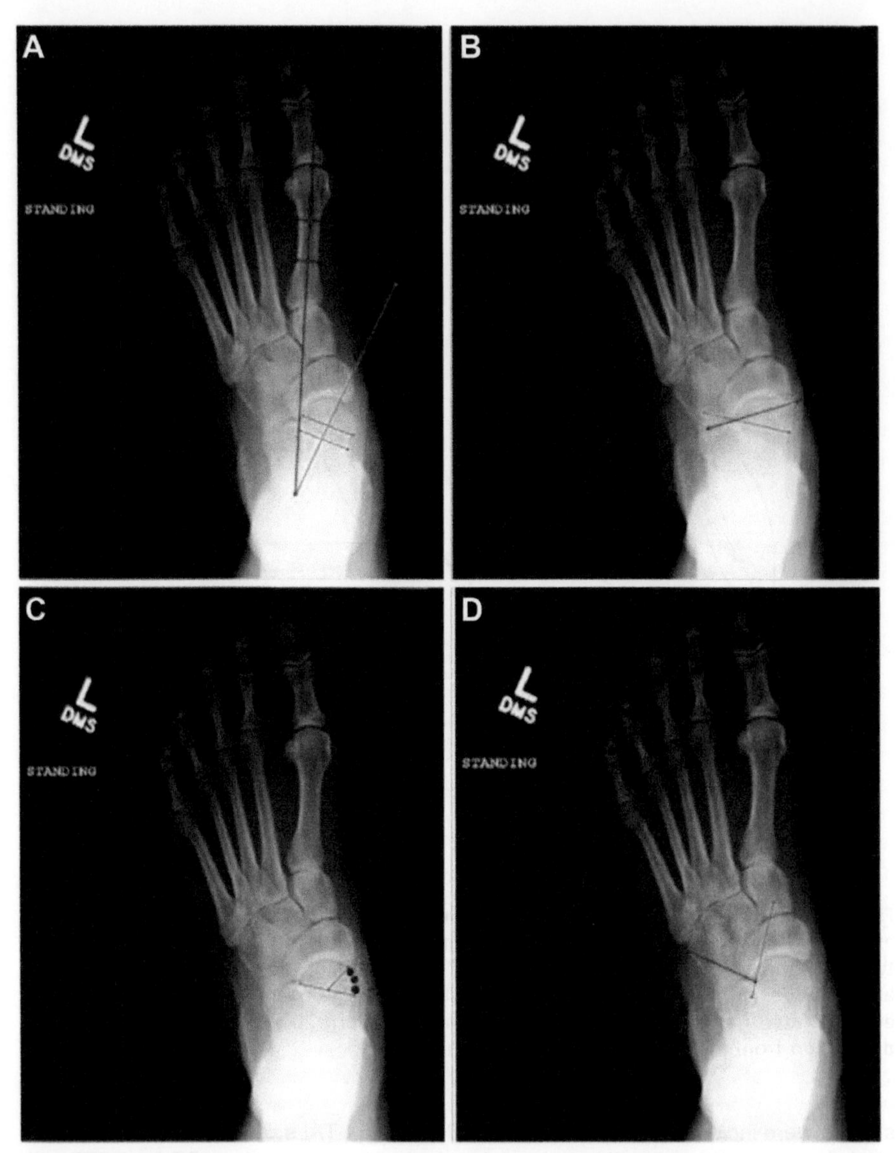

Fig. 2. Anteroposterior foot radiographs showing the anterior talo–first metatarsal angle, the talonavicular coverage angle, the talonavicular uncoverage percentage, and the lateral incongruency angle.[19–21] (*A*) Anteroposterior view of the anterior talo–first metatarsal angle, which is the angle between the longitudinal axes of the talus and first metatarsal (normal, 0° to 20°). (*B*) The talonavicular coverage angle, which is the angle between 2 lines, 1 between the medial and lateral articular margins of the talus and 1 between the medial and lateral articular margins of the navicular (normal<7°). (*C*) The talonavicular uncoverage percentage, in which small circles represent the amount of talar head uncovered by the navicular (normal, 10% to 30%). (*D*) The lateral incongruency angle, which is the angle between 2 lines, 1 connecting the lateral articular surface of the talus and navicular and 1 between the lateral articular surface of the talus and the lateral talar neck at its narrowest part (normal, 5° ± 26°). (*From* Abousayed et all JBJS review article - **reproduced with permission** from JBJS reviews Abousayed MM, Alley MC, Shakked R, Rosenbaum AJ. Adult-Acquired Flatfoot Deformity: Etiology, Diagnosis, and Management. JBJS Rev. 2017;5(8):e7. https://doi.org/10.2106/JBJS.RVW.16.00116.)

corrective foot procedures (ie, flexor digitorum longus [FDL] transfer, medializing calcaneal osteotomy, and hindfoot arthrodesis) in cases of PCFD.

Within the systematic review, complications rates typically were low. In patients undergoing GR, there was a 9% complication rate, which included neuritis of sural nerve (3%), decreased plantar flexor power (3%), and stiffness (4%). In patients undergoing TAL, there was a 10% complication rate, which included neuritis of sural nerve (8%) and Achilles tendon rupture (2%). The review concluded that the available evidence suggests GSC contracture is a common finding in PCFD and both GR and TAL, in combination with other corrective procedures, may improve postoperative radiographic parameters with a relatively low complication rate and improvements in postoperative range of motion and plantar flexion power. Included studies in the review, however, were retrospective and generally of lower quality. Therefore, the direct impact of GR and TAL on clinical and radiographic outcomes remains difficult to separate from the concomitant procedures that patients undergo in PCFD correction. Despite this, the authors believe there is strong evidence that GSC contracture plays an important role in PCFD. Clinical equinus should be evaluated in all cases of PCFD and, if present in the authors' practice, GSC lengthening performed to help correct hindfoot position and deformity—often combined with a medializing calcaneal osteotomy to shift the axis of the Achilles tendon.[42]

FLEXOR TENDONS AND INVERSION

The new PCFD classification does not negate the contribution of the PTT to medial column stability but rather attempts to explicitly highlight the other anatomic soft tissue structures that can be more involved frequently and more severely than the tendon itself.[1,6,7] The PTT functions to plantarflex and invert the subtalar joint thereby locking the transverse tarsal joints to generate a rigid platform during heel rise and enable push off during gait.[19,42] In PTTD, when explicitly interpreted to describe a malfunctioning PTT, the hindfoot remains relatively everted during the gait cycle. With the hindfoot in valgus, the forefoot must, in turn, develop a compensatory varus, leading to the medial collapse often seen in PCFD.[42] An extended array of medial soft tissues structures often are involved, including the superomedial and inferomedial bands of the spring, talocalcaneal interosseous, anterior component of the superficial deltoid, plantar metatarsal, and plantar naviculocuneiform ligaments, with the spring ligament complex affected most commonly.[6] Numerous studies have focused on the role of the reconstitution of PTT function with an associated hindfoot realignment. A review by Myerson and colleagues[42] of 129 patients with a painful flexible PCFD evaluated at an average of 5.2 years postoperatively and treated with a FDL tendon transfer into the navicular and medializing calcaneal osteotomy. They concluded that in cases of PCFD due largely in part to PTTD and with a flexible deformity, a medializing calcaneal osteotomy and transfer of the FDL to the navicular, along with other indicated adjunct procedures (GSC lengthening and limited medial column fusion), yielded excellent functional results with high patient satisfaction. Much of the literature similarly focuses on a tendon transfer to reconstitute PTT function while buttressing and protecting this transfer with a bony realignment.

In a recent review article by Dunham and colleagues[9] discusses the historic norm of routinely excising the PTT in cases of flexible PTTD and argue that the PTT should be assessed critically in each case and possibly débrided and/or repaired when indicated. They contend the PPT was mischaracterized as the main "pain generator" in PTTD, which led to its routine excision in the past. Furthermore, they argue that tendon excision rarely is first-line treatment of other areas of pain and deformity in the body.

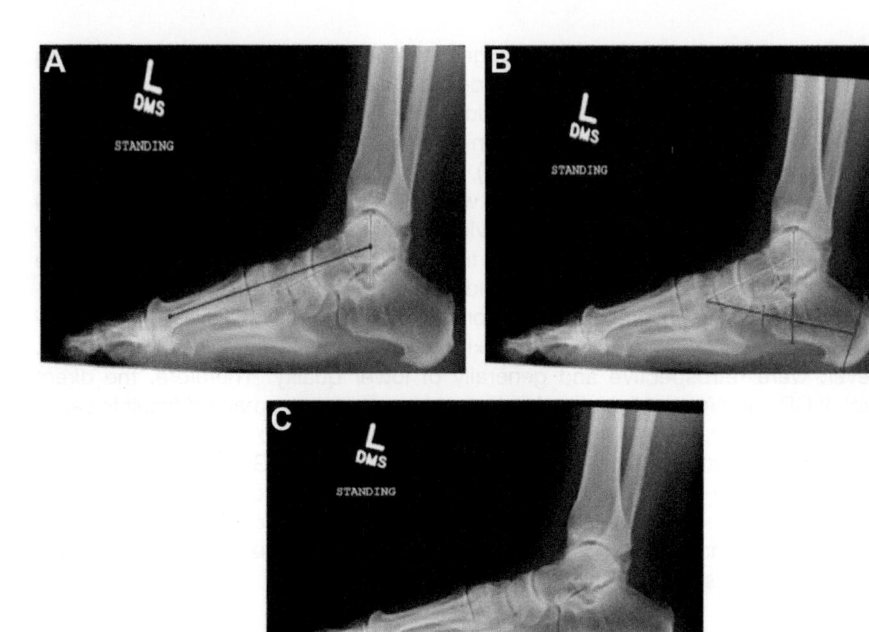

Fig. 3. Lateral foot radiographs showing the lateral talo–first metatarsal angle, the lateral talocalcaneal angle, and the calcaneal pitch.[19,22,23] (*A*) The lateral talo–first metatarsal (Meary) angle, which is the angle between the longitudinal axes of the talus and first metatarsal (normal, $0 \pm 4^\circ$). (*B*) The lateral talocalcaneal angle, which is the angle between a line bisecting the talus and a line bisecting the calcaneus (normal, 25° to 45°). (*C*) Calcaneal pitch, which is the angle between a line drawn along the most inferior part of the calcaneus and the supporting surface or the transverse plane (normal, 10° to 20°). (*From* Abousayed et all JBJS review article - **reproduced with permission** from JBJS reviews Abousayed MM, Alley MC, Shakked R, Rosenbaum AJ. Adult-Acquired Flatfoot Deformity: Etiology, Diagnosis, and Management. JBJS Rev. 2017;5(8):e7. https://doi.org/10.2106/JBJS.RVW.16.00116.)

Although studies have shown equivalent good results with regard to pain relief with PTT resection or the tendon being left in situ,[43] the review argues that in their experience, PTT retention may lead to better functional results and gait as retained healthy and springy PTT add power to the FDL tendon transfer and may prevent against long-term progressive foot collapse. The authors follow a similar practice of retention of the PTT except in cases of appearing unsalvageable or thought to be the primary pain generator. Additionally, in cases of flexible flatfoot reconstruction with involvement of the PTT, the authors invariably transfer the FDL to augment the PTT or replace it in cases of resection. Valderrabano and colleagues[44] demonstrated that surgical reconstruction of the completely ruptured PTT (end-to-end anastomosis or side-to-side augmentation with the FDL) led to "excellent" clinical outcomes in 12 of 14 patients and postoperative MRI demonstrated an intact PTT in all patients. In this study, the PTT was excised only in cases of substantially torn, fibrotic, or demonstrated limited excursion and retention if the tendon appeared healthy and maintained springiness. Other studies have demonstrated the PTT excision and FDL transfer (along with medializing calcaneal osteotomy) leads to FDL hypertrophy and complete PTT fatty degeneration but retention of the PTT leads to some muscle preservation and ability to power hindfoot inversion.[45]

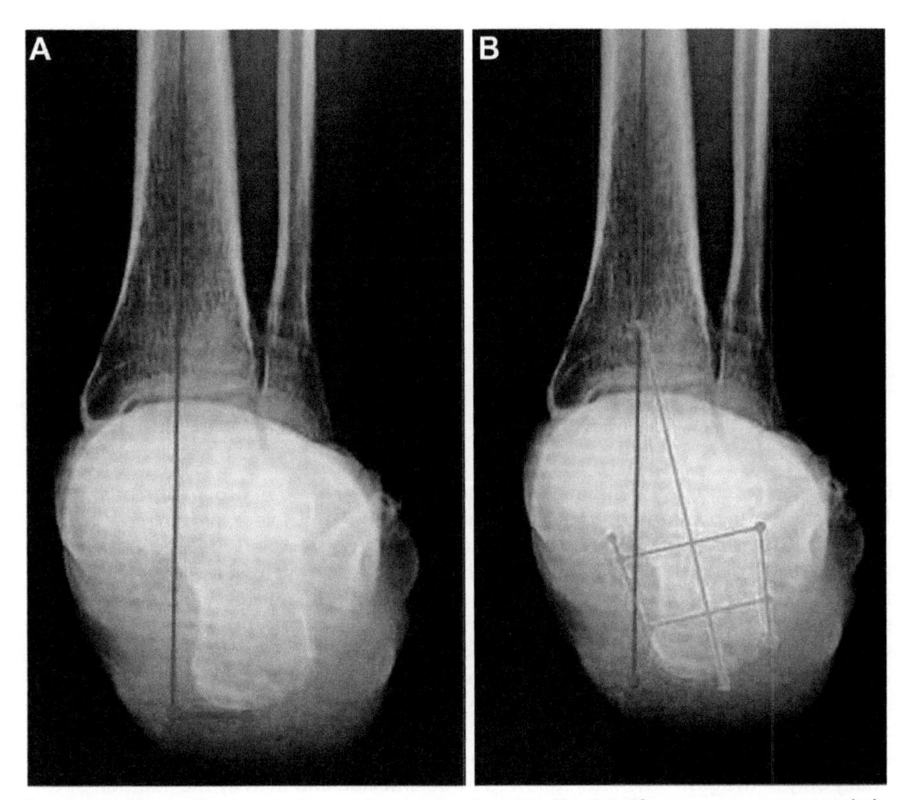

Fig. 4. Hindfoot alignment view radiographs showing the hindfoot moment arm and the hindfoot alignment angle.[19,24] (*A*) The hindfoot moment arm, which is the shortest distance between the longitudinal axis of the tibia and the most inferior part of the calcaneus (normal averages 3.2 mm in varus). (*B*) The hindfoot alignment angle, which is the angle between the longitudinal axis of the tibia and the axis of the calcaneal tuberosity. The axis of the calcaneal tuberosity is defined as the bisector of 2 transverse lines connecting the medial and lateral osseous contours of the calcaneus (normal, 5.6° ± 5.4°). (*From* Abousayed et all JBJS review article - **reproduced with permission** from JBJS reviews Abousayed MM, Alley MC, Shakked R, Rosenbaum AJ. Adult-Acquired Flatfoot Deformity: Etiology, Diagnosis, and Management. JBJS Rev. 2017;5(8):e7. https://doi.org/10.2106/JBJS.RVW.16.00116.)

PERONEAL TENDONS AND EVERSION

Deformity in the foot and ankle can be precipitated either by an overstretch or an overpull of a muscular attachment. Although much has been written about the contribution of attenuated hindfoot inverters toward PCFD, much less has been written about the role of overactive everters. The peroneus brevis muscle is the primary evertor of the foot, which opposes the PTT.[46] In some cases of PCFD, muscle imbalance due to prolonged hindfoot valgus, eversion, and forefoot abduction may lead to functional shortening and overpull of the laterally based peroneal tendons, especially the peroneal brevis, which can exacerbate the underlying deformity.[47] In a cadaver study comparing the eversion effect of the peroneal longus and peroneal brevis, Otis and colleagues[48] demonstrated that in a simulated gait model the loaded peroneal brevis rotated the navicular 2° more than the peroneus longus. Additionally, at the subtalar joint, the peroneus brevis loading resulted in 1° more calcaneus valgus compared

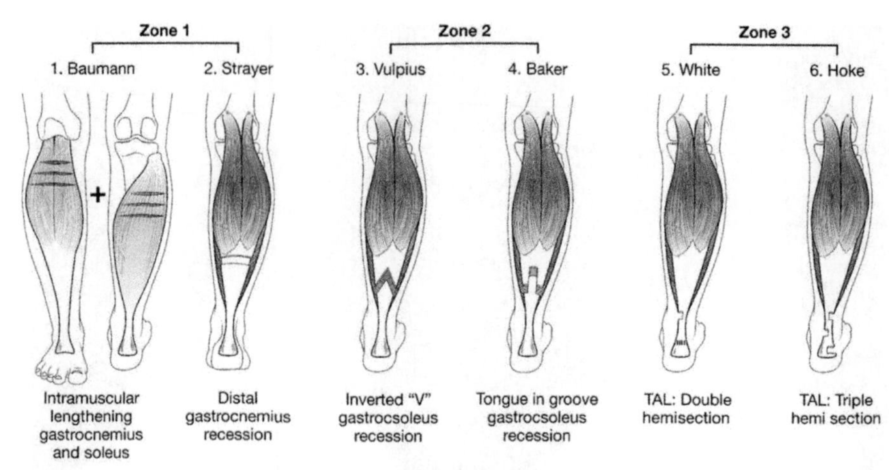

Fig. 5. The 6 procedures investigated in randomized trials, listed in order from proximal to distal, were intramuscular tenotomy of the gastrocnemius and soleus, as described by Baumann and Koch; distal GR, as described by Strayer; GSC (gastrocsoleus) recessions described by Vulpius and by Baker; and TAL by double hemisection, as described by White, and by triple hemisection, as described by Hoke. Note that the tongue-in-groove cut was performed as described by Baker but sutures were not inserted. The Strayer procedure was performed as a single transverse division of the gastrocnemius aponeurosis, in accordance with the original description of the procedure; following application of the dorsiflexion force and testing, a single transverse cut then was made in the underlying soleus fascia. This procedure sometimes is referred to a modified Strayer procedure or a Strayer procedure plus soleal fascial lengthening. The Baumann procedure also was performed as a series of cuts located initially only in the gastrocnemius, followed by dorsiflexion and then by the addition of cuts in the soleus fascia and repeated dorsiflexion. The midline raphe was divided during both the Baker and Vulpius GSC recessions. (**Reproduced with permission** from Firth GB, McMullan M, Chin T, et al. Lengthening of the gastrocnemius-soleus complex: an anatomical and biomechanical study in human cadavers. J Bone Joint Surg Am 2013;95(16):1489–1496.)

to the peroneus longus. Given its function as the strongest antagonist to the PTT, the role sof the peroneus brevis and as the peroneal longus are important to consider in rebalancing cases of PCFD due to PTTD.

Although distinct from PCFD, peroneal spastic flatfoot, a rare condition resulting in a painful rigid valgus hindfoot deformity due to peroneal muscle spasm, illustrates the important role of the peroneal tendons in functional hindfoot muscle imbalance. Multiple case reports exist in the literature of peroneal spastic flatfoot, without bony coalition, having been successfully treated with botulinum toxin injection and casting, leading to resolution of the deformity.[49–51] To better understand the role of the peroneal tendon function toward precipitating hindfoot valgus and pes planus deformity, Mizel and colleagues[46] evaluated 10 patients with traumatic, complete common peroneal nerve palsies who previously had undergone transfer of the PTT to the midfoot. Despite transfer of the PTT, in the absence of peroneal tendon function, patients did not demonstrated clinical or weight-bearing radiographic changes consistent with PCFD nor did Harris mat study demonstrate loss of the longitudinal arch compared with the contralateral foot. The investigators argue that PCFD likely requires a functioning peroneal brevis tendon to exacerbate deformity and that future surgical treatments may better address the dynamic functional imbalance caused by the peroneus brevis tendon through release or partial weakening of this PTT antagonist.

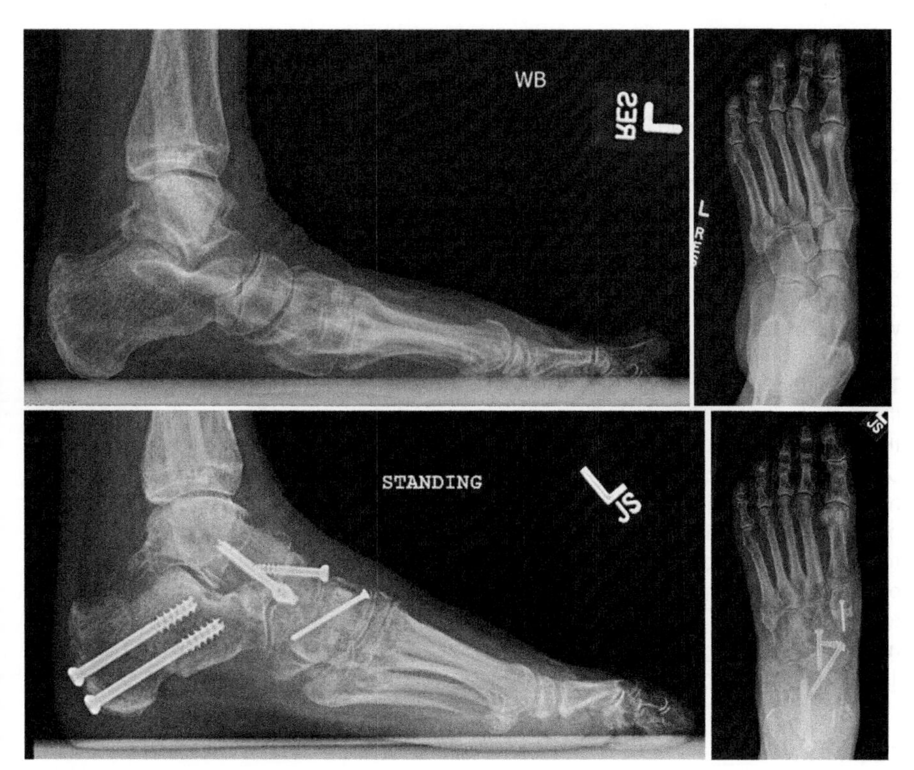

Fig. 6. First ray hypermobility stabilized with an opening wedge osteotomy to the medial cuneiform. Note the resolution of plantar gapping and first TMT subluxation. (*A*). (*top left*) Pre-operative lateral foot radiograph. (*B*) (*top right*) Pre-operative AP foot radiograph. (*C*) (*bottom left*) Post-operative lateral foot radiograph. (*D*) (*bottom right*) Post-operative AP foot radiograph.

Although FDL tendon transfer remains the most common tendon transfer in cases of PCFD due to degeneration of the PTT and weakness for inversion, addition of a peroneus brevis transfer could be considered.[52] By transferring the peroneus brevis to the navicular or medial side of the hindfoot, a potentially significant deforming force in PCFD is redirected to become an invertor of the hindfoot, helping to rebalance the foot. Song and Deland[52] studied 13 patients who underwent peroneus brevis tendon transfer in cases of PCFD where they felt the FDL tendon was particularly small (normally only one-half to one-third the size of the PTT) or previously was harvested. They compared the patients to age-matched controls who underwent a standard FDL tendon transfer without addition of peroneus brevis tendon transfer with an averaged follow-up of 21 months. Their results showed both groups did well, with an average American Orthopaedic Foot and Ankle Society score of 75.8 in the peroneus brevis tendon transfer group compared with 71.5 for the standard control group. Additionally, inversion and eversion strengths in the peroneus brevis tendon transfer group were rated good or excellent in 12 of 13 patients. The investigators concluded that peroneus brevis tendon transfer can be used to augment the FDL tendon transfer in cases of PCFD when the FDL is small, with good clinical outcomes and without compromising eversion strength.

The role of the peroneal tendons in PCFD likely is overlooked and almost certainly understudied, especially relative to the amount of biomechanical and clinical research devoted to the role of the FDL tendon transfer and medializing calcaneal osteotomy during correction of flexible PCFD. In cases of PCFD with hindfoot valgus, the contribution of the peroneal tendons as a deforming force requiring lengthening or rebalancing should be analyzed critically. Additionally, the peroneal brevis is a viable adjunct tendon transfer to the medial hindfoot to aid inversion force when the FDL tendon is small.

The contribution of the peroneus longus tendon toward plantar flexing the first ray also must be considered given that the first TMT joint frequently is involved in the deformity and medial column instability. Traditionally, surgical treatment of PCFD with associated first ray hypermobility often incorporates a first TMT fusion, preferentially resecting the inferior aspect of the medial cuneiform to plantarflex the first ray. The extent of plantarflexion achievable is controlled by the amount of the plantar cuneiform that can be resected. Conversely, the ability to add a bony or implant wedge through an opening Cotton osteotomy allows significant dorsal lengthening. In cases of first ray hypermobility, an opening wedge may be able to stabilize an otherwise hypermobile TMT joint by stretching the soft tissue attachments, including the peroneus longus (**Fig. 6**). There also may be a role for peroneus brevis to peroneus longus tendon transfer in cases of PCFD with hindfoot valgus to eliminate the primary evertor of the foot while simultaneously strengthening the peroneus longus, which contributes to the medial arch of the foot. Although the authors do not routinely perform a peroneus brevis to longus transfer in cases of PCFD, it is an intriguing concept that may 1 day become standard in flexible PCFD reconstructions and warrants further study.

SUMMARY

In summary, management of muscle and tendon balancing in the PCFD is an evolving area of research. The new terminology and classification system of PCFD, which replaces PTTD and AAFD, better accounts for the different etiologies and varying degrees of hindfoot valgus, forefoot abduction, forefoot varus, peritalar subluxation, and medial column collapse or hypermobility that comprise a flatfoot. Research related to muscle and tendon balancing in the setting of PCFD relies mostly on the prior study of PTTD but remains pertinent to surgical correction of flexible cases of PCFD with at least some degree of PTT compromise. GSC contracture is an important component of hindfoot valgus and the need for gastrocnemius or Achilles lengthening should be evaluated in each case. More distal procedures are better able to lengthen the GSC but with a likely trade off of heightened weakness, and care must be taken to not over-lengthen to the point of tendon failure. Failure of the PTT is studied more extensively than overpull of the peroneus brevis, but the latter also may have a contributing role in PCFD. The ability of the peroneus longus to plantarflex the first ray and shore up medial and plantar soft tissues also deserves additional study.

CLINICS CARE POINTS

- Many patients with PCFD can be managed successfully with nonoperative treatments, including orthotics, bracing, and physical therapy.
- History and physical examination focused on each patient's symptoms attributable to PCFD remain critically important to developing a customized treatment approach.

- Physical examination should include gait assessment, single toe raise, standing hindfoot alignment, and assessment of equinus, along with passive and active ankle and foot range of motion.
- Silfverskiöld testing should be performed in each patient to assess the contribution of the gastrocnemius with regard to equinus. The need for gastrocnemius or achilles lengthening should be evaluated in each case.
- At minimum, weight-bearing radiographs of the foot and ankle are required for each patient with PCFD.
- Surgical treatment of PCFD invariably involves a customized approach for each individual patient with consideration for bony osteotomies (ie, medializing calcaneal osteotomy and cotton osteotomy) and musculotendinous rebalancing (ie, gastrocnemius lengthening, FDL transfer to the medial navicular, and peroneus brevis to longus transfer).

DISCLOSURE

The authors have nothing to disclose.

REFERENCES

1. Myerson MS, Thordarson D, Johnson JE, et al. Classification and nomenclature: progressive collapsing foot deformity. Foot Ankle Int 2020;41(10):1271–6.
2. de Cesar Netto C, Deland JT, Ellis SJ. Guest editorial: expert consensus on adult-acquired flatfoot deformity. Foot Ankle Int 2020;41(10):1269–71.
3. Johnson KA, Strom DE. Tibialis posterior tendon dysfunction. Clin Orthop Relat Res 1989;239:196–206.
4. Bluman EM, Title CI, Myerson MS. Posterior tibial tendon rupture: a refined classification system. Foot Ankle Clin 2007;12(2):233–49, v.
5. Myerson MS. Adult acquired flatfoot deformity: treatment of dysfunction of the posterior tibial tendon. Instr Course Lect 1997;46:393–405.
6. de Cesar Netto C, Saito GH, Roney A, et al. Combined weightbearing CT and MRI assessment of flexible progressive collapsing foot deformity. Foot Ankle Surg 2020. https://doi.org/10.1016/j.fas.2020.12.003.
7. Deland JT, de Asla RJ, Sung I-H, et al. Posterior tibial tendon insufficiency: which ligaments are involved? Foot Ankle Int 2005;26(6):427–35.
8. Niki H, Ching RP, Kiser P, et al. The effect of posterior tibial tendon dysfunction on hindfoot kinematics. Foot Ankle Int 2001;22(4):292–300.
9. Dunham AM, de Cesar Netto C, Godoy-Santos AL, et al. Should it stay or should it go? Thinking critically about posterior tibial tendon excision in flatfoot correction. Tech Foot Ankle Surg 2019;18(4):166–73.
10. Myerson MS, Badekas A. Hypermobility of the first ray. Foot Ankle Clin 2000;5(3):469–84.
11. Sangeorzan BJ, Hintermann B, de Cesar Netto C, et al. Progressive collapsing foot deformity: consensus on goals for operative correction. Foot Ankle Int 2020;41(10):1299–302.
12. Chang SH, Abdelatif NMN, Netto CC, et al. The effect of gastrocnemius recession and tendo-achilles lengthening on adult acquired flatfoot deformity surgery: a systematic review. J Foot Ankle Surg 2020;59(6):1248–53.
13. Chan JY, Williams BR, Nair P, et al. The contribution of medializing calcaneal osteotomy on hindfoot alignment in the reconstruction of the stage II adult acquired flatfoot deformity. Foot Ankle Int 2013;34(2):159–66.

14. Anderson JG, Bohay DR, Eller EB, et al. Gastrocnemius recession. Foot Ankle Clin 2014;19(4):767–86.
15. Abdulmassih S, Phisitkul P, Femino JE, et al. Triceps surae contracture: implications for foot and ankle surgery. J Am Acad Orthop Surg 2013;21(7):398–407.
16. Aronow MS, Diaz-Doran V, Sullivan RJ, et al. The effect of triceps surae contracture force on plantar foot pressure distribution. Foot Ankle Int 2006;27(1):43–52.
17. DiGiovanni CW, Kuo R, Tejwani N, et al. Isolated gastrocnemius tightness. J Bone Joint Surg Am 2002;84(6):962–70.
18. Arangio G, Rogman A, Reed JF. Hindfoot alignment valgus moment arm increases in adult flatfoot with Achilles tendon contracture. Foot Ankle Int 2009; 30(11):1078–82.
19. Abousayed MM, Alley MC, Shakked R, et al. Adult-acquired flatfoot deformity: etiology, diagnosis, and management. JBJS Rev 2017;5(8):e7.
20. Chan JY, Greenfield ST, Soukup DS, et al. Contribution of lateral column lengthening to correction of forefoot abduction in stage IIb adult acquired flatfoot deformity reconstruction. Foot Ankle Int 2015;36(12):1400–11.
21. Chu IT, Myerson MS, Nyska M, et al. Experimental flatfoot model: the contribution of dynamic loading. Foot Ankle Int 2001;22(3):220–5.
22. Arangio GA, Wasser T, Rogman A. Radiographic comparison of standing medial cuneiform arch height in adults with and without acquired flatfoot deformity. Foot Ankle Int 2006;27(8):636–8.
23. Arangio GA, Wasser T, Rogman A. The use of standing lateral tibial-calcaneal angle as a quantitative measurement of Achilles tendon contracture in adult acquired flatfoot. Foot Ankle Int 2006;27(9):685–8.
24. Saltzman CL, el-Khoury GY. The hindfoot alignment view. Foot Ankle Int 1995; 16(9):572–6.
25. Singh D. Nils Silfverskiöld (1888-1957) and gastrocnemius contracture. Foot Ankle Surg 2013;19(2):135–8.
26. Adiputra LS, Parasuraman S, khan MKAA, et al. Bio mechanics of desending and ascending walk. Proced Computer Sci 2015;76:264–9.
27. Protopapadaki A, Drechsler WI, Cramp MC, et al. Hip, knee, ankle kinematics and kinetics during stair ascent and descent in healthy young individuals. Clin Biomech (Bristol, Avon) 2007;22(2):203–10.
28. Firth GB, McMullan M, Chin T, et al. Lengthening of the gastrocnemius-soleus complex: an anatomical and biomechanical study in human cadavers. J Bone Joint Surg Am 2013;95(16):1489–96.
29. Hatt RN, Lamphier TA. Triple hemisection: a simplified procedure for lengthening the Achilles tendon. N Engl J Med 1947;236(5):166–9.
30. Hoke M. An operation for the correction of extremely relaxed flat feet. J Bone Joint Surg Am 1931;13(4):773–83.
31. Graham HK, Fixsen JA. Lengthening of the calcaneal tendon in spastic hemiplegia by the White slide technique. A long-term review. J Bone Joint Surg Br 1988; 70(3):472–5.
32. Strayer LM. Recession of the gastrocnemius; an operation to relieve spastic contracture of the calf muscles. J Bone Joint Surg Am 1950;32-A(3):671–6.
33. Baker LD. Triceps surae syndrome in cerebral palsy; an operation to aid in its relief. AMA Arch Surg 1954;68(2):216–21.
34. Banks HH, Green WT. The correction of equinus deformity in cerebral palsy. J Bone Joint Surg Am 1958;40(6):1359–79.
35. Baumann J, Koch H. [Lengthening of the anterior aponeurosis of the gastrocnemius muscle]. Oper Orthop Traumatol 1989;1:254–8.

36. Herzenberg JE, Lamm BM, Corwin C, et al. Isolated recession of the gastrocnemius muscle: the Baumann procedure. Foot Ankle Int 2007;28(11):1154–9.
37. Lamm BM, Paley D, Herzenberg JE. Gastrocnemius soleus recession: a simpler, more limited approach. J Am Podiatric Med Assoc 2005;95(1):18–25.
38. Vulpius O, Stoffe A. Tenotomie der endschnen der mm. gastrocnemius el soleus. In: Orthopadische operationslehre. Stuttgart: Ferdinand Enke; 1913.
39. White J. Torsion of the achilles tendon; its surgical significance. Arch Surg 1943; 46(5):748–87.
40. Kou JX, Balasubramaniam M, Kippe M, et al. Functional results of posterior tibial tendon reconstruction, calcaneal osteotomy, and gastrocnemius recession. Foot Ankle Int 2012;33(7):602–11.
41. Saxena A, Widtfeldt A. Endoscopic gastrocnemius recession: preliminary report on 18 cases. J Foot Ankle Surg 2004;43(5):302–6.
42. Myerson MS, Badekas A, Schon LC. Treatment of stage II posterior tibial tendon deficiency with flexor digitorum longus tendon transfer and calcaneal osteotomy. Foot Ankle Int 2004;25(7):445–50.
43. Demetracopoulos CA, DeOrio JK, Easley ME, et al. Equivalent pain relief with and without resection of the posterior tibial tendon in adult flatfoot reconstruction. J Surg Orthop Adv 2014;23(4):184–8.
44. Valderrabano V, Hintermann B, Wischer T, et al. Recovery of the posterior tibial muscle after late reconstruction following tendon rupture. Foot Ankle Int 2004; 25(2):85–95.
45. Rosenfeld PF, Dick J, Saxby TS. The response of the flexor digitorum longus and posterior tibial muscles to tendon transfer and calcaneal osteotomy for stage II posterior tibial tendon dysfunction. Foot Ankle Int 2005;26(9):671–4.
46. Mizel MS, Temple HT, Scranton PE Jr, et al. Role of the peroneal tendons in the production of the deformed foot with posterior tibial tendon deficiency. Foot Ankle Int 1999;20(5):285–9.
47. Mann RA, Baumgarten M. Subtalar fusion for isolated subtalar disorders. Preliminary report. Clin Orthop Relat Res 1988;(226):260–5.
48. Otis JC, Deland JT, Lee S, Gordon J. Peroneus brevis is a more effective evertor than peroneus longus. Foot & ankle international 2004;25(4):242–6.
49. Harris RI, Beath T. Etiology of peroneal spastic flat foot. J Bone Joint Surg Br 1948;30B(4):624–34.
50. Page JC. Peroneal spastic flatfoot and tarsal coalitions. J Am Podiatr Med Assoc 1987;77(1):29–34.
51. Xu J, Muhammad H, Wang X, et al. Botulinum toxin type A injection combined with cast immobilization for treating recurrent peroneal spastic flatfoot without bone coalitions: a case report and review of the literature. J Foot Ankle Surg 2015;54(4):697–700.
52. Song SJ, Deland JT. Outcome following addition of peroneus brevis tendon transfer to treatment of acquired posterior tibial tendon insufficiency. Foot Ankle Int 2001;22(4):301–4.

Spring and Deltoid Ligament Insufficiency in the Setting of Progressive Collapsing Foot Deformity. An Update on Diagnosis and Management

Kurt Krautmann, MD[a], Anish R. Kadakia, MD[b,*]

KEYWORDS

- Deltoid • Tibiospring • Spring ligament • Adult acquired flatfoot
- Deltoid reconstruction • Spring ligament reconstruction
- Progressive collapsing foot deformity • PCFD

KEY POINTS

- Failure of the spring ligament is required for deformity to progress in PCFD.
- The deltoid ligament may become incompetent even in cases of flexible hindfoot deformity.
- The deltoid and spring ligament, while individually described, are so intimately related in form and function that incompetence in one likely causes incompetence in the other and therefore combined reconstruction techniques are becoming more popular.
- Progressive valgus deformity may progress to lateral ankle instability that requires correction.
- Staged procedures may be necessary to adequately address severe deformity safety, especially when attempting ankle arthroplasty.

INTRODUCTION

Adult acquired flatfoot deformity is now more appropriately termed progressive collapsing foot deformity (PCFD) and is a complex process that results from successive compromise of tendinous, ligamentous, and osseous structures within the foot, ultimately leading to progressive deformity and dysfunction.[1,2] The original classification in 1989 by Johnson & Strom[3] has been expanded, most notably by Bluman in

[a] Northwestern Medicine Department of Orthopedics, 259 East Erie Street, 13th Floor, Chicago, IL 60611, USA; [b] Orthopedic Foot and Ankle, Northwestern Medicine Department of Orthopedics, 259 East Erie Street, 13th Floor, Chicago, IL 60611, USA
* Corresponding author.
E-mail address: kadak259@gmail.com

Foot Ankle Clin N Am 26 (2021) 577–590
https://doi.org/10.1016/j.fcl.2021.05.004
foot.theclinics.com

2007[4] to incorporate a broader spectrum of pathologies. As with all classification systems, they attempt to create an algorithmic approach to treatment that fits as many patients as possible, but often falls short in many cases. Two components of PCFD that are often overlooked in classification systems are the spring and deltoid ligament.

Although dysfunction of the posterior tibial tendon (PTT) is often the focus of PCFD, the spring ligament is almost universally compromised in PCFD if deformity is present.[5–8] The deltoid ligament, while recognized as a component of the later stages of severe flatfoot deformity, is often overlooked in the earlier stages, even though it may be compromised early in the deformity and go unrecognized. Therefore, the evaluation and treatment of the spring ligament and deltoid complex in PCFD must be evaluated regardless of the disease stage and appropriately addressed during any reconstruction. This becomes particularly important when attempting joint sparing procedures to avoid the complications associated with extended fusions of the ankle and hindfoot.[9,10]

ANATOMY

The deltoid and spring ligament form a complex along the medial ankle and foot that stabilize the talus. The spring ligament is composed of several distinct structures that extend from the calcaneus to the navicular and serve to stabilize the talar head. The most important component of the spring ligament, the superomedial calcaneonavicular ligament (SMCN), contains both ligamentous and fibrocartilaginous components that together create an acetabulum tali that stabilizes the talar head.[11] The inferior calcaneonavicular ligament (ICN) was also described more lateral and plantar to the SMCN. Taniguchi and colleagues in 2003[12] described a third distinct component between the two previously described and again highlighted the fibrocartilaginous nature of the SMCN.

The deltoid ligament is a complex of structures on the medial ankle that includes two main components, the superficial and deep deltoid. The deep deltoid extends from the medial malleolus to the medial talus, whereas the superficial deltoid contains components that originate from the medial malleolus and insert on both the navicular and calcaneus.[13] The superficial component includes the tibiospring ligament, which originates from the medial malleolus and inserts on the plantar calcaneonavicular ligament. This highlights the intimate relationship between the deltoid and spring ligament.[13–15] The function of the deltoid is to resist lateral talar translation, rotation, and valgus talar tilt.[13,14,16] Ultimately, the superficial deltoid and spring ligament cannot easily be separated anatomically, and therefore incompetence in one should be a cause for concern in the other. This is particularly true with the spring ligament and superficial deltoid that are intimately interconnected along the sustentaculum tali.

EVALUATION

Proper treatment of PCFD requires evaluation of both the spring and deltoid ligament before surgical management. The spring ligament is almost invariably involved in PCFD if there is deformity present.[6,8,17] Spring ligament injury can also occur in isolation and lead to progressive flatfoot deformity. Currently, MRI is the gold standard for evaluation of the spring ligament. Toye and colleagues in 2005[18] looked at MRI findings in surgically proven cases of spring ligament tear compared with intact ligaments and found full-thickness gaping to be unique to surgically confirmed cases. Menigiardi and Zanetti in 2016[19] determined that increased signal on T2 or proton-density sequences, thickening above 5 mm or thinning below 2 mm, and partial or complete discontinuity were the best criteria to diagnose spring ligament tear on MRI. Deland and colleagues in 2005[6] used MRI to evaluate 31 patients with posterior tibial tendon insufficiency compared with age-matched controls and found significant pathology in the SMCN, ICN, talocalcaneal interosseous ligament, anterior superficial deltoid, plantar metatarsal ligaments, and plantar naviculocuneiform ligaments. Ultrasound may also be useful in the diagnosis of spring ligament pathology, although it is significantly more user-dependent than MRI. Tryfonidis and colleagues[20] reported on isolated spring ligament injuries in 9 patients with normal PTTs. They used ultrasound to evaluate the spring ligament, using a thickness of greater than 5.5 mm or less than 2.5 mm, loss of fibrillary echo pattern, and increased vascularity to be indicative of spring ligament incompetence. In 2020, de Cesar Netto and colleagues[8] used weight-bearing CT and MRI to correlate degeneration of the soft tissue structures as seen on MRI with deformity on MRI. Degeneration of the PTT correlated with sinus tarsi impingement, spring ligament degeneration correlated with subtalar subluxation, and talocalcaneal interosseous ligament correlated with subfibular impingement.

As deformity progresses, ankle pathology becomes a more important component, with valgus ankle instability or valgus deformity developing.[21] Although MRI is preferred for evaluation of ligamentous structures, weight-bearing CT may be the preferred evaluation for significant osseous deformity of the tibia and fibula that can be seen in severe deformity.[22,23]

ISOLATED SPRING LIGAMENT INJURY AS A CAUSE OF COLLAPSING DEFORMITY

Although the spring ligament is mainly involved in the pathology of PCFD, isolated injury to the spring ligament may be sufficient to cause a collapsing deformity. Although rare in the literature, several case reports and case series suggest that the spring ligament alone can be a cause of PCFD. These patients can present very similarly to PCFD but with several subtle differences. Tryfonidis and colleagues in 2007[20] presented 9 cases of PCFD with normal posterior tibialis tendon function. In their cohort, they found that patients maintained the ability to perform single-leg heel rise with partial arch restoration. They also had maintained inversion strength and had tenderness anterior to the medial malleolus as opposed to over the PTT. Only 3 of their cases had surgery, with one presenting acutely and undergoing repair of both the deltoid and spring ligament. The other two cases underwent flexor digitorum longus (FDL) transfer and medializing calcaneal osteotomy, along with spring ligament repair. Borton and Saxby in 1997[24] described a single case in a triple jump athlete who sustained a spring ligament injury with normal PTT. The patient underwent FDL transfer and spring ligament repair with return to sporting activity. Chen and Allen in 1997[25] reported on the MRI diagnosis of a spring ligament tear in a pole vaulter who was confirmed at surgery to have both spring ligament and deep deltoid cause subluxation of the talonavicular joint. Repair of the ligaments allowed the patient to return to prior level of competition. Orr and Nunley in 2013[26] reported on 6 operatively treated patients with unilateral PCFD and surgically proven spring ligament tears in the setting of a normal posterior tibialis tendon. The patients in this study localized pain to the medial arch as opposed to the medial malleolus described by Tryfonidis. MRI was performed in 5 of those patients and showed abnormalities in the spring ligament later confirmed at surgery. All 6 patients were treated with ligament repair, and a combination of either lateral column lengthening (LCL), medial sliding calcaneal osteotomy, or cuneiform osteotomy as dictated by the deformity. Kadakia et al in 2013[27] described the use of a hamstring allograft along with LCL to reconstruct the spring ligament and avoid fusion in a patient with traumatic fracture dislocation of the Chopart joint. In their case report, the LCL was successful in correcting the abduction deformity, but unable to restore talonavicular instability. They then used a hamstrings allograft, anchored in the talar neck, passed deep to the PTT, and then passed through a bone tunnel in the medial cuneiform. At 1-year postinjury, the patient was at full activity, without significant complaints, and with full range of motion of the ankle and hindfoot. Ultimately, there is limited evidence to guide treatment. Whether a graft is necessary or if a suture tape reconstruction can be performed is difficult to determine given the small sample sizes and discrepancy in treatment in the literature. Our current algorithm is to perform a suture tape reconstruction of the Deltoid/Spring Ligament complex with imbrication of the native tissue as the primary surgical procedure. If the patient has persistent hindfoot valgus after the reconstruction compared with the contralateral lower extremity, an additional medial slid calcaneal osteotomy is considered. In all cases, a cotton osteotomy is performed if residual forefoot supination is present.

FLEXIBLE PROGRESSIVE COLLAPSING FOOT DEFORMITY AND THE SPRING LIGAMENT

Currently, most of the research on spring ligament reconstruction has been performed for patients presenting with a flexible PCFD. Flexible deformity, now PCFD stage I, is characterized by hindfoot valgus (Class A) and flattening of the arch, with varying degrees of forefoot abduction (Class B).[2–4] Historically, PCFD stage I was treated with FDL transfer, medial displacement calcaneal osteotomy (MDCO), or LCL. More recently, there has been more interest in soft tissue reconstructions, specifically the spring ligament, in the correction of flexible flatfoot deformity. Although there is little debate about the use of FDL transfer and MDCO in the treatment of flexible PCFD, the addition of the LCL is more controversial. LCL is effective at reducing forefoot abduction,[28–30] but is known to contribute to lateral column overload.[31,32] Conti and colleagues in 2015[33] showed that overcorrection of forefoot abduction from LCL led to worse patient outcomes, and that special attention should be paid to the extent of LCL performed to avoid overcorrection.

Owing to the potential complications of LCL, many surgeons are looking to spring ligament reconstruction as a potential method to correct forefoot abduction and restore medial column stability. Myerson and colleagues in 1995[34] combined tendon transfer, calcaneal osteotomy, and repair of talonavicular capsule in 18 patients with PCFD. The contribution of the capsular imbrication could not be determined, although later studies looking at isolated repair of the spring ligament have been successful when done in an acute setting. In the chronic setting of PCFD, most of the current interest is in reconstruction or augmentation of the spring ligament and deltoid complex. Many different reconstruction options have been described in the literature. Tan and colleagues in 2010[35] performed graft augmentation from the talar head through the navicular in a cadaveric model and obtained significant correction of the AP talo-first metatarsal angle, lateral talo-first metatarsal ankle, and medial cuneiform height.

Acevedo and Vora in 2013[36] performed a repair of the native spring ligament, with internal brace augmentation from the sustentaculum tali to the navicular. Their technique was performed in 25 patients with overall good results. The authors noted that in their experience, this technique reduced the need for LCL, which was only performed in two of the patients in the study, while adequate correction of talonavicular uncoverage was achieved with medial augmentation alone. Baxter and colleagues in 2014[37] used a cadaveric flatfoot model to assess 3 different configurations of spring ligament reconstruction. They compared an anatomic reconstruction, similar to Acevedo and Vora, with an isolated talonavicular reconstruction and a tibionavicular reconstruction. They found that the more proximal fixation from navicular to tibia gave more powerful correction. Pasapula and colleagues in 2017[38] studied the spring ligament reconstruction using FiberTape to recreate a plantar and dorsal limb of the spring ligament and found that the plantar limb of the reconstruction was the primary stabilizer. Aynardi and colleagues in 2019[39] performed a biomechanical analysis using FiberTape augmentation in a cadaveric model and showed that augmentation improved load to failure without significant change in the contact pressure at the talonavicular joint. Nery and colleagues in 2018[40] described a combined reconstruction of the spring ligament and deltoid complex that was used in 10 patients. Their technique involves primary ligament repair with FDL transfer and FiberTape augmentation. The FiberTape augments both the deep and superficial deltoid, as well as the spring ligament. They had significant correction of talo-first metatarsal angle, talonavicular ankle, talar pitch, and calcaneal pitch. Improvement in VAS and AOFAS scores at mean follow-up of 20 months was also seen. Brodell and colleagues in 2019[41] reported on 14 feet that had combined deltoid and spring ligament reconstruction using allograft with two limbs, one passed from the medial malleolus to the sustentaculum tali and the other passed through the navicular. They showed improvement in FAAM activities of daily living, PROMIS, and SF-36, as well as improved AP talo-first metatarsal ankle, talonavicular coverage ankle, and Meary's angle. Of note, all the patients in this study also had an LCL, so contribution of the medial reconstruction to overall outcomes could not be isolated. Most recently, Hayes and colleagues 2020[42] compared spring ligament reconstruction with hamstring allograft to reconstruction with synthetic ligament augmentation. They found that while both provided excellent radiographic correction, patient outcomes were better with synthetic ligament augmentation.

Without long-term studies on the efficacy of spring ligament reconstructions, as well as confounding from concomitant LCL procedures, it is difficult to determine what role the medial soft tissue reconstruction plays in the overall PCFD correction. Historically, more than 30% uncoverage of the talar head was used as the indication for LCL, but with current results from medial reconstruction techniques, the LCL may be reserved for greater deformity, or for patient with deformity that is not adequately addressed with spring ligament reconstruction.[36,43] When balancing the risks and benefits of an LCL compared with a spring ligament reconstruction, with the known fact that the lateral column is not short in patients with PCFD,[44] we believe that a spring ligament reconstruction should be the preferred technique in PCFD patients with either significant abduction (Class B) or marked peritalar subluxation (Class D) given the low morbidity and recent literature demonstrating its efficacy. The consensus statements from Deland and colleagues in 2020[21] concluded that spring ligament reconstruction or TN fusion should be considered if LCL does not adequately correct abduction. They also concluded that medial soft tissue reconstructions, encompassing spring ligament, deep deltoid, and superficial deltoid should be considered as a joint sparing operation in valgus ankle deformity with more than 50% lateral cartilage remaining.

AUTHOR'S PREFERRED TECHNIQUE

Owing to the intimate relationship of the spring and superficial deltoid ligament,[11] we developed our current technique to reconstruct both the calcaneonavicular and tibiospring components of the superficial deltoid ligament, while still allowing for independent tensioning of both limbs. Given the superior radiographic results with synthetic ligament reconstruction as opposed to allograft reconstruction,[42] we use synthetic tape for our preferred reconstruction technique.

Using a standard medial approach over the PTT, the PTT is excised, leaving enough distal insertion to allow for suturing of the transferred FDL. If the PTT is felt to be viable, the tendon may be left intact with a direct side to side tenodesis performed of the FDL to the PTT with distal transection of the FDL. The spring ligament is then incised transversely, and a wedge resected for later imbrication to tighten the native ligament after reconstruction. The sustentaculum tali of the calcaneus is then identified, just distal to the tip of the medial malleolus and just deep to the previously harvested FDL tendon. Using the canulated Internal Brace System (Arthrex), a guidewire is placed into the sustentaculum (**Fig. 1**). This is then confirmed on fluoroscopy with an axial view of the calcaneus (**Fig. 2**) and the 2.7 mm drill for a 3.5 mm PEEK anchor is passed over the wire, followed by the cannulated tap. A 3.5 mm anchor, loaded with a suture tape, is then inserted into the sustentaculum. A wire is then placed from plantar to dorsal within the navicular. This wire position is again confirmed with fluoroscopy (**Fig. 3**), and the 2.7 mm drill for a 3.5 mm anchor is passed over the wire. The suture tape from the sustentaculum is then routed from plantar to dorsal through the navicular (**Fig. 4**). Our technique can be modified using a larger tunnel in the navicular and passing both the suture anchor and FDL tendon through the navicular, but it is our preference to suture the FDL into the remaining stump of the PT tendon. Tensioning of the spring ligament component of the reconstruction is then performed. The ankle is held in neutral dorsiflexion and the hindfoot in neutral adduction, tension is pulled on the suture tape as it exits the dorsal navicular, and a 3.5 mm anchor is placed into the navicular tunnel to affix the suture tape. A guidewire is then placed into the tip of the medial malleolus, confirmed on fluoroscopy, and overdrilled with the 3.4 mm drill followed by the appropriate tap (**Figs. 5** and **6**). The suture tape from the navicular is then loaded onto a 4.75 mm PEEK anchor. The ankle is again held in neutral dorsiflexion and the hindfoot in neutral adduction and the anchor is marked to provide appropriate tensioning and inserted into the medial malleolar tunnel, completing the suture augmentation (**Fig. 7**). Finally, the native spring ligament is imbricated in a pants-over-vest fashion using 0-vicryl sutures.

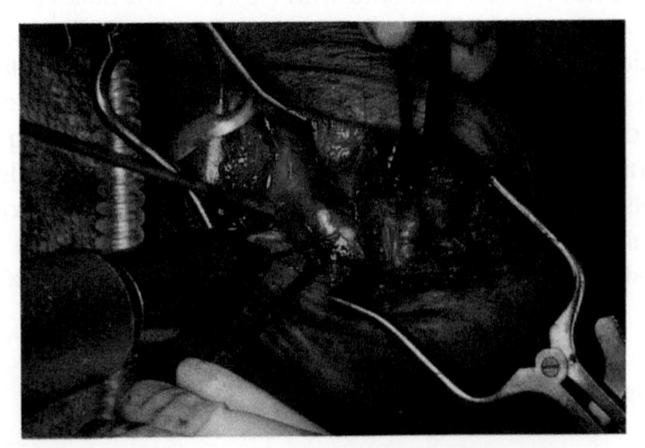

Fig. 1. Intraoperative photograph demonstrating the placement of a K-wire into the sustentaculum tali for placement of the initial 3.5 mm PEEK anchor.

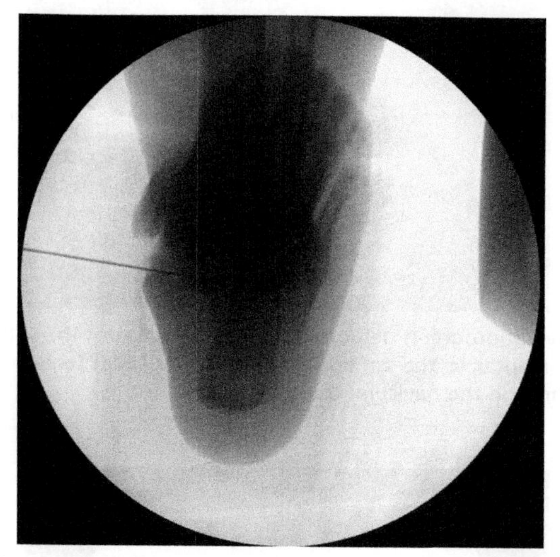

Fig. 2. An axial view of the calcaneus demonstrates appropriate fluoroscopy image to confirm placement of the guidewire into the sustentaculum tali. Care must be taken to place the wire from proximal to distal to avoid violation of the subtalar joint.

PROGRESSIVE COLLAPSING FOOT DEFORMITY AND DELTOID INSUFFICIENCY

As PCFD progresses, the medial arch collapses, the foot abducts, and the deltoid ligament fails. Although deltoid insufficiency can be seen in stage II flatfoot deformity,[45] it is the hallmark of stage IV deformity. This stage was added to the original classification by Myerson[46] and subdivided into IV-A and IV-B by Bluman in 2007.[45] Stage IV-A represented a flexible ankle valgus without significant arthritis, whereas stage IV-B was either a rigid hindfoot valgus or significant tibiotalar arthritis. Historically,

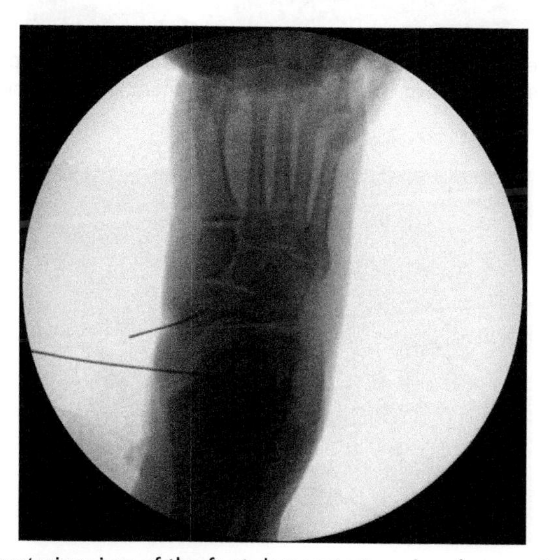

Fig. 3. An anteroposterior view of the foot demonstrates wire placement within the navicular for creation of the navicular tunnel.

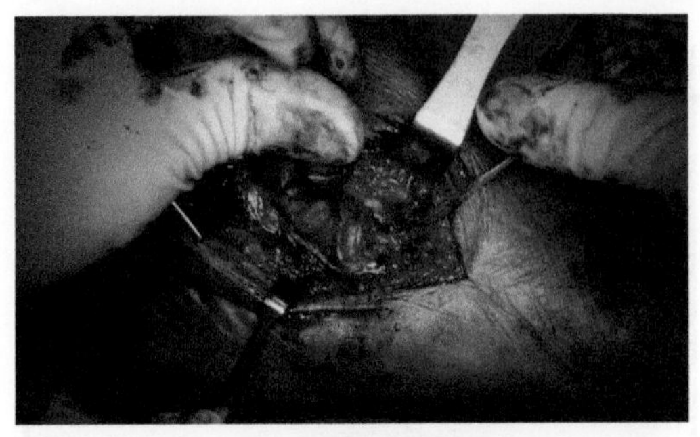

Fig. 4. Intraoperative photograph demonstrating the passage of the suture tape from the sustentaculum tali, plantar to the stump of the posterior tibial tendon, and routed from plantar to dorsal through the navicular tunnel.

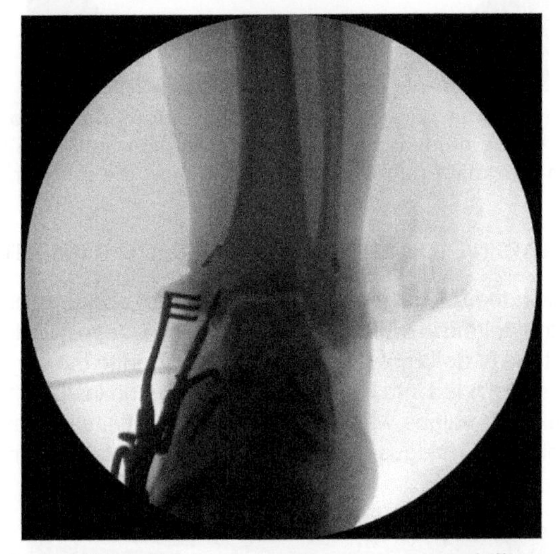

Fig. 5. A mortice view of the ankle demonstrating appropriate drilling position within the medial malleolus for insertion of the tibiospring component of the reconstruction.

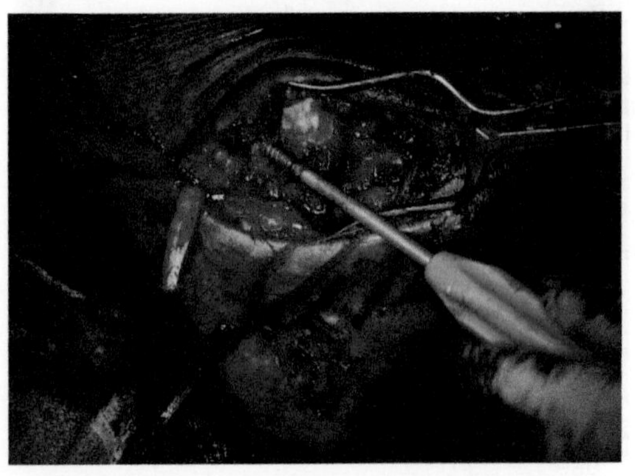

Fig. 6. Intraoperative photograph demonstrating the tap insertion into the tip of the medial malleolus.

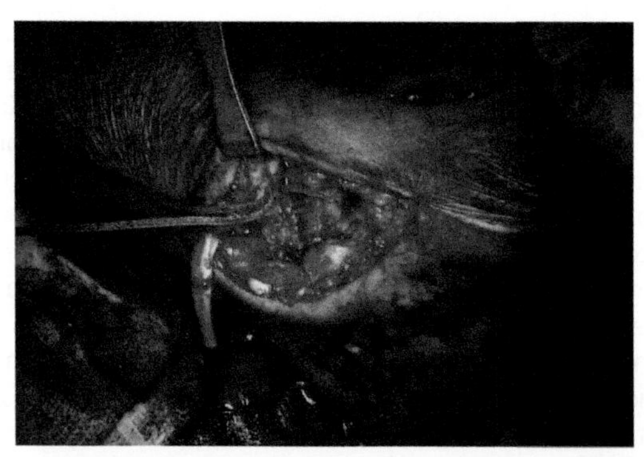

Fig. 7. Intraoperative photograph demonstrating the tibiospring component of the reconstruction with the suture tape now anchored into the medial malleolus.

reconstruction of the deltoid was performed for stage IV-A deformity, along with the required hindfoot and forefoot procedures necessary to correct the deformity. Often this entailed a triple arthrodesis, as the hindfoot deformity is typically rigid. Stage IV-B was generally treated with a pantalar arthrodesis.[4]

A new classification of PCFD has just been developed, which allows for a more thorough description of the inherent variability in PCFD presentation. The consensus group classification from Myerson and colleagues[2] classifies PCFD as either stage 1 (flexible) or stage II (rigid). It then assigns the deformity a letter A–E, with A representing hindfoot valgus, B representing midfoot or forefoot abduction, C representing forefoot varus or medial column instability, D representing peritalar subluxation, and E representing valgus ankle instability. This classification allows for easier classification of flexible deformity even in historically later-stage disease, and highlights that although PCFD is a progressive disease, it does not always progress from one stage to another and will commonly skip steps such as abduction deformity and progress directly to valgus ankle instability. Owing to the morbidity associated with extended hindfoot fusions, joint sparing whenever possible is the goal of current management.[10,21] The ability to salvage or replace the ankle joint in severe flatfoot deformity depends on many factors.

First, appropriate hindfoot correction must be obtained. Friedman and colleagues in 2001[47] showed in a cadaveric model that flatfoot deformity causes significant lateral shift of the tibiotalar contact area as well as 35% reduction in contact area. Rohm and colleagues[48] showed good results with talonavicular and subtalar fusion for correction of patients with primarily stage III disease, but Song and colleagues[49] showed in a cadaveric model that triple arthrodesis increased deltoid strain significantly and likely contributes to progressive tibiotalar arthritis after hindfoot arthrodesis. In 2017, Miniaci-Coxhead et al[50] reported on 187 patients who underwent hindfoot arthrodesis, of which 51 (27%) developed valgus tibiotalar tilt postoperatively. Without appropriate alignment, stress on the medial ankle, especially with a stiffened hindfoot, will result in deltoid failure and progression to stage IV disease.

Second, in patients with existing deltoid dysfunction but intact cartilage, appropriate realignment of the talus within the ankle mortise must be obtained. Many different techniques for deltoid reconstruction have been described. Deland and colleagues in 2004[51] used a peroneus longus autograft passed through the talus and anchored into the tibia through the medial malleolus to restore the deep deltoid.

Haddad and colleagues in 2010[52] performed a cadaveric study using anterior tibial tendon to reconstruct both the deep and superficial deltoid. Their technique restored biomechanical function compared with testing of the native deltoid. Jeng and colleagues in 2011[53] performed a deltoid reconstruction using hamstring allograft anchored with interference screws in the tibia, talus, and sustentaculum tali. Of their 8 patients, 5 had successful outcomes with reduction of tibiotalar valgus angle and maintenance of lateral ankle joint space. As the anatomy of the deltoid complex is more thoroughly understood, there had been a trend toward combining deltoid and spring ligament reconstructions. The entire medial ligamentous complex works together to prevent valgus talar tilting as well as flattening of the foot. Although each of these pathologies can be seen in isolation, they are often present concomitantly within the flat foot deformity. As a result, the more recent procedures published, such as those by Nery[40] and Brodell,[41] are designed to effectively reconstruct the superficial and deep deltoid as well as the spring ligament.

Finally, recognition of concomitant lateral ankle instability is necessary. Persaud and colleagues in 2018[54] showed MRI evidence of lateral ligament injury in 74 of 118 (62.7%) of patients with stages II and III flatfoot deformity. PCFD increases stress on the lateral ankle and can lead to fibular insufficiency fracture,[55] syndesmotic instability,[56] lateral malleolus valgus deformity, and distal tibial valgus that must be addressed.[22]

Stages II-E is of special concern regarding joint sparing procedures. As the tibiotalar joint is rigid and arthritic, surgical options are limited to fusion and joint replacement. Historically, total ankle replacement (TAR) was contraindicated with significant deformity, but with newer implants as well as more robust soft tissue reconstruction options described earlier, TAR in the setting of stage II-E flatfoot deformity is possible. Most authors would recommend a staged procedure to correct deformity and restore ankle stability in one stage and then perform ankle replacement after soft tissues have recovered.[22] Current research also suggests that TAR has better outcomes to ankle fusion in patients with complex end-stage ankle arthritis.[57]

AUTHORS' PREFERRED TECHNIQUE

For patients with stage II-E, it is preferable to avoid a hindfoot fusion if possible because of the increased strain on the deltoid ligament that is seen after a triple fusion.[49,50] In these cases, both the deep and superficial deltoid ligament must be adequately reconstructed to provide talar stability. Nery and colleagues[40] describe a technique that combines deep and superficial deltoid with spring ligament reconstruction using suture tape augmentation. This is done by first anchoring a suture tape into the medial malleolus. One limb of this suture tape is anchored into the talus to reconstruct the deep deltoid, whereas the other limb is anchored into the sustentaculum tali, along with a second suture tape. This reconstructs the superficial deltoid, while providing two new suture tape limbs that are then routed through a tunnel into the navicular to reconstruct the spring ligament. This reconstruction is combined with an MDCO to medialize the force of the Achilles.

If a hindfoot fusion must be performed due to significant subtalar arthritis, then a concomitant MDCO should be performed to further medialize the forces on the ankle, as the increased rigidity after a hindfoot fusion will increase the valgus stress on the ankle if any residual hindfoot valgus is present. The deltoid ligament must also be reconstructed. The native deltoid ligament is elevated from the distal tip of the medial malleolus, leaving a cuff of proximal periosteum. Although this aspect of the case may seem counterintuitive, the deltoid is lax and patulous in this case and therefore must be shortened if the ankle is to be reduced to a neutral position. Augmentation is required and this is performed by inserting a double-loaded 4.75 mm PEEK anchor into the medial malleolus. One pair of limbs is then anchored into the talus 5 mm distal and 5 mm anterior to the tip of the medial malleolus. The other is anchored into the sustentaculum, thus reconstructing both the deep and superficial deltoid. Fusion of the subtalar and talonavicular joint obviates the need for soft tissue reconstruction of the spring ligament in these cases. Tensioning is performed with ankle in neutral dorsiflexion with a reduced mortise, ensuing the suture tape is maximally tensioned in this position to avoid recurrence of deformity. The deltoid ligament should then be reconstructed/imbricated with the use of anchors and additional number 0 vicryl to the periosteum.

In all cases, patients must use an ASO and an arch support for 3 to 6 months to protect the soft tissue repair. Recurrence of talar tilt is common, especially if there is significant lateral joint wear in combination with medial ligament laxity. Total ankle arthroplasty is often required in these cases, but the improved medial soft tissue provided by the repair may limit the need for medial reconstruction at the time of total ankle arthroplasty and overall good patient outcomes have been reported.[58]

CLINICS CARE POINTS

- Failure of the spring ligament is required for deformity to progress in PCFD
- The deltoid ligament may become incompetent even in cases of flexible hindfoot deformity
- The deltoid and spring ligament, while individually described, are so intimately related in form and function that incompetence in one likely causes incompetence in the other, and therefore combined reconstruction techniques are becoming more popular
- Progressive valgus deformity may lead to overload of the lateral ankle, and consequently cause syndesmotic and lateral ankle instability, which may require correction
- Staged procedures may be necessary to adequately address severe deformity safety, especially when attempting ankle arthroplasty

DISCLOSURE

The author K. Krautmann has no relevant disclosures. The author A.R. Kadakia is an Arthrex consultant and receives royalties from Depuy, Acumed, and Elsevier.

REFERENCES

1. de Cesar Netto C, Deland JT, Ellis SJ. Guest editorial: expert consensus on adult-acquired flatfoot deformity. Foot Ankle Int 2020;41(10):1269–71.
2. Myerson MS, Thordarson DB, Johnson JE, et al. Classification and nomenclature: progressive collapsing foot deformity. Foot Ankle Int 2020;41(10):1271–6.
3. Johnson KA, Strom DE. Tibialis posterior tendon dysfunction. Clin Orthop Relat Res 1989;239:196–206.
4. Bluman EM, Title CI, Myerson MS. Posterior tibial tendon rupture: a refined classification system. Foot Ankle Clin 2007;12(2):233–49, v.
5. Deland JT. The adult acquired flatfoot and spring ligament complex: pathology and implications for treatment. Foot Ankle Clin 2001;6(1):129–35.
6. Deland JT, de Asla RJ, Sung IH, et al. Posterior tibial tendon insufficiency: which ligaments are involved? Foot Ankle Int 2005;26(6):427–35.

7. Williams G, Widnall J, Evans P, et al. Could failure of the spring ligament complex be the driving force behind the development of the adult flatfoot deformity? J Foot Ankle Surg 2014;53(2):152–5.
8. de Cesar Netto C, Saito GH, Roney A, et al. Combined weightbearing CT and MRI assessment of flexible progressive collapsing foot deformity. Foot Ankle Surg 2020; S1268-7731(20):30262–9.
9. Colin F, Zwicky L, Barg A, et al. Peritalar instability after tibiotalar fusion for valgus unstable ankle in stage IV adult acquired flatfoot deformity: case series. Foot Ankle Int 2013;34(12):1677–82.
10. Taylor R, Sammarco VJ. Minimizing the role of fusion in the rigid flatfoot. Foot Ankle Clin 2012;17(2):337–49.
11. Davis WH, Sobel M, DiCarlo EF, et al. Gross, histological, and microvascular anatomy and biomechanical testing of the spring ligament complex. Foot Ankle Int 1996;17(2):95–102.
12. Taniguchi A, Tanaka Y, Takakura Y, et al. Anatomy of the spring ligament. J Bone Joint Surgery-American 2003;85(11):2174–8.
13. Campbell KJ, Michalski MP, Wilson KJ, et al. The ligament anatomy of the deltoid complex of the ankle: a qualitative and quantitative anatomical study. J Bone Joint Surg Am 2014;96(8):e62.
14. Harper MC. Deltoid ligament: an anatomical evaluation of function. Foot Ankle 1987;8(1):19–22.
15. Cromeens BP, Kirchhoff CA, Patterson RM, et al. An attachment-based description of the medial collateral and spring ligament complexes. Foot Ankle Int 2015; 36(6):710–21.
16. Alshalawi S, Galhoum AE, Alrashidi Y, et al. Medial ankle instability: the deltoid dilemma. Foot Ankle Clin 2018;23(4):639–57.
17. Gazdag AR, Cracchiolo A. Rupture of the posterior tibial tendon. Evaluation of injury of the spring ligament and clinical assessment of tendon transfer and ligament repair. J Bone Joint Surg (American Volume) 1997;79(5):675–81.
18. Toye LR, Helms CA, Hoffman BD, et al. MRI of spring ligament tears. AJR Am J Roentgenol 2005;184(5):1475–80.
19. Mengiardi B, Pinto C, Zanetti M. Spring ligament complex and posterior tibial tendon: MR anatomy and findings in acquired adult flatfoot deformity. Semin Musculoskelet Radiol 2016;20(1):104–15.
20. Tryfonidis M, Jackson W, Mansour R, et al. Acquired adult flat foot due to isolated plantar calcaneonavicular (spring) ligament insufficiency with a normal tibialis posterior tendon. Foot Ankle Surg 2008;14(2):89–95.
21. Deland JT, Ellis SJ, Day J, et al. Indications for deltoid and spring ligament reconstruction in progressive collapsing foot deformity. Foot Ankle Int 2020;41(10): 1302–6.
22. Dodd A, Daniels TR. Total ankle replacement in the presence of talar varus or valgus deformities. Foot Ankle Clin 2017;22(2):277–300.
23. de Cesar Netto C, Myerson MS, Day J, et al. Consensus for the use of weightbearing CT in the assessment of progressive collapsing foot deformity. Foot Ankle Int 2020;41(10):1277–82.
24. Borton DC, Saxby TS. Tear of the plantar calcaneonavicular (spring) ligament causing flatfoot. A case report. J Bone Joint Surg Br 1997;79(4):641–3.
25. Chen JP, Allen AM. MR diagnosis of traumatic tear of the spring ligament in a pole vaulter. Skeletal Radiol 1997;26(5):310–2.
26. Orr JD, Nunley JA 2nd. Isolated spring ligament failure as a cause of adult-acquired flatfoot deformity. Foot Ankle Int 2013;34(6):818–23.

27. Kadakia AR, Ho BS, Molloy AP. A new technique of treatment of fracture-subluxation of chopart joint. Tech Foot Ankle Surg 2013;12(4):201–9.
28. Chan JY, Greenfield ST, Soukup DS, et al. Contribution of lateral column lengthening to correction of forefoot abduction in stage IIB adult acquired flatfoot deformity reconstruction. Foot Ankle Int 2015;36(12):1400–11.
29. Sangeorzan BJ, Mosca V, Hansen ST Jr. Effect of calcaneal lengthening on relationships among the hindfoot, midfoot, and forefoot. Foot Ankle 1993;14(3): 136–41.
30. Dumontier TA, Falicov A, Mosca V, et al. Calcaneal lengthening: investigation of deformity correction in a cadaver flatfoot model. Foot Ankle Int 2005;26(2): 166–70.
31. Oh I, Imhauser C, Choi D, et al. Sensitivity of plantar pressure and talonavicular alignment to lateral column lengthening in flatfoot reconstruction. J Bone Joint Surg Am 2013;95(12):1094–100.
32. Benthien RA, Parks BG, Guyton GP, et al. Lateral column calcaneal lengthening, flexor digitorum longus transfer, and opening wedge medial cuneiform osteotomy for flexible flatfoot: a biomechanical study. Foot Ankle Int 2007;28(1):70–7.
33. Conti MS, Chan JY, Do HT, et al. Correlation of postoperative midfoot position with outcome following reconstruction of the stage II adult acquired flatfoot deformity. Foot Ankle Int 2015;36(3):239–47.
34. Myerson MS, Corrigan J, Thompson F, et al. Tendon transfer combined with calcaneal osteotomy for treatment of posterior tibial tendon insufficiency: a radiological investigation. Foot Ankle Int 1995;16(11):712–8.
35. Tan GJ, Kadakia AR, Ruberte Thiele RA, et al. Novel reconstruction of a static medial ligamentous complex in a flatfoot model. Foot Ankle Int 2010;31(8): 695–700.
36. Acevedo J, Vora A. Anatomical reconstruction of the spring ligament complex: "internal brace" augmentation. Foot Ankle Spec 2013;6(6):441–5.
37. Baxter JR, LaMothe JM, Walls RJ, et al. Reconstruction of the medial talonavicular joint in simulated flatfoot deformity. Foot Ankle Int 2014;36(4):424–9.
38. Pasapula C, Devany A, Fischer NC, et al. The resistance to failure of spring ligament reconstruction. Foot, The. 2017;33:29–34.
39. Aynardi MC, Saloky K, Roush EP, et al. Biomechanical evaluation of spring ligament augmentation with the fibertape device in a cadaveric flatfoot model. Foot Ankle Int 2019;40(5):596–602.
40. Nery C, Lemos A, Raduan F, et al. Combined spring and deltoid ligament repair in adult-acquired flatfoot. Foot Ankle Int 2018;39(8):903–7.
41. Brodell JD Jr, MacDonald A, Perkins JA, et al. Deltoid-spring ligament reconstruction in adult acquired flatfoot deformity with medial peritalar instability. Foot Ankle Int 2019;40(7):753–61.
42. Heyes G, Swanton E, Vosoughi AR, et al. Comparative study of spring ligament reconstructions using either hamstring allograft or synthetic ligament augmentation. Foot Ankle Int 2020;41(7):803–10.
43. Kadakia AR. Valgus malalignment: what joints to address? Foot Ankle Int 2012; 33(2):161–3.
44. Kang S, Charlton TP, Thordarson DB. Lateral column length in adult flatfoot deformity. Foot Ankle Int 2013;34(3):392–7.
45. Bluman EM, Myerson MS. Stage IV posterior tibial tendon rupture. Foot Ankle Clin 2007;12(2):341–62, viii.
46. Myerson MS. Adult acquired flatfoot deformity: treatment of dysfunction of the posterior tibial tendon. Instr Course Lect 1997;46:393–405.

47. Friedman MA, Draganich LF, Toolan B, et al. The effects of adult acquired flatfoot deformity on tibiotalar joint contact characteristics. Foot Ankle Int 2001;22(3): 241–6.
48. Rohm J, Zwicky L, Horn Lang T, et al. Mid- to long-term outcome of 96 corrective hindfoot fusions in 84 patients with rigid flatfoot deformity. Bone Joint J 2015; 97-b(5):668–74.
49. Song SJ, Lee S, O'Malley MJ, et al. Deltoid ligament strain after correction of acquired flatfoot deformity by triple arthrodesis. Foot Ankle Int 2000;21(7):573–7.
50. Miniaci-Coxhead SL, Weisenthal B, Ketz JP, et al. Incidence and radiographic predictors of valgus tibiotalar tilt after hindfoot fusion. Foot Ankle Int 2017; 38(5):519–25.
51. Deland JT, de Asla RJ, Segal A. Reconstruction of the chronically failed deltoid ligament: a new technique. Foot Ankle Int 2004;25(11):795–9.
52. Haddad SL, Dedhia S, Ren Y, et al. Deltoid ligament reconstruction: a novel technique with biomechanical analysis. Foot Ankle Int 2010;31(7):639–51.
53. Jeng CL, Bluman EM, Myerson MS. Minimally invasive deltoid ligament reconstruction for stage IV flatfoot deformity. Foot Ankle Int 2011;32(1):21–30.
54. Persaud S, Hentges MJ, Catanzariti AR. Occurrence of lateral ankle ligament disease with stage 2 to 3 adult-acquired flatfoot deformity confirmed via magnetic resonance imaging: a retrospective study. J Foot Ankle Surg 2019;58(2):243–7.
55. Srinivasan S, Kurup H. Fibular insufficiency fracture: an under-reported complication of advanced tibialis posterior dysfunction. BMJ Case Rep 2017;2017. bcr2017221206.
56. Auch E, Barbachan Mansur NS, Alexandre Alves T, et al. Distal tibiofibular syndesmotic widening in progressive collapsing foot deformity. Foot Ankle Int 2021;42(6):768–75.
57. Penner M, Wing K, Glazebrook M, et al. The effect of deformity and hindfoot arthritis on midterm outcomes of ankle replacement and fusion: a prospective COFAS multi-centre study of 890 patients. Foot & Ankle Orthopaedics 2018;3. 2473011418S2473010009.
58. Nayak R, Patel M, Kadakia AR. Outcomes after tibiocalcaneonavicular ligament reconstruction in stage IIB and stage IV adult acquired flatfoot deformity. Foot & Ankle Orthopaedics 2020;5(4). 2473011420S2473000366.

Spare the Talonavicular Joint! The Role of Isolated Subtalar Joint Fusion in the Treatment of Progressive Collapsing Foot Deformity

Matthew S. Conti, MD[a], Scott J. Ellis, MD[b,*]

KEYWORDS

- Talonavicular arthrodesis • Subtalar arthrodesis • Adult-acquired flatfoot deformity
- Progressive collapsing foot deformity • Weight-bearing CT scans
- Subtalar impingement • Subfibular impingement

KEY POINTS

- Arthrodesis of the talonavicular joint has been shown in cadaveric models to lead to very little residual motion at the subtalar and calcaneocuboid joints and, consequently, may accelerate adjacent-joint arthrosis.
- Subtalar arthrodesis may be combined with reconstructive procedures, such as a medializing calcaneal osteotomy, first tarsometatarsal fusion, Cotton osteotomy, and/or soft tissue procedures to address the midfoot abduction and hindfoot valgus deformities in a patient with a severe flexible or rigid progressive collapsing foot deformities.
- Preoperative weight-bearing computed tomography scans may guide surgical management, and patients with sinus tarsi and subfibular impingement deformities may benefit from a subtalar fusion in addition to traditional reconstructive procedures.

INTRODUCTION

Progressive collapsing foot deformity (PCFD), more commonly referred to as adult-acquired flatfoot deformity, is a condition that results from failure of the ligaments, tendons, and bony structures that support the arch of the foot.[1] The condition has been described as peritalar subluxation due the deformities that occur around the talus, such as subluxation of the middle facet of the subtalar joint, hindfoot valgus, and a

[a] Academic Training Department, Hospital for Special Surgery, 535 East 70th Street, New York, NY 10021, USA; [b] Foot and Ankle Service, Hospital for Special Surgery, 523 East 72nd Street, 5th Floor, New York, NY 10021, USA
* Corresponding author.
E-mail address: elliss@hss.edu
Twitter: @matthew_conti (M.S.C.)

Foot Ankle Clin N Am 26 (2021) 591–607
https://doi.org/10.1016/j.fcl.2021.05.005

more valgus-oriented subtalar joint compared with control patients. In addition, plantar sag and midfoot abduction at the talonavicular joint may develop.[2–5]

PCFD is complex, with a wide variation in the site and severity of the deformity.[5] Previously, the disease was divided into 4 stages based on early work focusing on PCFD.[6] A new classification has been proposed, however, that first divides patients into 2 stages based on whether their deformity is flexible (stage I) or rigid (stage II).[7] Once the stage is determined, additional classes (A–E) denote different types and patterns of deformity, and these classes may be used in isolation or combined together. The classes and deformities are as follows: class A describes a hindfoot valgus deformity, class B describes a midfoot/forefoot abduction deformity, class C describes a forefoot varus deformity or medial column instability, class D describes peritalar subluxation or dislocation, and class E describes ankle instability.[7] A patient with a flexible PCFD with hindfoot valgus and midfoot/forefoot abduction is classified as having a stage I, class AB deformity. This new classification may help guide treatment.

Hindfoot valgus in patients with flexible deformity is caused, in part, by failure of the talocalcaneal interosseous ligament.[5] The midfoot/forefoot deformity has been attributed to compromise of the superomedial calcaneonavicular (spring) ligament.[1] In rigid PCFD deformities, passive inversion of the talonavicular, subtalar, and calcaneocuboid joints does not result in a neutral plantigrade position of the foot and occurs due to long-standing contractures or arthritis of the triple joint complex.[1,5]

Historically, operative management of PCFD included either reconstruction of the foot in order to avoid fusion in patients with flexible (stage I) PCFD or a triple arthrodesis in rigid (stage II) patients.[1,8] Recent studies, however, have begun to question that treatment paradigm.[9–12] The advent of weight-bearing computed tomography (CT) scans has helped to describe new findings, such as sinus tarsi and subfibular impingement.[13,14] These deformities may be present in patients with flexible PCFD and potentially could result in poor outcomes following reconstructive procedures, such as a medializing calcaneal osteotomy or lateral column lengthening do not address deformity at the subtalar joint in cases of sinus tarsi impingement or where the calcaneus contacts the fibula in the case of subfibular impingement. Although no studies to date have investigated outcomes of patients with sinus tarsi or subfibular impingement, these patients instead may benefit from an isolated subtalar arthrodesis, which can address extra-articular degenerative changes due to sinus tarsi impingement or shift the calcaneus to improve subfibular impingement at the same time they eliminated impingement.

Sequential fusion of additional joints of the triple joint complex has been shown to decrease motion of the remaining unfused joints.[15] Triple arthrodesis affects gait and hindfoot motion and leads to adjacent joint degeneration at long-term follow-up; therefore, selective fusions in the foot may avoid the need for a triple arthrodesis.[15–17] In particular, arthrodesis of the talonavicular joint has a significant effect on motion at the hindfoot.[15] Long-term gait and clinical outcomes data at an average of 9.5 years' follow-up (range, 2.5–21 y) found that isolated talonavicular arthrodesis resulted in satisfactory pain relief but adjacent joint arthrosis in 27% of patients and difficulty with walking on irregular ground.[18]

The purpose of this review article is to discuss the role of arthrodesis in the treatment of PCFD, specifically, why surgeons may choose to avoid arthrodesis of the talonavicular joint by employing selective fusions of the naviculocuneiform, first tarsometatarsal, and subtalar joints. The article reviews currents indications and outcomes of triple arthrodesis, selective fusions of the hindfoot, and isolated subtalar arthrodesis. A case example at the end of the article demonstrates a more recent treatment algorithm for patients with severe flexible PCFD disease.

TRIPLE ARTHRODESIS

For a rigid PCFD, a triple arthrodesis has been considered the treatment of choice.[19] Triple arthrodesis provides excellent correction of the PCFD and may be indicated in patients with multiple arthritic, unstable, or stiff joints.[20] Arthrodesis allows a surgeon to completely mobilize joints, even in cases of dislocation, and achieve powerful and lasting correction at the cost of motion. One study retrospectively reviewed 22 adult patients who underwent a triple arthrodesis due to hindfoot pain and deformity resulting from conditions, such as posterior tibial tendon rupture or painful pes planus.[21] At a minimum of 3 years' follow-up, they reported good results in 36% of patients and fair results in 59% of patients with 95% of patients stating that they were improved overall.[21] Radiographic evidence of adjacent-joint arthrosis at the tibiotalar joint or midfoot developed in 11 patients and 11 patients, respectively.[21] In another study with 25-year and 40-year average follow-up in 57 patients with neuromuscular imbalance of the hindfoot who were treated with a triple arthrodesis, 45% of feet were painful at 25 years, and 55% of feet were painful at 40 years[17]; 69% of patients had radiographic evidence degenerative changes at the tibiotalar joint at 25 years, and all patients had evidence of tibiotalar arthritis at 40 years.[17] Despite their symptoms and radiographic changes in the tibiotalar joint, 95% of patients stated that they were satisfied with their outcome.[17] Other studies also have reported acceptable clinical outcomes in patients undergoing triple arthrodesis for rigid PCFD.[22,23]

Results of triple arthrodesis for rigid PCFD have not been uniformly excellent. Deland and colleagues (2006)[24] showed that patients with rigid disease treated with a triple arthrodesis had significantly lower 2-year American Orthopaedic Foot and Ankle Society (AOFAS) outcome scores than patients with flexible PCFD treated with osteotomies. Additionally, triple arthrodesis have been found to limit hindfoot motion considerably.[15,16] Gait analysis was performed at an average of 5.2 years postoperatively in 13 patients who underwent a double or triple arthrodesis to determine altered motion at the knee and ankle joints.[16] Patients who underwent a double or triple arthrodesis had an average of 8° to 10° less ankle plantarflexion as well as 50% reduction in ankle plantarflexion power generation in the limb that underwent a double or triple arthrodesis.[16] These patients often compensated with an average increase of 5° of ipsilateral knee flexion during the third rocker.[16] As a result of significant changes in gait, lower patient-reported outcome measures, and radiographic evidence of adjacent joint arthrosis, selective arthrodesis for the treatment of severe flexible and rigid PCFD recently have been employed.

DOUBLE AND ISOLATED TALONAVICULAR ARTHRODESIS

Sag of the medial longitudinal arch and forefoot abduction in patients with PCFD often is seen at the talonavicular joint.[25] In a study of 23 patients with flexible PCFD, Haleem and colleagues[25] (2014) showed that sagittal plane deformity notably was found at the talonavicular joint on weight-bearing CT scans. Thus, many investigators have proposed, including the talonavicular joint in selective fusions of the hindfoot for PCFD and have reported acceptable clinical results.[11,26–28] Indications for fusing the talonavicular joint the setting of PCFD include severe deformity, an arthritic and stiff talonavicular joint, or substantial sagittal place sagging of the joint.[20] In patients with nonarthritic talonavicular joints, significant forefoot abduction deformities may be corrected using joint-preserving procedures, such as a lateral column lengthening or spring ligament repair[20,29]; however, if the abduction deformity cannot be adequately corrected intraoperatively, then an isolated talonavicular arthrodesis may be considered to correct residual deformity.[12]

Röhm and colleagues (2015)[11] reported their experience in 84 patients with symptomatic rigid PCFD who were treated using talonavicular and subtalar joint fusions with a minimum of 1 year follow-up (average 4.7 years). They reported no loss of correction in 90.5% of feet, and 81% of patients stated that they would have the procedure again.[11] Eight patients had a nonunion of the talonavicular joint, and 7 patients had a nonunion of the subtalar joint.[11] Four patients required a total ankle replacement or ankle fusion at a mean of 17 months following their talonavicular and subtalar fusion.[11] In a study of 16 feet in 14 patients who underwent arthrodesis of the talonavicular and subtalar joints for hindfoot malalignment, Sammarco and colleagues (2006)[30] reported that all patients were satisfied with the result of the procedure. At a minimum follow-up of 18 months, evidence of radiographic arthritis had increased in 6 ankles, 6 calcaneocuboid joints, and 5 midfoot joints.[30] Using an isolated medial approach to perform subtalar and talonavicular fusions for severe PCFD deformity of the foot, Knupp and colleagues (2009)[28] demonstrated significant improvements in radiographic parameters with no evidence of malunions or nonunions on postoperative radiographs. Complications included superficial wound healing issues in 3 patients, removal of hardware in 4 patients, and hardware failure at the talonavicular fusion site in 1 patient.[28]

An early study by Clain and colleagues (1994)[27] investigated the results of a double arthrodesis of the talonavicular and calcaneocuboid joints in 16 patients with various hindfoot disorders, including 7 patients with PCFD. Although no patients were dissatisfied, 6 were satisfied with major reservations, and there was 1 asymptomatic nonunion of the talonavicular joint.[27] Six patients had progression of ankle arthritis, and 7 patients had increased radiographic degenerative arthritis of the naviculocuneiform joint.[27]

Increased degenerative changes in the midfoot including the naviculocuneiform joint after double arthrodesis may be due to higher load across the midfoot region.[31] Schuh and colleagues (2012)[31] compared 16 feet in 14 patients who were treated with arthrodesis of the subtalar and talonavicular joints for PCFD deformities with 14 healthy control patients who were matched to the treatment group based on age and sex. At a minimum follow-up of 18 months postoperatively, they found that patients who underwent a double arthrodesis for the treatment of PCFD had increased loads across the midfoot foot region and decreased push-off force compared with healthy control patients.[31]

There is evidence that an isolated talonavicular arthrodesis can be used for the treatment of PCFD.[26,32,33] O'Malley and colleagues (1995)[32] using 5 cadaveric specimens demonstrated that an isolated talonavicular fusion was able to correct all of the PCFD deformities, including hindfoot valgus in their flatfoot model. In the largest case series of isolated talonavicular arthrodesis to treat PCFD, Harper and Tisdel (1996)[33] reported their results of talonavicular arthrodesis in 26 consecutive patients with PCFD and found that no patient was dissatisfied with the procedure. One patient required additional surgery to address a nonunion at the arthrodesis site, and 5 patients had progressive radiographic arthrosis of adjacent joints.[33] They did not report radiographic changes in hindfoot alignment or collapse along the medial longitudinal arch.[33] Complications of isolated arthrodesis of the talonavicular joint include lateral midfoot pain, malunion, a higher rate of nonunion compared with an isolated fusion of the subtalar joint, and adjacent joint arthrosis in the ankle, subtalar, and remaining midfoot joints.[26]

SELECTIVE ARTHRODESES THAT SPARE THE TALONAVICULAR JOINT

In addition to the complications associated with talonavicular arthrodesis, fusion of the talonavicular joint significantly limits motion at the remaining hindfoot joints, and there is clinical evidence that the talonavicular joint may be preserved in the treatment of severe PCFD.[9,15,34] Astion and colleagues (1997)[15] performed simulated arthrodeses of the talonavicular, calcaneocuboid, and subtalar joints in 10 cadaveric specimens. Fusion of the subtalar joint left an average of 26% of prearthrodesis motion in the talonavicular joint and 56% of prearthrodesis motion in the calcaneocuboid joint.[15] Fusion of the calcaneocuboid joint resulted in an average of 67% of prearthrodesis motion in the talonavicular joint and almost full motion of the subtalar joint.[15] Arthrodesis of the talonavicular joint, however, reduced range of motion of the subtalar and calcaneocuboid joints to approximately 2% of their prearthrodesis values.[15] Consequently, arthrodesis of the talonavicular joint essentially results in no postoperative motion of the hindfoot, and, therefore, incorporating the talonavicular joint in the fusion construct may result in increased rates of adjacent joint arthrosis at the ankle and midfoot.

Additionally, the location of medial longitudinal arch collapse may not be centered at the talonavicular joint.[35] In contrast to Haleem and colleagues (2014),[25] Greisberg and colleagues (2003),[35] using simulated weight-bearing CT scans in 23 feet, found that 65% of patients had more than 10° of collapse at the naviculocuneiform joint whereas only 20% of patients had more than 10° of collapse at the talonavicular joint. There was only 1 patient (5%) in the study who had more than 10° of collapse through both the naviculocuneiform and talonavicular joints.[35]

Some investigators have advocated for naviculocuneiform fusion as an alternative to talonavicular fusion for the management severe PCFD.[9,34] Ajis and Geary (2014)[9] reported their results of 28 patients who had a naviculocuneiform fusion as their only arthrodesis procedure, with 20 patients having the procedure for symptomatic PCFD. In the PCFD subgroup, 2 patients had medial displacement osteotomies, 8 had a split tibialis anterior reconstruction of a degenerative posterior tibial tendon, and 7 had gastrocnemius recessions.[9] The mean time to union of the naviculocuneiform fusion was 21.7 weeks with 1 symptomatic nonunion that required revision and went on to heal at approximately 14 months after the index procedure.[9] Other complications included 2 superficial wound infections. Meary's angle improved from a preoperative value of 12.3° to 5.2° at final follow-up.[9] The mean talonavicular coverage angle improved by approximately 7°; 32 of 33 patients described satisfactory improvement in pain and deformity.[9]

Steiner and colleagues (2019)[34] proposed using a naviculocuneiform fusion in combination with a subtalar arthrodesis for the treatment of PCFD. The investigators retrospectively identified 34 feet in 31 patients with rigid PCFD and collapse of the medial arch at the level of the naviculocuneiform joint[34]; 15 feet underwent a concomitant medializing calcaneal osteotomy because subtalar fusion did not achieve a neutral hindfoot alignment, and five feet required a flexor digitorum longus transfer.[34] There were significant improvements in Meary angle from 25.3° to 14.3° apex plantar as well as substantial improvements in midfoot abduction parameters, such as talonavicular coverage angle from 37.4° to 23.8° and anteroposterior (AP) talo–first metatarsal angle from 16.2° to 6.8°.[34] Complications included 2 patients with asymptomatic nonunions with 1 occurring at the subtalar joint and the other occurring at the naviculocuneiform joint.[34] One patient underwent a total ankle replacement at 1 year postoperatively due to avascular necrosis of the lateral talus.[34]

In order to treat collapse at the naviculocuneiform joint, other investigators have suggested that arthrodesis of the medial longitudinal column may be avoided or limited to a first tarsometatarsal fusion.[36,37] Aiyer and colleagues (2015)[36] reviewed 67 patients who underwent an opening wedge plantarflexing medial cuneiform (Cotton) osteotomy to improve residual forefoot supination in addition to a lateral column lengthening, medializing calcaneal osteotomy, and/or flexor digitorum longus transfer in patients with PCFD, flexible planovalgus deformity, or accessory navicular syndrome. At an average radiographic follow-up was 13 months (range, 2.1–53 mo), the investigators found that the Cotton osteotomy did not significantly affect the postoperative Meary angle but did significantly improve the medial arch sag angle.[36] They reported no evidence of adjacent joint disease or radiographic instability in their cohort at final follow-up and concluded that the Cotton osteotomy may be sufficient without additional medial longitudinal column fusions.[36] A similar study investigated the effect of a subtalar arthrodesis with a concomitant first tarsometatarsal fusion on naviculocuneiform deformity in 40 patients with severe PCFD.[37] They found that the first tarsometarsal fusion did not significantly affect deformity at the naviculocuneiform joint at a minimum of 6 months postoperatively.[37] Additionally, patients who developed increased collapse at the naviculocuneiform joint did not have significantly worse patient-reported outcomes at 1 year postoperatively compared with patients who had improvements in sag at the naviculocuneiform joint.[37] The investigators suggested that patients may tolerate more deformity at the naviculocuneiform joint that at other joints along the medial column.[37] No patients underwent subsequent naviculocuneiform arthrodesis in this cohort.[37]

These studies suggest that the deformities associated with severe PCFD, such as sag at the medial longitudinal arch, forefoot abduction, and residual forefoot supination, can be addressed through limited fusions or reconstructive procedures that spare the talonavicular joint.

ROLE OF ISOLATED SUBTALAR ARTHRODESIS TO AVOID FUSION OF THE TALONAVICULAR JOINT

Isolated subtalar fusions have been successfully used to treat PCFD while avoiding arthrodesis of the talonavicular joint.[38–40] Although this technique may preserve hindfoot motion and decrease the rate of development of ankle and midfoot adjacent-joint arthrosis compared with double or triple arthrodeses, isolated subtalar fusions lead to nonphysiologic stresses at the talonavicular and calcaneocuboid joints, possibly resulting in arthritic changes.[39] Studies with short-term follow-up, however, have found low rates of clinically significant talonavicular and calcaneocuboid arthritis following isolated subtalar arthrodesis.[38–40]

Indications and Contraindications

In patients with PCFD, isolated subtalar joint arthrodesis is indicated in patients with a flexible forefoot deformity and a fixed subtalar joint deformity or degenerative changes of the subtalar joint or in patients with severe peritalar subluxation/dislocation.[41,42] If the forefoot deformity is fixed, then correction of hindfoot valgus through the subtalar joint may result in a forefoot in persistent varus leading to increased pressure on the lateral border of the foot.[39] One series of 21 patients treated with an isolated subtalar fusion for pes planus reported that 3 patients developed painful calluses under the fifth metatarsal.[39] Mann and colleagues (1998)[40] found that transverse tarsal motion was diminished by 40% in patients who underwent an isolated subtalar fusion, and they recommended that an isolated subtalar fusion is contraindicated in patients who had greater than 10° to 15° of forefoot varus or transverse tarsal joint hypermobility. Hypermobility of the transverse tarsal joints may result in midfoot collapse.[43] Another study in cadaveric specimens demonstrated a similar loss of adjacent joint motion as Mann and colleagues (1998),[40] with a 41% loss of inversion and 39% loss of inversion with relative preservation of plantarflexion and dorsiflexion at the transverse tarsal joints.[44]

Additionally, isolated subtalar fusions may not adequately correct all the deformities associated with a severe PCFD.[45] O'Malley and colleagues (1995)[45] demonstrated in a cadaveric flatfoot model that an isolated subtalar arthrodesis failed to fully correct the hindfoot valgus and forefoot abduction deformities. A clinical study, however, demonstrated acceptable correction of the forefoot abduction deformity using a subtalar arthrodesis in combination with other bony or soft tissue reconstructive procedures.[46] Johnson and colleagues (2000)[46] retrospectively reviewed 16 patients with flexible PCFD who failed nonoperative management and underwent a flexor digitorum longus transfer to the navicular, spring ligament repair, and subtalar arthrodesis. They reported improvements in radiographic measures of forefoot abduction, including AP talo–first metatarsal angle and talonavicular coverage angle.[46]

In cases of severe abduction deformity at the talonavicular joint not adequately addressed with a subtalar fusion alone, a spring ligament reconstruction may be performed.[47] This requires, however, that the talonavicular joint is able to be corrected intraoperatively by at least 50% in both the AP and sagittal planes.[47] A talonavicular arthrodesis is indicated when the abduction and plantar sag deformities at the talonavicular joint are not able to be corrected intraoperatively, patients have severe talonavicular arthritis, or they have a fixed deformity preoperatively.[47] In a study of 14 feet in which lateral column lengthening failed to adequately address talonavicular abduction intraoperatively, a spring ligament reconstruction using peroneus longus autograft resulted in good to excellent results in all patients at a mean follow-up of 8.9 years, and none of the patients underwent a subsequent talonavicular fusion.[48] Another study investigating the results of combined deltoid-spring ligament reconstruction using semitendinosus or peroneus longus allografts in 14 feet reported significant clinical and radiographic improvements at a minimum of 12 months follow-up.[49] The decision to proceed with the combined deltoid-spring ligament reconstruction was made intraoperatively if there was severe residual hindfoot valgus or an inadequately reduced talonavicular joint with a large spring ligament tear.[49] There are no studies to date, however, looking at the results of concomitant spring ligament reconstruction and subtalar arthrodesis.

Sinus Tarsi and Subfibular Impingement Deformities

Weight-bearing CT scans have provided new insight into the deformity at the subtalar joint in patients with PCFD.[2,3,13,14,50–52] PCFD patients often have a more valgus subtalar alignment than healthy control subjects.[2,53,54] A study of 45 patients with flexible PCFD and 17 control patients demonstrated that patients with flexible disease had, on average, 11° of additional valgus alignment of the posterior facet of the subtalar joint compared with normal patients.[2]

In addition to more innate valgus alignment of the subtalar joint, patients with PCFD often have significant subluxation of the subtalar joint.[3,50,51] Using weight-bearing CT scans, de Cesar Netto and colleagues (2019)[3] compared the alignment of the middle facet of the subtalar joint in 30 flexible PCFD deformity patients with 30 matched control patients. They found that patients with PCFD had a mean uncoverage of the middle facet of 45.3%, which was statistically significantly higher than control patients who had an average of only 4.8% uncoverage.[3] Similarly, Ananthakrisnan and colleagues (1999)[51] reported that only 68% of the posterior facet of the calcaneus was in contact with the talus in 8 patients with PCFD, including 1 patient with an acute rupture of the posterior tibial tendon on simulated weight-bearing CT scans compared with 92% in controls. This more recent understanding of the PCFD have led some to describe the disease as peritalar subluxation because the primary deformities of the disease occur at the talocalcaneal and talonavicular joints, which are subluxated.[51]

Consequently, by correcting subluxation of the talocalcaneal joint, the senior author (S.J.E.) believes that isolated arthrodesis of the subtalar joint has the potential to result in adequate correction of the peritalar deformities, including the abduction deformity at the talonavicular joint, without the need for fusion of additional joints. Future studies looking at long-term follow-up following isolated subtalar arthrodesis in PCFD are necessary, however, to determine if an isolated subtalar fusion provides durable deformity correction and improvements in patient-reported outcomes.

Weight-bearing CT scans also have identified deformities difficult to assess on plain radiographs, such as sinus tarsi and/or calcaneofibular (subfibular) impingement, which typically present with pain laterally at the sinus tarsi or at the anterior fibula, respectively.[13,14,52] Malicky and colleagues (2002)[13] used simulated weight-bearing CT scans in 19 patients with symptomatic PCFD to investigate subtalar and subfibular impingement and then compared their results to simulated weight-bearing CT scans in 5 patients with normal feet in neutral alignment. The prevalence of subtalar and subfibular impingement was 92% and 66%, respectively, in the PCFD group and 0 and 5%, respectively, in the control group.[13] All patients with subfibular impingement also had subtalar impingement.[13] Jeng and colleagues (2018)[14] used weight-bearing CT scans in 34 patients with flexible and rigid adult-acquired PCFD deformity to evaluate sinus tarsi and subfibular impingement. They reported a lower prevalence of subfibular and subtalar impingement in patients at 35 and 38%, respectively, than Malicky and colleagues (2002)[13]; however, compared with normal control subjects, PCFD patients had a lower mean talocalcaneal and calcaneofibular distances on weight-bearing CT scans.[14]

These studies have expanded the indications for isolated subtalar fusions in the setting of PCFD. Patients with severe sinus tarsi and/or subfibular impingement may benefit from a subtalar fusion rather than joint-preserving reconstructive procedures to better address these deformities.[55] Sinus tarsi impingement may be an early indication of peritalar subluxation,[56] but, because it is an extra-articular deformity, flexible PCFD with signs of sinus tarsi impingement may be treated with reconstructive procedures rather than fusion as the subtalar joint is not necessarily arthritic. Subfibular impingement may be a sign of more severe disease.[56] In a study correlating findings of magnetic resonance imaging (MRI) and whole-body CT scans in patients with PCFD, subfibular impingement was associated with degeneration of the talocalcaneal interosseous ligament, and because all ligamentous attachments between the talus and calcaneus are incompetent, a translational deformity between the talus and calcaneus is created that may be correctable only by arthrodesis.[56]

Outcomes

There are few studies reporting the results of isolated subtalar arthrodesis for the treatment of PCFD.[38–40] Kitaoka and Patzer (1997)[39] reported their experience of 21 patients who were treated with a realignment subtalar arthrodesis for posterior tibial tendon dysfunction and pes planus. In addition to improvements in radiographic parameters, they reported good to excellent results in 16 patients, fair results in 4 patients, and poor results in 1 patient with union in all feet. There was no significant progression of adjacent joint arthrosis.

Mangone and colleagues (1997)[38] reviewed 32 patients who underwent 34 isolated subtalar fusions for various conditions, including PCFD. Eighteen patients had adequate postoperative radiographs to evaluate degenerative changes in adjacent joints, and 3 patients had signs of progression of adjacent joint arthrosis.[38] More than 80% of patients stated that they would have the surgery again at an average follow-up on 30.8 months.[38]

Similarly, Mann and colleagues (1998)[40] described the results of 48 isolated subtalar arthrodeses in 44 patients for multiple diagnoses, including 11 patients with PCFD with a mean follow-up of almost 5 years.[40] At final follow-up, 41 patients were satisfied or very satisfied, and 3 patients were dissatisfied with their surgery[40]; 36% and 41% of patients developed evidence of mild adjacent-joint arthrosis of the ankle and transverse tarsal joints, respectively.[40]

Stephens and colleagues (1999)[57] retrospectively reviewed 25 isolated repositional subtalar arthrodeses in 24 patients with adult-acquired PCFD deformity with middle to late flexible disease and lateral sinus tarsi pain. Clinical outcomes were measured at an average of 49.4 months postoperatively, and radiographic outcomes were measured at a mean of 21.1 months postoperatively.[57] In their study, all patients would have chosen to undergo the procedure again, and all patients had union of their subtalar fusion.[57] Meary angle improved preoperative to postoperatively from 21° to 7° apex plantar, and the talonavicular uncoverage percentage decreased from 36% to 18% postoperatively. They reported no evidence of adjacent-joint arthrosis in their study.[57]

These studies suggest that an isolated subtalar arthrodesis for the treatment of PCFD results in acceptable postoperative clinical outcomes at short to midterm follow-up. Taken with the studies discussed previously, isolated subtalar arthrodesis without concomitant talonavicular fusion for the treatment of PCFD provides a powerful tool for correcting collapse at the medial longitudinal arch as well as the forefoot abduction and hindfoot valgus deformities. Further investigation is needed, however, to determine the longevity of this procedure and better define specific indications.

CASE STUDY

History and Physical Examination

A 60-year-old woman presented with a chief complaint of left foot pain that had been present for approximately 1 year. Her symptoms were located primarily at her medial arch, but she complained of pain laterally at the sinus tarsi. She has noticed progressive collapse of the left foot. The pain began insidiously, and she denied any specific trauma. The patient worked as a dance instructor and previously danced 25 hours to 30 hours per week, but her left foot had limited her activities significantly. The patient had tried an Arizona brace with only mild relief of her symptoms, and she continued to have considerable pain in her left foot. Her past medical history was notable for migraines and previous débridement of her posterior tibial tendon by an outside provider.

On physical examination, she had an antalgic gait and swelling around the medial arch. The hindfoot was noticeably in valgus on the left, but the deformity was passively correctible. Clinically, her forefoot abduction was not significant, but she did have residual forefoot supination. She had a large hallux valgus deformity with hypermobility at the first tarsometarsal joint. The patient had tenderness to palpation along the course of the posterior tibial tendon, throughout the medial longitudinal arch, and in the sinus tarsi. She was unable to do a single or double heel rise without difficulty. She was neurovascularly intact.

Imaging

Plain radiographs of the left demonstrated a collapse of the medial longitudinal arch with a Meary angle of 12.2° apex plantar (**Fig. 1**A). Lateral radiographs of the left foot also demonstrated plantar-gapping at the first tarsometarsal joint and beaking

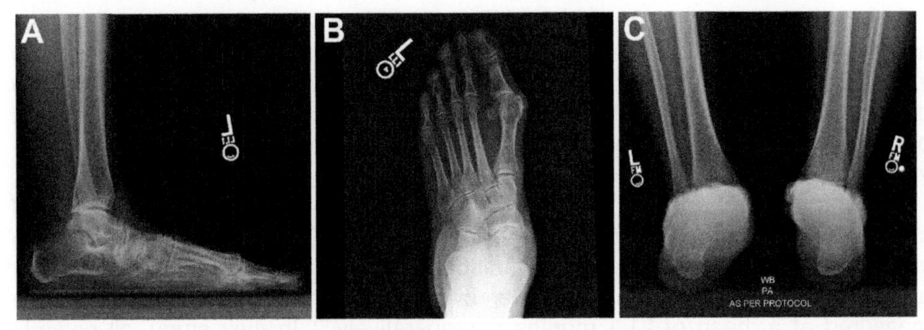

Fig. 1. Preoperative weight-bearing radiographs of the left foot. (*A*) A lateral radiograph of the left foot showing the patient's preoperative medial longitudinal arch collapse, sclerosis of the subtalar joint suggesting impingement, beaking at the talonavicular joint without evidence of tarsal coalition on advanced imaging, and plantar-gapping of the first tarsometatarsal joint. (*B*) An AP radiograph of the left foot illustrating the abduction deformity at the talonavicular joint and hallux valgus. (*C*) A Saltzman hindfoot alignment view showing the patient's severe hindfoot valgus deformity.

of the talus at the talonavicular joint. There was no evidence of tarsal coalition on advanced imaging. There was sclerosis in the subtalar joint suggestive of subtalar impingement. On the AP view of the left foot, she had approximately 50% to 60% talonavicular uncoverage, a first–second intermetatarsal angle of 15.4°, and a hallux valgus angle of 25.3° (**Fig. 1**B). On the Saltzman hindfoot alignment view, she had a hindfoot moment arm of 32.1 mm (**Fig. 1**C).[58]

MRI showed evidence of degeneration of the posterior tibial tendon with fluid in the tendon sheath (**Fig. 2**A) on axial proton density–weighted imaging. On sagittal inversion recovery sequences, there was sclerosis in the calcaneus at the angle of Gissane with edema in the lateral talar process (**Fig. 2**B). Sagittal proton-density sequences showed a tear of the superomedial fibers of the spring ligament (**Fig. 2**C). There was evidence of subfibular impingement of coronal proton-density sequences (**Fig. 2**D).

Weight-bearing CT scans again demonstrated subtalar impingement on sagittal sequences with sclerosis of the calcaneus at the angle of Gissane, plantar-gapping and subluxation of the first tarsometatarsal joint, and early degenerative changes at the talonavicular joint (**Fig. 3**A–C). Coronal weight-bearing CT scan images demonstrate subluxation of the middle facet of the subtalar joint with 59.3% uncoverage (**Fig. 3**D), an angle of 41.2° between the inferior and superior facets of the talus (**Fig. 3**E), and a calcaneofibular distance of 3.2 (**Fig. 3**F).[2,3,14] There was no evidence of a tarsal coalition on weight-bearing CT scans or MRIs.

Surgical Management

Despite early arthritic changes at the talonavicular joint, the decision was made to avoid arthrodesis of the talonavicular joint because her hindfoot deformity was flexible, and fusion of the talonavicular joint would limit hindfoot motion significantly.[15] The senior author also typically avoids fusion of the talonavicular joint in patients with flexible PCFD as a result of its higher nonunion and complication rate.[26] Correction of the abduction and sag deformities at the talonavicular joint can often be obtained with subtalar and first tarsometatarsal arthrodeses.[37] Deformities along the medial longitudinal arch commonly are found at the naviculocuneiform joint, and patients typically

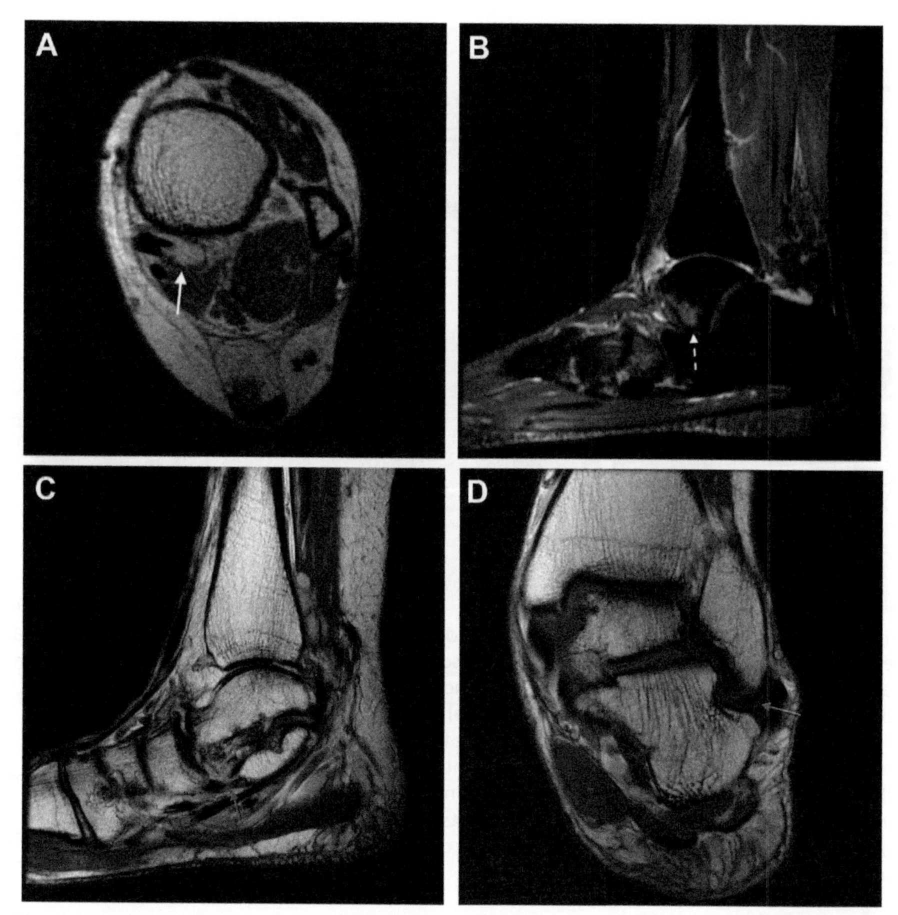

Fig. 2. Preoperative MRI of the left foot. (*A*) The arrow shows fluid in the posterior tibial tendon sheath on axial proton density–weighted imaging. (*B*) On the sagittal inversion recovery sequence, the arrow in indicates edema in the lateral talar process. (*C*) A sagittal proton density–weighted image, with the arrow pointing to tearing of the superomedial spring ligament. (*D*) A coronal proton density weighted image; the orange arrow indicates subfibular mpingement.

tolerate more severe deformities at this articulation.[35,37] Consequently, fusion of the talonavicular joint frequently may be spared during the reconstruction of the PCFD.

The patient's significant subtalar impingement, moderate subfibular impingement, and subluxation of the middle facet of the subtalar joint evident on both MRI and weight-bearing CT scan images led the senior author to perform a subtalar fusion. The patient also required a medializing calcaneal osteotomy due her sizable hindfoot valgus deformity.[59] As a result of the hypermobility of her first tarsometatarsal joint, seen clinically as well as on weight-bearing radiographs and CT scans, her hallux valgus deformity was corrected using a first tarsometatarsal fusion and modified McBride procedure. Additionally, the flexor digitorum longus was transferred to the navicular, and a gastrocnemius recession was performed.

Postoperatively, the patient was placed in a short-leg splint for 2 weeks and discharged with appropriate deep vein thrombosis prophylaxis for a total duration of

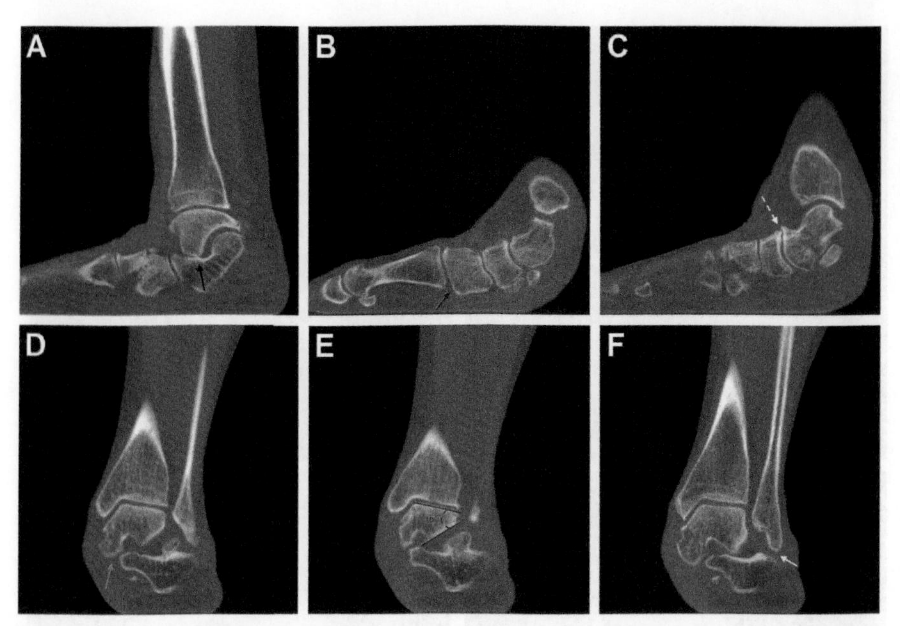

Fig. 3. Preoperative weight-bearing CT scans of the left foot. (*A–C*) Sagittal images of the left foot. (*C*) The solid black arrow points to sclerosis in the calcaneus at the angle of Gissane. (*C*) The arrow points to subluxation and plantar-gapping of the first tarsometarsal joint. (*C*)The arrow points to beaking of the talus indicative of early arthrosis of the talonavicular joint, although there was no evidence of tarsal coalition on a weight-bearing CT scan or MRI. (*D*) A coronal image of the left foot, and the arrow points to subluxation of the middle facet of the subtalar joint. (*E*) Also, a coronal image of the left foot demonstrating the angle between the inferior and superior facets of the talus at the middle of the posterior facet of the talus in the sagittal plane. (*F*) A coronal image of the left foot with an arrow pointing to subfibular impingement.

8 weeks. At the 2-week postoperative visit, the splint was taken down, the sutures removed, and the patient placed in a short-leg fiberglass for an additional 2 weeks. The patient was transitioned to a CAM walker boot 4 weeks postoperative and made non–weight bearing for an additional 4 weeks.

Follow-up

At her 1-year follow-up appointment, the patient noted that she was pleased with her result. She has had a 95% resolution of her symptoms. She does not complain of pain at the talonavicular joint or in her left ankle. Physical examination demonstrated improved alignment from her preoperative state with persistent flattening of the medial arch with mild forefoot abduction. She was able to perform a single heel rise but could not sustain it for prolonged periods of time. One-year weight-bearing postoperative radiographs demonstrate improvement of the first-second intermetatarsal angle to 2° and talonavicular uncoverage to 32.1% on an AP radiograph (**Fig. 4**A). A lateral radiograph shows partial restoration of the medial longitudinal arch with a postoperative Meary angle of 9.1° apex plantar and fusion of the subtalar and first tarsometatarsal joints (**Fig. 4**B). A Saltzman view reveals a postoperative hindfoot moment of 19.8 mm (**Fig. 4**C). A previous CT scan demonstrated evidence of bony union across the subtalar and first tarsometatarsal joints.

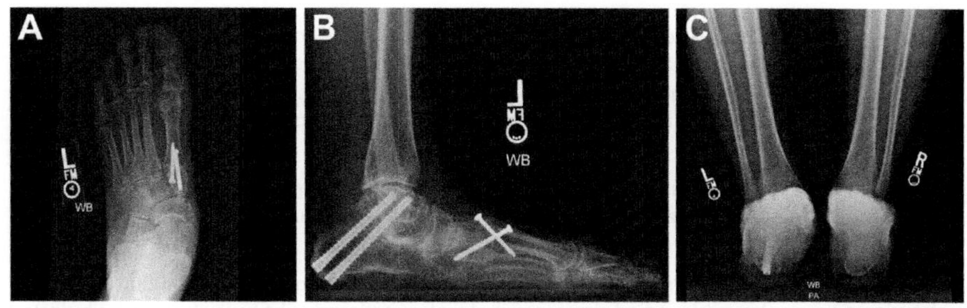

Fig. 4. One-year postoperative weight-bearing radiographs of the left foot. (*A*) An AP radiograph of the left foot showing improvement in talonavicular abduction and improvement in the hallux valgus deformity. (*B*) A lateral radiograph of the left foot with improvement in the medial longitudinal arch deformity and solid fusion of the subtalar and first tarsometatarsal joints. (*C*) A Saltzman hindfoot view illustrating the final postoperative correction of the hindfoot valgus deformity.

SUMMARY

As PCFD is better understood, surgical management will continue to evolve. Triple arthrodesis remains a useful tool for patients with severe and rigid hindfoot deformities who are not amenable to reconstruction.[19] Nevertheless, concerns regarding changes in gait, adjacent-joint arthrosis, need to obtain fusion across 3 joints, and lower patient-reported outcome measures have led surgeons to find alternative treatment options, such as selective hindfoot arthrodesis with or without concomitant reconstructive procedures.[15–17,24]

Arthrodesis of the talonavicular joint, in particular, has reportedly high rates of nonunion and considerable loss of hindfoot motion, which may accelerate adjacent joint arthrosis.[15,26] Consequently, recent literature has supported using alternative arthrodesis constructs that spare the talonavicular joint, such as naviculocuneiform or isolated subtalar fusions that have the potential to both maintain some degree of hindfoot motion and adequately address the patient's deformity.[9,34,57] PCFD patients with significant subluxation of the middle facet of the subtalar joint or with sinus tarsi and/or subfibular impingement deformities with flexible deformity may benefit from a subtalar arthrodesis to more appropriately treat these deformities. In addition to addressing the subtalar joint, isolated subtalar arthrodesis may be a useful tool for correcting midfoot abduction deformities.[57,59] Concomitant reconstructive procedures, such as a medializing calcaneal osteotomy, first tarsometatarsal fusion, Cotton osteotomy, and/or flexor digitorum longus transfer, may be used in addition to a subtalar fusion to address severe deformities.[37] Further work is necessary to identify specific indications for these procedures. In order to optimize patient results and minimize complications, meticulous preoperative history, physical examination, and imaging are essential to developing an appropriate surgical plan.

CLINICS CARE POINTS

- Fusion of the talonavicular joint results in almost no motion at the subtalar and calcaneocuboid joints, and, therefore, may accelerate adjacent-joint arthrosis.
- Isolated subtalar arthrodesis can be used to correct both hindfoot valgus and midfoot abduction deformities with acceptable postoperative clinical outcomes at short-term to midterm follow-up.

- Subtalar arthrodesis may be combined with reconstructive procedures, including medializing calcaneal osteotomy, first tarsometatarsal fusion, Cotton osteotomy, and/or flexor digitorum longus transfer in order to address severe flexible or rigid PCFD. Some investigators have used a naviculocuneiform arthrodesis in combination with a subtalar fusion to treat PCFD and have reported good clinical results.
- Studies using weight-bearing CT scans have demonstrated that patients with PCFD typically have a more valgus subtalar joint as well as more middle facet uncoverage than healthy control patients.
- Preoperative weight-bearing CT scans may be useful guide surgical management. Weight-bearing CT scans have identified sinus tarsi (talocalcaneal) and subfibular (calcaneofibular) impingement deformities in patients with PCFD. Severe sinus tarsi or subfibular impingement deformities may be indications to use a subtalar fusion in addition to traditional reconstructive procedures.

DISCLOSURE

M.S. Conti: this author has nothing to disclose. S.J. Ellis: this author reports consulting fees from Paragon 28 and Wright Medical.

REFERENCES

1. Deland JT. Adult-acquired flatfoot deformity. J Am Acad Orthop Surg 2008;16(7):399–406.
2. Cody EA, Williamson ER, Burket JC, et al. Correlation of Talar Anatomy and Subtalar Joint Alignment on Weightbearing Computed Tomography with Radiographic Flatfoot Parameters. Foot Ankle Int 2016;37(8):874–81.
3. De Cesar Netto C, Godoy-Santos AL, Saito GH, et al. Subluxation of the Middle Facet of the Subtalar Joint as a Marker of Peritalar Subluxation in Adult Acquired Flatfoot Deformity: A Case-Control Study. J Bone Joint Surg Am 2019;101(20):1838–44.
4. Oh I, Williams BR, Ellis SJ, et al. Reconstruction of the Symptomatic Idiopathic Flatfoot in Adolescents and Young Adults. Foot Ankle Int 2011;32(03):225–32.
5. Ellis SJ. Determining the Talus Orientation and Deformity of Planovalgus Feet Using Weightbearing Multiplanar Axial Imaging. Foot Ankle Int 2012;33(5):444–9.
6. Johnson KA, Strom DE. Tibialis posterior tendon dysfunction. Clin Orthop Relat Res 1989;239:196–206.
7. Myerson MS, Thordarson DB, Johnson JE, et al. Classification and Nomenclature: Progressive Collapsing Foot Deformity. Foot Ankle Int 2020;41(10):1271–6.
8. Pomeroy GC, Manoli A. A new operative approach for flatfoot secondary to posterior tibial tendon insufficiency: a preliminary report. Foot Ankle Int 1997;18(4):206–12.
9. Ajis A, Geary N. Surgical technique, fusion rates, and planovalgus foot deformity correction with naviculocuneiform fusion. Foot Ankle Int 2014;35(3):232–7.
10. Barg A, Brunner S, Zwicky L, et al. Subtalar and naviculocuneiform fusion for extended breakdown of the medial arch. Foot Ankle Clin 2011;16(1):69–81.
11. Rohm J, Zwicky L, Horn Lang T, et al. Mid- to long-term outcome of 96 corrective hindfoot fusions in 84 patients with rigid flatfoot deformity. Bone Joint J 2015;97-B(5):668–74.
12. Taylor R, Sammarco VJ. Minimizing the Role of Fusion in the Rigid Flatfoot. Foot Ankle Clin 2012;17(2):337–49.

13. Malicky ES, Crary JL, Houghton MJ, et al. Talocalcaneal and subfibular impingement in symptomatic flatfoot in adults. J Bone Joint Surg Am 2002;84(11):2005–9.
14. Jeng CL, Rutherford T, Hull MG, et al. Assessment of Bony Subfibular Impingement in Flatfoot Patients Using Weight-Bearing CT Scans. Foot Ankle Int 2019; 40(2):152–8.
15. Astion DJ, Deland JT, Otis JC, et al. Motion of the hindfoot after simulated arthrodesis. J Bone Joint Surg Am 1997;79(2):241–6.
16. Beischer AD, Brodsky JW, Polio FE, et al. Functional outcome and gait analysis after triple or double arthrodesis. Foot Ankle Int 1999;20(9):545–53.
17. Saltzman CL, Fehrle MJ, Cooper RR, et al. Triple arthrodesis: Twenty-five and forty-four-year average follow-up of the same patients. J Bone Joint Surg Am 1999;81(10):1391–402.
18. Fogel GR, Katoh Y, Rand JA, et al. Talonavicular arthrodesis for isolated arthrosis: 9.5-year results and gait analysis. Foot Ankle 1982;3(2):105–13.
19. Erard MUE, Sheean MAJ, Sangeorzan BJ. Triple Arthrodesis for Adult-Acquired Flatfoot Deformity. Foot Ankle Orthop 2019;4(3):1–12.
20. Sangeorzan BJ, Hintermann B, de Cesar Netto C, et al. Progressive Collapsing Foot Deformity: Consensus on Goals for Operative Correction. Foot Ankle Int 2020;41(10):1299–302.
21. Bennett GL, Graham CE, Mauldin DM. Triple arthrodesis in adults. Foot Ankle 1991;12(3):138–43.
22. Fortin PT, Walling AK. Triple arthrodesis. Clin Orthop Relat Res 1999;365:91–9.
23. Graves SC, Mann RA, Graves KO. Triple arthrodesis in older adults. Results after long-term follow-up. J Bone Joint Surg Am 1993;75(3):355–62.
24. Deland JT, Page A, Sung I-H, et al. Posterior tibial tendon insufficiency results at different stages. HSS J 2006;2(2):157–60.
25. Haleem AM, Pavlov H, Bogner E, et al. Comparison of deformity with respect to the talus in patients with posterior tibial tendon dysfunction and controls using multiplanar weight-bearing imaging or conventional radiography. J Bone Joint Surg Am 2014;96(8):e63.
26. Fortin PT. Posterior tibial tendon insufficiency. Isolated fusion of the talonavicular joint. Foot Ankle Clin 2001;6(1):137–51.
27. Clain MR, Baxter DE. Simultaneous calcaneocuboid and talonavicular fusion. Long-term follow-up study. Bone Joint J 1994;76(1):133–6.
28. Knupp M, Schuh R, Stufkens SAS, et al. Subtalar and talonavicular arthrodesis through a single medial approach for the correction of severe planovalgus deformity. Bone Joint J 2009;91(5):612–5.
29. Ellis SJ, Johnson JE, Day J, et al. Titrating the Amount of Bony Correction in Progressive Collapsing Foot Deformity. Foot Ankle Int 2020;41(10):1292–5.
30. Sammarco VJ, Magur EG, Sammarco GJ, et al. Arthrodesis of the subtalar and talonavicular joints for correction of symptomatic hindfoot malalignment. Foot Ankle Int 2006;27(9):661–6.
31. Schuh R, Salzberger F, Wanivenhaus AH, et al. Kinematic changes in patients with double arthrodesis of the hindfoot for realignment of planovalgus deformity. J Orthop Res 2013;31(4):517–24.
32. O'Malley MJ, Deland JT, Lee KT. Selective hindfoot arthrodesis for the treatment of adult acquired flatfoot deformity: an in vitro study. Foot Ankle Int 1995;16(7): 411–7.
33. Harper MC, Tisdel CL. Talonavicular Arthrodesis for the Painful Adult Acquired Flatfoot. Foot Ankle Int 1996;17(11):658–61.

34. Steiner CS, Gilgen A, Zwicky L, et al. Combined Subtalar and Naviculocuneiform Fusion for Treating Adult Acquired Flatfoot Deformity With Medial Arch Collapse at the Level of the Naviculocuneiform Joint. Foot Ankle Int 2019;40(1):42–7.
35. Greisberg J, Hansen ST, Sangeorzan B. Deformity and degeneration in the hindfoot and midfoot joints of the adult acquired flatfoot. Foot Ankle Int 2003;24(7): 530–4.
36. Aiyer A, Dall GF, Shub J, et al. Radiographic Correction Following Reconstruction of Adult Acquired Flat Foot Deformity Using the Cotton Medial Cuneiform Osteotomy. Foot Ankle Int 2016;37(5):508–13.
37. Day J, Conti MS, Ellis SJ, et al. Contribution of First Tarsometatarsal Joint Fusion to Deformity Correction in the Treatment of Adult Acquired. Flatfoot Deformity 2020;5(3):1–8.
38. Mangone PG, Fleming LL, Fleming SS, et al. Treatment of acquired adult planovalgus deformities with subtalar fusion. Clin Orthop Relat Res 1997;341:106–12.
39. Kitaoka HB, Patzer GL. Subtalar arthrodesis for posterior tibial tendon dysfunction and pes planus. Clin Orthop Relat Res 1997;345:187–94.
40. Mann RA, Beaman DN, Horton GA. Isolated subtalar arthrodesis. Foot Ankle Int 1998;19(8):511–9.
41. Johnson JE Yu JR. Arthrodesis techniques in the management of stage II and III acquired adult flatfoot deformity. Instr Course Lect 2006;55:531–42.
42. Hintermann B, Deland JT, de Cesar Netto C, et al. Consensus on Indications for Isolated Subtalar Joint Fusion and Naviculocuneiform Fusions for Progressive Collapsing Foot Deformity. Foot Ankle Int 2020;41(10):1295–8.
43. Kadakia AR, Haddad SL. Hindfoot arthrodesis for the adult acquired flat foot. Foot Ankle Clin 2003;8(3):569–94.
44. Gellman H, Lenihan M, Halikis N, et al. Selective tarsal arthrodesis: an in vitro analysis of the effect on foot motion. Foot Ankle 1987;8(3):127–33.
45. O'Malley M-J, Deland JT, Lee K-T. Selective Hindfoot Arthrodesis for the Treatment. Foot Ankle Int 1995;16(7):411–7.
46. Johnson JE, Cohen BE, DiGiovanni BF, et al. Subtalar arthrodesis with flexor digitorum longus transfer and spring ligament repair for treatment of posterior tibial tendon insufficiency. Foot Ankle Int 2000;21(9):722–9.
47. Deland JT, Ellis SJ, Day J, et al. Indications for Deltoid and Spring Ligament Reconstruction in Progressive Collapsing Foot Deformity. Foot Ankle Int 2020; 41(10):1302–6.
48. Ellis SJ, Williams BR, Wagshul AD, et al. Deltoid ligament reconstruction with peroneus longus autograft in flatfoot deformity. Foot Ankle Int 2010;31(9):781–9.
49. Brodell JD, MacDonald A, Perkins JA, et al. Deltoid-Spring Ligament Reconstruction in Adult Acquired Flatfoot Deformity With Medial Peritalar Instability. Foot Ankle Int 2019;40(7):753–61.
50. Kunas GC, Probasco W, Haleem AM, et al. Evaluation of peritalar subluxation in adult acquired flatfoot deformity using computed tomography and weightbearing multiplanar imaging. Foot Ankle Surg 2018;24(6):495–500.
51. Ananthakrisnan D, Ching R, Tencer A, et al. Subluxation of the talocalcaneal joint in adults who have symptomatic flatfoot. J Bone Joint Surg Am 1999;81(8): 1147–54.
52. de Cesar Netto C, Myerson MS, Day J, et al. Consensus for the Use of Weightbearing CT in the Assessment of Progressive Collapsing Foot Deformity. Foot Ankle Int 2020;41(10):1277–82.
53. Colin F, Horn Lang T, Zwicky L, et al. Subtalar joint configuration on weightbearing CT scan. Foot Ankle Int 2014;35(10):1057–62.

54. Apostle KL, Coleman NW, Sangeorzan BJ. Subtalar joint axis in patients with symptomatic peritalar subluxation compared to normal controls. Foot Ankle Int 2014;35(11):1153–8.
55. Ellis SJ. Peritalar Symposium: determining the talus orientation and deformity of planovalgus feet using weightbearing multiplanar axial imaging. Foot Ankle Int 2012;33(5):444–9.
56. de Cesar Netto C, Saito GH, Roney A, et al. Combined weightbearing CT and MRI assessment of flexible progressive collapsing foot deformity. Foot Ankle Surg 2020. Online ahead of print.
57. Stephens HM, Walling AK, Solmen JD, et al. Subtalar repositional arthrodesis for adult acquired flatfoot. Clin Orthop Relat Res 1999;365:69–73.
58. Saltzman CL, el-Khoury GY. The hindfoot alignment view. Foot Ankle Int 1995; 16(9):572–6.
59. Davies J, Garfinkel J, Ma X, et al. Subtalar Fusion for Correction of Forefoot Abduction in Stage II Adult Acquired Flatfoot Deformity. Foot Ankle Spec 2020. Online ahead of print.

Is Arthrodesis Sufficient in the Setting of Complex, Severe and Rigid Progressive Collapsing Foot Deformities?

Michelle M. Coleman, MD, PhD[a], Gregory P. Guyton, MD[b,*]

KEYWORDS

- Flatfoot deformity • Progressive collapsing foot deformity • Complex foot deformity
- Triple arthrodesis • Hindfoot fusion • Flatfoot undercorrection
- Flatfoot overcorrection

KEY POINTS

- Arthrodesis procedures provide excellent correction and maintenance of deformity in most of the patients with severe progressive collapsing foot deformity.
- Patients with congenital or acquired bony abnormalities, tendon contractures, flexible ankle ligamentous instability, or concomitant deformities of the proximal extremity may require additional procedures in addition to joint fusion.
- Although there are many surgical options for addressing individual challenges in the severe and complex progressive collapsing foot deformities, limited objective data are available to guide decisions regarding the need for concomitant procedures. Specific indications are up to individual surgeon judgment and discretion.

INTRODUCTION

Arthrodesis is the most common treatment of rigid and/or arthritic progressive collapsing foot deformity (PCFD).[1] Although severe and complex deformities are not always rigid, the stability provided and the degree of correction afforded by arthrodesis procedures also make fusion the most common method of treatment in severe flexible deformity.

Arthrodesis is sufficient in the treatment of many, but not all, complex and severe deformities. Arthrodesis procedures include triple arthrodesis (subtalar, talonavicular, and calcaneocuboid fusion), double arthrodesis (2 of the previous 3 joints), isolated

[a] Emory University School of Medicine, 59 Executive Park South, Suite 2000, Atlanta, GA 30329, USA; [b] Department of Orthopaedic Surgery, MedStar Union Memorial Hospital, 3333 North Calvert Street, Suite 400, Baltimore, MD 21218, USA
* Corresponding author.
E-mail address: gpguyton@gmail.com

Foot Ankle Clin N Am 26 (2021) 609–617
https://doi.org/10.1016/j.fcl.2021.06.006

arthrodesis (1 of the previous 3 joints), or pantalar fusion (tibiotalar, subtalar, and talonavicular fusion). Unfortunately, there are no published papers that describe the degree of correction possible with particular joint fusion procedures. However, a thorough understanding of the unique deformities associated with a particular patient's flatfoot case does allow targeted reduction and fixation of the contributing pathologic joint malalignment in most of the cases. Fusion procedures provide excellent correction of alignment,[2,3] which seems to be maintained at mid-term to long-term follow-up.[4]

When Is Arthrodesis Insufficient?

Although freeing up the necessary ligamentous connections between the target joints allows manual reduction to a physiologic alignment in many cases, there are some instances where fusion procedures alone are not sufficient to treat severe or complex PCFD (**Box 1**). In these instances, supplemental procedures may be necessary to aid in achieving appropriate reduction and/or stabilization of the deformity (**Table 1**).

Specific Congenital Deformities

A variety of congenital deformities may be associated with the planovalgus foot. Most common is a hindfoot coalition.[5] Even in the setting of significant planovalgus, hindfoot arthrodesis remains a mainstay of treatment, particularly for talocalcaneal coalitions in adult patients or in adolescents with very significant involvement of the posterior facet. More problematic is the ball-and-socket ankle, a rare condition in which the tibiotalar articulation acquires a hemispheric shape during early development. Although the precise cause remains unclear, it has been hypothesized that it is a result of excessive loads through the ankle as a result of other pathology including fibular deficiency, hindfoot coalition, or clubfoot.[6] When accompanied by a planovalgus deformity, the ball-and-socket ankle presents special challenges (**Fig. 1**). The deformity is usually accompanied by severe ligamentous laxity that can prove difficult to manage. When possible, hindfoot arthrodesis should be avoided, given the likelihood that end-stage tibiotalar arthritis may develop and fusion rather than total ankle replacement may be mandated due to the bony deformity. If hindfoot fusion is undertaken, residual dynamic valgus may result from the instability of the tibiotalar joint itself, and long-term brace use may still be required.

The congenital vertical talus is an irreducible congenital dorsal dislocation of the navicular relative to the talar head. The rigid rocker-bottom foot is typically recognized and treated shortly after birth, but neglected cases require significant tendon balancing in addition to hindfoot fusion. The deformity includes elevation of the medial column of the foot and contractures both of the anterior tibialis and flexor hallucis longus. In addition to hindfoot fusion, adult cases have been successfully treated with

Box 1
Instances in which fusion procedures alone may not be sufficient to treat severe or complex deformities

- Congenital/developmental bone abnormality
- Acquired bone loss
- Tendon contracture or spasticity
- Ligamentous instability of the ankle
- Alignment abnormalities in the proximal limb

Table 1
Adjunctive procedures to aid in correction of severe and complex flatfoot deformities

Procedure Type	Examples
Extraarticular osteotomy	Medial displacement calcaneal osteotomy Cotton osteotomy Evans osteotomy
Intraarticular osteotomy	Wedge osteotomy with fusion Medial column shortening with fusion
Bone block arthrodesis with a wedge	Subtalar joint bone block arthrodesis Calcaneocuboid joint bone block arthrodesis
Tendon procedures	Tendoachilles lengthening Peroneal tendon lengthening Peroneal tendon transfer Anterior tibialis lengthening Flexor hallucis longus transfer
Proximal limb correction of alignment	Proximal tibial osteotomy Distal tibial osteotomy Total knee arthroplasty

z-lengthening of the anterior tibialis and transfer of the flexor hallucis longus to the plantar aspect of the first metatarsal to assist in plantarflexing the first ray.[7]

Spasticity and Contracture

In some instances of severe deformity, tendon contracture or spasticity may prevent appropriate reduction of the targeted joints. The most common example of this is an Achilles tendon contracture, which may prevent correction of hindfoot alignment. Achilles tendon lengthening or gastrocnemius recession is commonly indicated in a long-standing PCFD.[8] Less commonly, the peroneal musculature may be severely contracted in the case of a long-standing deformity. If a triple arthrodesis is being performed, a peroneal tenotomy may be performed through a small incision behind the lateral malleolus at the beginning of the surgery to facilitate joint access and

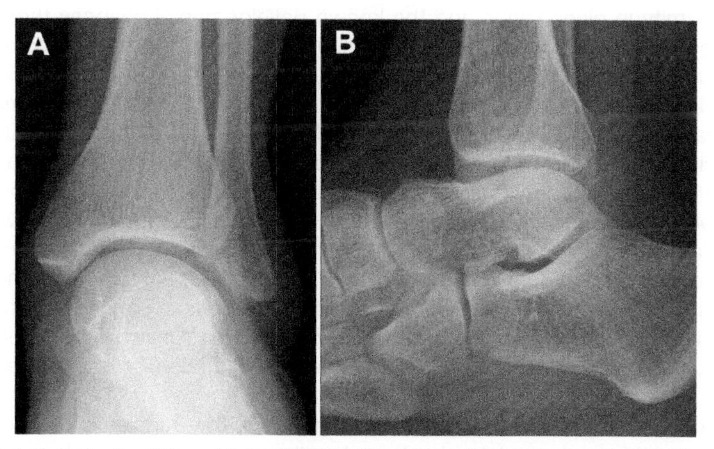

Fig. 1. Anteroposterior (*A*) and lateral (*B*) radiographs of a patient with a ball-and-socket ankle joint. This deformity commonly requires long-term brace management despite subtalar or triple arthrodesis due to valgus instability from the tibiotalar joint itself.

reduction.[9] This maneuver may be especially helpful in the case of a planned medial-only incision technique.

Spasticity or motor imbalance represents a less-common cause of an uncontrollable hindfoot requiring arthrodesis. Cases of spastic planovalgus are rare but may occur in the setting of cerebral palsy or focal dystonia. Motor imbalance is more commonly seen. Poliomyelitis affects the anterior horn cells in the spinal cord and commonly results in the sparing of motor levels below the affected portions of the cord. Because the peroneals draw innervation from more distal nerve roots than both the anterior and posterior tibialis, this may result in neurogenic planovalgus deformity. As a practical matter, most such cases seen today are due to failed lumbar disk surgery or injury.

There is no evidence that normal motor units can overpower the alignment achieved from arthrodesis, but the situation in spasticity may be different. In particular, the spastic peroneal tendon may still lead to dysfunction even if a hindfoot arthrodesis is performed to control the deformity. Spasticity may lead to deformity through the naviculocuneiform level or tarsometatarsal level (**Fig. 2**).[10] If adequate dorsiflexion power remains in the foot, the peroneals may simply be released. If the anterior tibialis has poor function and the peroneus brevis or longus represents the most appropriate tendon to transfer for dorsiflexion power, it can be brought subcutaneously around the anterior aspect of the fibula to the third cuneiform. In this position, continued spasticity of the motor unit may yield dorsiflexion but will not forcibly evert the foot.

Bony Defects and Dysplasia

Planovalgus in both the adult and the adolescent is not solely a result of soft tissue deficiency. Recent surveys of bone shape in adult humans indicate that structural changes are present in the calcaneus of subjects with a planovalgus foot[11]; this includes the relationship of the calcaneocuboid joint relative to the long axis of the bone and the angular relationship of the middle and posterior facets of the subtalar joint to each other.[12] These studies have been performed using analysis of plain radiographs and could likely be refined using weight-bearing computed tomography surveys. In addition, the morphology of hindfoot bones changes with growth. The anteroposterior talocalcaneal angle normally decreases by 6° from birth to adulthood, as the arch assumes a less planovalgus position.[13] The combination of demonstrated bony deformity in planovalgus and the known developmental changes the hindfoot bones undergo mean that some patients will have significant dysplasia that does not neatly fit into other categories of congenital disease.

Arthrodesis alone is insufficient in these patients if there is residual deformity such as residual and excessive hindfoot valgus, forefoot abduction, or forefoot varus. Leaving a residual deformity may result in a nonplantigrade foot, continued pathologic stress on the ankle, and/or impingement within the sinus tarsi impingement or subfibular region. Intraoperatively, the surgeon should manually reduce and provisionally hold the affected joints in position. Overall alignment should be accessed in each plane clinically and radiographically. Gapping or significant subluxation at nonfused joints on radiographs is a clue to residual deformity. For example, in the setting of a double arthrodesis of the subtalar and talonavicular joints, significant calcaneocuboid gapping or plantar subluxation suggests either malreduction or baseline anatomic variation.

In the case of significant calcaneocuboid gapping, the addition of a bone-block arthrodesis of this joint or a lateral column lengthening procedure such as an Evans procedure may provide additional stability and correction of deformity. Less commonly, a medial column shortening may be performed by subtly removing bone

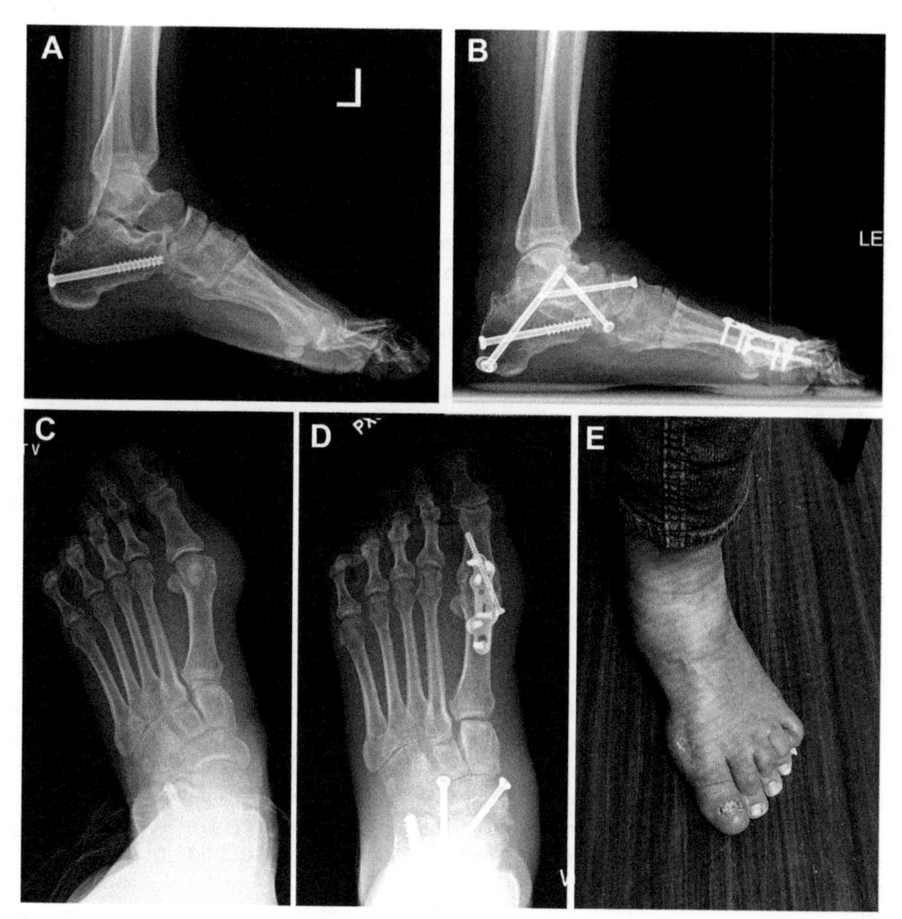

Fig. 2. A 42-year-old patient with a brain stem injury and a spastic planovalgus foot. Anteroposterior and lateral radiographs (*A* and *C*) of the patient after undergoing a medial displacement calcaneal osteotomy. This failed to control the patient's deformity (*B* and *D*). The patient subsequently underwent salvage with a triple arthrodesis. Two years after a successful correction and fusion, the patient's baclofen pump was removed due to complications and she experienced a dramatic increase in peroneal spasticity. Clinical photograph (*E*) demonstrates secondary abduction and planus deformity through the midfoot, which ultimately required treatment with peroneal tendon transfer.

from the talar head to match the lateral column length. In the setting of residual medial instability and sag after maximal talonavicular correction, a plantarflexion opening wedge osteotomy of the medial cuneiform (Cotton osteotomy) may be considered in lieu of a more extended medial column fusion.[14] In the case of residual hindfoot valgus deformity, a medial displacement calcaneal osteotomy (MDCO) may be considered in addition to a subtalar fusion.

Significant loss of normal bone stock may occur in the setting of inflammatory disease, avascular necrosis, or other pathologic processes. Significant erosion of a joint surface may make anatomic reduction impossible without the assistance of adjunctive techniques. For example, in a patient with a PCFD complicated by rheumatoid arthritis–related erosion of the subtalar joint, addition of a bone block to the subtalar arthrodesis may be necessary.[15] In a collapsing deformity caused by midfoot Charcot neuroarthropathy, a biplanar osteotomy may be needed to achieve flat surfaces for bony fusion.[16]

Ligamentous Instability of the Ankle

Correction of severe or complex PCFD may be associated with ligamentous instability of the ankle. Although obvious valgus deformity of the tibiotalar joint may be present in some patients, in some instances dynamic deltoid insufficiency may not be recognized clinically or radiographically until an intraoperative talar tilt test is performed. Therefore, the surgeon must be prepared to perform a deltoid reefing or reconstruction in these instances of flexible instability.[17] Despite recognition of the problem, there remains no long-term data on the efficacy of these reconstructions in severe disease.

In addition, ankle instability due to attenuation of the anterior talofibular or calcaneofibular ligaments may occasionally be present in severe flatfoot deformities.[1,18] Although most associated with the cavovarus rather than the planovalgus foot shape, a concomitant lateral ankle ligament reconstruction may be required in instances of gross instability.

Proximal Bony Deformity

In addition to intrinsic alignment abnormalities in the foot or ankle, more proximal bony deformities may also be present. For example, in the instances of a patient with ipsilateral genu valgum and pes planovalgus alignment, correction of the foot alignment alone may be insufficient to produce a plantigrade foot, as the foot may still strike in a valgus position. In a patient with ipsilateral genu varum and a compensatory pes planovalgus alignment, correction of the foot alignment alone may cause lateral overload due to the foot striking on the lateral border of the foot. Hallux valgus associated with planovalgus has also been associated with knee deformities. Careful evaluation of the entire limb is important in patients with severe flatfoot deformity, and additional procedures to address more proximal deformity may be required in a separate setting.[19–21]

What Evidence Is There to Support Concomitant Procedures?

Although concomitant procedures may be considered during the fusion of complex, severe, and rigid PCFD, there are minimal published data to guide these decisions. During the surgical treatment of PCFD in general, experts in the field caution against both overcorrection of deformity[22] and undercorrection.[23] Lateral column lengthening increases lateral forefoot pressures,[24] which may lead to symptomatic overload.[25] In fact, in patients with flexible PCFD overcorrection of forefoot position into a relatively adducted position was significantly associated with lower postoperative improvement in Foot and Ankle Outcomes Score (FAOS) daily activities and quality of life subscales compared with maintenance of relative abduction.[26] Similarly, excessive plantarflexion of the medial column has been conjectured to increase medial forefoot pressures that can be symptomatic.[22] In patients who undergo double arthrodesis (subtalar and talonavicular fusion) for a rigid PCFD, overcorrection of coronal plane alignment has caused symptomatic lateral foot overload.[4] However, one study has demonstrated that overcorrection of the heel into a position of slight varus (0–5° varus) was associated significantly with improved FAOS pain subscale scores compared with patients with postoperative valgus or moderate varus alignment.

Level V expert consensus does offer general guidelines for titrating the amount of bony correction in progressive collapsing foot deformities.[27] However, this is not specifically in the context of concomitant fusion procedures. In our experience, lateral column lengthening procedures (such as an Evans calcaneal osteotomy) are recommended when the amount of talonavicular uncoverage is greater than 40%. Stabilizing the first ray may assist in avoiding a subsequent valgus moment on the ankle, although data are lacking. The Cotton osteotomy is recommended if the surgeon determines intraoperatively that there is residual forefoot supination as judged by imbalance of the medial and lateral rays when palpating the plantar aspect of the metatarsal heads.[14] The Cotton osteotomy is not considered to be strictly contraindicated in the setting of instability of the first ray, but recent evidence suggests that the long-term correction it affords may be unpredictable.[28] Despite this concern, the Cotton procedure avoids further fusion of the medial column when a triple arthrodesis is also being performed. It should be strongly considered except in extreme cases of first tarsometatarsal instability.

Concomitant triple arthrodesis and deltoid ligament reconstruction has been described more commonly than many other procedures, given the relative frequency of deltoid insufficiency in patients with severe collapsing deformity (eg, adult acquired flatfoot stage IV-A; PCFD with a class 1E).[29–32] Flexible tibiotalar tilt of 3° or more has been suggested as an indication for this procedure.[30] To date, however, long-term follow-up has yet to establish the efficacy and durability of these procedures.

In one cadaver study exploring the role for concomitant MDCO in the setting of triple arthrodesis, simulated specimens with “irreducible peritalar subluxation/dislocation” had decreased forces across the deltoid ligament with concomitant MDCO in addition to in situ triple arthrodesis compared with the arthrodesis alone.[33] The investigators concluded that if the subtalar joint cannot be properly positioned intraoperatively and there is residual valgus deformity, an MDCO may decrease the risk for abnormal forces across the deltoid and potentially prevent subsequent deterioration of deltoid integrity. In fact, one study reported that 27% of their patients treated with hindfoot fusion (subtalar, double, or triple arthrodesis) developed valgus tibiotalar tilt within the first 10 months after operative treatment.[34] In this study, development of postoperative tibiotalar tilt was significantly associated with worsened preoperative Meary angle (first talometatarsal angle) using a Cox proportional hazards regression model.

Although Achilles tendon lengthening and gastrocnemius recession procedures are described in the context of triple arthrodesis, there are no current consensus guidelines regarding their indications due to a lack of data and difficulty reaching expert agreement.[35]

SUMMARY

Arthrodesis procedures are typically used for the correction of severe, complex, and arthritic PCFD. Although most deformities may be treated with arthrodesis alone, concomitant procedures should be considered in some instances. For example, associated bony or soft tissue procedures may be helpful in patients with congenital or acquired bony abnormalities, spasticity, ankle instability, or deformities of the proximal extremity. Additional research is needed to provide an evidence-based guideline for the indications for concomitant procedures during arthrodesis in the setting of PCFD correction.

CLINICS CARE POINTS

- Always be aware that neuromuscular imbalance has the potential to overwhelm the correction achieved from a hindfoot fusion by acting on the ankle or the midfoot.

- Evaluation of the entire leg is necessary when addressing cavus or planus deformities because proximal limb malalignment can drive progressive deformities in the foot or ankle.
- Although adding concomitant osteotomy procedures in the setting of a triple arthrodesis is rarely discussed, it may be required in severe cases to achieve a plantigrade foot.

DISCLOSURE

The authors have nothing to disclose.

REFERENCES

1. Myerson MS, Kadakia AR. Triple arthrodesis. In: Reconstructive foot and ankle surgery: management of complications. 3rd ed. Philadelphia: Elsevier; 2019. p. 480–509.
2. Pell RF, Myerson MS, Schon LC. Clinical outcome after primary triple arthrodesis. J Bone Joint Surg Am 2000;82(1):47–57.
3. Frost NL, Grassbaugh JA, Baird G, et al. Triple arthrodesis with lateral column lengthening for the treatment of planovalgus deformity. J Pediatr Orthop 2011;31(7):773–82.
4. Rohm J, Zwicky L, Horn Lang T, et al. Mid- to long-term outcome of 96 corrective hindfoot fusions in 84 patients with rigid flatfoot deformity. Bone Joint J 2015;97-B(5):668–74.
5. Klammer G, Espinosa N, Iselin LD. Coalitions of the tarsal bones. Foot Ankle Clin 2018;23(3):435–49.
6. Takakura Y, Tamai S, Masuhara K. Genesis of the ball-and-socket ankle. J Bone Joint Surg Br 1986;68(5):834–7.
7. Lui TH. Correction of neglected vertical talus deformity in an adult. BMJ Case Rep 2015;2015.
8. Jeng CL, Vora AM, Myerson MS. The medial approach to triple arthrodesis. Indications and technique for management of rigid valgus deformities in high-risk patients. Foot Ankle Clin 2005;10(3):515–vii.
9. Minor PD. An Introduction to poliovirus: pathogenesis, vaccination, and the endgame for global eradication. Methods Mol Biol 2016;1387:1–10.
10. Cohen JC, de Freitas Cabral E. Peroneus longus transfer for drop foot in Hansen disease. Foot Ankle Clin 2012;17(3). 425-436, vi.
11. Heard-Booth AN. Morphological and functional correlates of variation in the human longitudinal arch. Available at: https://repositories.lib.utexas.edu/handle/2152/60398 [Dissertation]. 2017. Accessed June 4, 2021.
12. Agoada D, Kramer PA. Radiographic measurements of the talus and calcaneus in the adult pes planus foot type. Am J Phys Anthropol 2020;171(4):613–27.
13. McCarthy DJ. The developmental anatomy of pes valgo planus. Clin Podiatr Med Surg 1989;6:491–509.
14. Hirose CB, Johnson JE. Plantarflexion opening wedge medial cuneiform osteotomy for correction of fixed forefoot varus associated with flatfoot deformity. Foot Ankle Int 2004;25(8):568–74.
15. Jackson JB 3rd, Jacobson L, Banerjee R, et al. Distraction subtalar arthrodesis. Foot Ankle Clin 2015;20(2):335–51.
16. Sammarco VJ, Sammarco GJ, Walker EW Jr, et al. Midtarsal arthrodesis in the treatment of Charcot midfoot arthropathy. J Bone Joint Surg Am 2009;91(1):80–91.

17. Alshalawi S, Galhoum AE, Alrashidi Y, et al. Medial ankle instability: the deltoid dilemma. Foot Ankle Clin 2018;23(4):639–57.
18. Wirth SH, Viehofer AF, Singh S, et al. Anterior talofibular ligament lesion is associated with increased flat foot deformity but does not affect correction by lateral calcaneal lengthening. BMC Musculoskelet Disord 2019;20(1):496.
19. Golightly YM, Hannan MT, Dufour AB, et al. Factors associated with hallux valgus in a community-based cross-sectional study of adults with and without osteoarthritis. Arthritis Care Res (Hoboken) 2015;67(6):791–8.
20. Steinberg N, Finestone A, Noff M, et al. Relationship between lower extremity alignment and hallux valgus in women. Foot Ankle Int 2013;34(6):824–31.
21. Lin CJ, Lai KA, Kuan TS, et al. Correlating factors and clinical significance of flexible flatfoot in preschool children. J Pediatr Orthop 2001;21(3):378–82.
22. Irwin TA. Overcorrected flatfoot reconstruction. Foot Ankle Clin 2017;22(3): 597–611.
23. Hunt KJ, Farmer RP. The undercorrected flatfoot reconstruction. Foot Ankle Clin 2017;22(3):613–24.
24. Oh I, Imhauser C, Choi D, et al. Sensitivity of plantar pressure and talonavicular alignment to lateral column lengthening in flatfoot reconstruction. J Bone Joint Surg Am 2013;95(12):1094–100.
25. Kou JX, Balasubramaniam M, Kippe M, et al. Functional results of posterior tibial tendon reconstruction, calcaneal osteotomy, and gastrocnemius recession. Foot Ankle Int 2012;33(7):602–11.
26. Conti MS, Chan JY, Do HT, et al. Correlation of postoperative midfoot position with outcome following reconstruction of the stage II adult acquired flatfoot deformity. Foot Ankle Int 2015;36(3):239–47.
27. Ellis SJ, Johnson JE, Day J, et al. Titrating the amount of bony correction in progressive collapsing foot deformity. Foot Ankle Int 2020;41(10):1292–5.
28. Abousayed MM, Coleman MM, Wei L, et al. Radiographic outcomes of Cotton osteotomy in treatment of adult-acquired flatfoot deformity. Foot Ankle Int 2021. [Epub ahead of print].
29. Bluman EM, Title CI, Myerson MS. Posterior tibial tendon rupture: a refined classification system. Foot Ankle Clin 2007;12(2). 233-249, v.
30. Jeng CL, Bluman EM, Myerson MS. Minimally invasive deltoid ligament reconstruction for stage IV flatfoot deformity. Foot Ankle Int 2011;32(1):21–30.
31. Deland JT, de Asla RJ, Segal A. Reconstruction of the chronically failed deltoid ligament: a new technique. Foot Ankle Int 2004;25(11):795–9.
32. Ellis SJ, Williams BR, Wagshul AD, et al. Deltoid ligament reconstruction with peroneus longus autograft in flatfoot deformity. Foot Ankle Int 2010;31(9):781–9.
33. Resnick RB, Jahss MH, Choueka J, et al. Deltoid ligament forces after tibialis posterior tendon rupture: effects of triple arthrodesis and calcaneal displacement osteotomies. Foot Ankle Int 1995;16:14–20.
34. Miniaci-Coxhead SL, Weisenthal B, Ketz JP, et al. Incidence and radiographic predictors of valgus tibiotalar tilt after hindfoot fusion. Foot Ankle Int 2017; 38(5):519–25.
35. de Cesar Netto C, Deland JT, Ellis SJ. Guest editorial: Expert consensus on adult-acquired flatfoot deformity. Foot Ankle Int 2020;41(10):1269–71.

Moving?

Make sure your subscription moves with you!

To notify us of your new address, find your **Clinics Account Number** (located on your mailing label above your name), and contact customer service at:

Email: journalscustomerservice-usa@elsevier.com

800-654-2452 (subscribers in the U.S. & Canada)
314-447-8871 (subscribers outside of the U.S. & Canada)

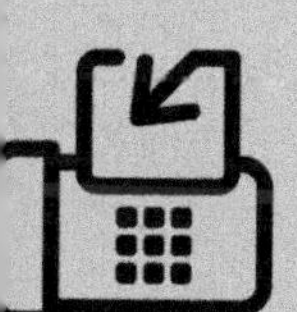

Fax number: 314-447-8029

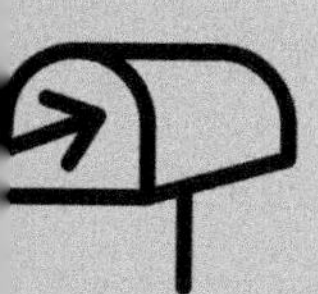

Elsevier Health Sciences Division
Subscription Customer Service
3251 Riverport Lane
Maryland Heights, MO 63043

*To ensure uninterrupted delivery of your subscription, please notify us at least 4 weeks in advance of move.

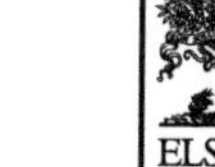

Printed and bound by CPI Group (UK) Ltd, Croydon, CR0 4YY
08/05/2025
01864697-0001